7 55503A

30

94 2P

APS

Advances in Pharmacological Sciences

Radioactive Isotopes in Clinical Medicine and Research

Proceedings of the 22nd International Badgastein Symposium

Edited by
H. Bergmann
A. Kroiss
H. Sinzinger

Birkhäuser Verlag
Basel · Boston · Berlin

Editors:

Professor Dr. H. Bergmann
Institut für Biomedizinische Technik
und Physik
Allgemeines Krankenhaus Wien
Währinger Gürtel 18-20
A-1090 Wien

Prim. Dozent Dr. A. Kroiss
KA Rudolfstiftung
Nuklearmedizinisches Institut
Juchg. 25
A-1030 Wien

Professor Dr. H. Sinzinger
Universitäts-Klinik für Nuklearmedizin
Allgemeines Krankenhaus Wien
Währinger Gürtel 18-20
A-1090 Wien

A CIP catalogue record for this book is available from the Library of Congress,
Washington D.C., USA

Deutsche Bibliothek Cataloging-in-Publication Data
Radioactive isotopes in clinical medicine and research :
proceedings of the 22nd International Badgastein Symposium / ed. by
H. Bergmann ... - Basel ; Boston ; Berlin : Birkhäuser, 1997
  (Advances in pharmacological sciences)
  ISBN 3-7643-5645-6 (Basel ...)
  ISBN 0-8176-5645-6 (Boston)
NE: Bergmann, Helmar [Hrsg.]; Badgastein Symposium <22, 1996>

© 1997 Birkhäuser Verlag, P.O. Box 133, CH-4010 Basel, Switzerland
Camera-ready copy prepared by the editors and authors
Printed on acid-free paper produced from chlorine-free pulp. TCF ∞
Printed in Germany

ISBN 3-7643-5645-6
ISBN 0-8176-5645-6

9 8 7 6 5 4 3 2 1

Table of contents

The Badgastein Lecture
Clinical PET in Oncology

Oncology
Pretargeting: Improved Pharmacokinetics and Therapeutic Ratio

Brain Tumors – Effect of Radiation Therapy on Amino Acid Transport

Scintimammography with Technetium-99m-SESTAMIBI: Planar Scanning Vs. SPECT

How to Further Evaluate Indeterminate Mammograms. A Comparison between Semiquantitative Tc-99m SESTAMIBI Scintimammography and Dynamic MRI

The Use of Technetium-99m Methoxyisobutylisonitrile (Tc-99m-MIBI) Breast Scintigraphy For Early Detection of Breast Cancer

FDG SPECT to Monitor Lung Cancer Chemotherapy

Diagnosis and Therapy Control of Ocular Melanoma with 18-FDG-PET – A Pilot Study

FDG-PET, I-131 and MIBI-Scintigraphy in the Follow-Up of Differentiated Thyroid
Cancer

Preface

Once again, the proceedings of the Badgastein Symposium, this one being the 22nd in an uninterrupted series, offer a comprehensive record of the scientific events. Highlights at this meeting were certainly reports of the exciting new developments of positron imaging with Anger cameras, both with conventional high-energy collimators and with coincidence techniques. Preliminary clinical results are promising and seem to offer a true alternative to sophisticated PET-technology with its for many laboratories prohibitive costs.

The general nature of the symposium is documented by the large range of topics covered so that all major topics of interest in both the basic sciences of nuclear medicine and clinical application are found. In accordance with the general trends in nuclear medicine, there has been a substantial increase in oncological work compared to the more traditional topics. This is also reflected in the Badgastein lecture, given by Professor P. Rigo, who presented an excellent survey of nuclear oncology.

A major change to the structure of the symposium was the inclusion of the Austrian Nuclear Medicine Society as a co-organizer, jointly with the Departments of Nuclear Medicine and of Biomedical Engineering and Physics of the Medical Faculty of the University of Vienna. Also, the meeting was shortened in time by one day, but without decreasing the number of contributions. This was made possible by upgrading and expanding the poster sessions which made up for more concise but nevertheless informative contributions to both the meeting and the proceedings. Special thanks are due to our referees, who worked through all the manuscripts picking up inconsistencies, errors, omissions and the like, thereby improving substantially the quality of the proceedings.

It should be put on record that in spite of quite attractive weather attendance of the sessions was remarkably good. This is a promising outlook to future Badgastein meetings, the next one taking place from 13 to 16 January 1998, where we will again try to do our best in combining scientific exchange with an open and relaxed atmosphere for informal discussions and leisure activities.

H. Bergmann   A. Kroiss   H. Sinzinger

List of chairmen

W. Becker	(Göttingen)
H. Biersack	(Bonn)
A. Bischof-Delaloye	(Lausanne)
M.H. Bourguignon	(Paris)
K.E. Britton	(London)
P.J. Ell	(London)
J. Fettich	(Ljubljana)
H. Fritzsche	(Feldkirch)
G.F. Fueger	(Graz)
G. Galvan	(Salzburg)
D.A. Goodwin	(Palo Alto, U.S.A.)
E. Havlik	(Vienna)
E. Henze	(Kiel)
R. Höfer	(Vienna)
K. Kletter	(Vienna)
W.H. Knapp	(Leipzig)
H. Köhn	(Vienna)
J.T. Kuikka	(Kuopio)
G. Limouris	(Athens)
B. Markt	(Linz)
J. Martín-Comín	(Barcelona)
V.R. McCready	(Sutton)
E. Ogris	(Vienna)
R. Palumbo	(Perugia)
S.N. Reske	(Ulm)
G. Riccabona	(Innsbruck)
M. Šamal	(Prague)
A. Skretting	(Oslo)
A.E. Todd-Pokropek	(London)

List of participants

Agren Brita, Dept. of Radiology, Huddinge Hospital, 14186 Huddinge, S
Ahonen Aapo Kaarlo Aapeli, Dr., Division of Nuclear Medicine, Oulu University Hospital, Kajaanintie 50, Box 22, 90220 Oulu, FIN
Aigner Reingard, Dr., 8010 Graz, A
Albrecht W., BSM-Diagnostica GesmbH, Alser Str. 25, 1080 Vienna, A
Alexander Christof, Dr., Abteilung Nuklearmedizin, Universitätskliniken, 66421 Homburg, D
Als Claudine, Dr., Institute of Pathology, University of Berne, 3010 Berne, CH
Andreas Jörg, Dr., Klinik für Nuklearmedizin, Uni-Klinik Mainz, 55101 Mainz, D
Andreeff Michael, Dipl.-Phys., Klinik für Nuklearmedizin, Uni-Klinikum Carl Gustav Carus, Fetscherstraße 74, 01307 Dresden, D
Angelberger Peter, Dr., Austrian Research Center Seibersdorf, 2444 Seibersdorf, A
Antalfty Maria, Institute of Isotopes Co. Ltd., Konkoly Thege St 29-33, 1121 Budapest, H
Antonelli Tatiana, Via Romagnosi 88, 47023 Cesena, I
Aprile Carlo, Fond. "S. Maugeri", 26, V. Boezio, 27100 Pavia, I
Artner Christoph, IASON Labormedizin, Rechbauerstr. 3/2, 8010 Graz, A
Atefie Khosrow, Dr., Arnikaweg 99, 1220 Vienna, A
Auinger Christian, OA Dr., Department of Nuclear Medicine, Rudolfstiftung, Juchgasse 25, 1030 Vienna, A

Barthel Henryk, Klinik für Nuklearmedizin, Universität Leipzig, Liebigstraße 20a, 04103 Leipzig, D
Bauer Harald, Hanusch-KH, Department of Nuclear Medicine, Heinrich-Collinstr. 32, 1140 Vienna, A
Becherer Alexander, Dr., Department of Nuclear Medicine, Vienna University Hospital AKH, Währinger Gürtel 18-20, 1090 Vienna, A
Behr Thomas, Dr., Center for Molecular Medicine & Immunology, 1 Brook Street, New York, NY 09103-2763, U.S.A
Berberich Richard, Prof. Dr., Klinikum Wuppertal GmbH, Heusnerstraße 40, 42283 Wuppertal, D
Bergmann Helmar, Prof. Dr., Department of Biomedical Engineering and Physics, Vienna University Hospital AKH, Währinger Gürtel 18-20/4L, 1090 Vienna, A
Biersack Hans-Jürgen, Prof. Dr., Department of Nuclear Medicine, University of Bonn, Sigmund-Freud-Straße 25, 53127 Bonn, D
Bischof-Delaloye Angelika, Prof. Dr., Division Autonome de Médecine Nucléaire, Centre Hospitalier Universitaire Vaudois, 1011 Lausanne, CH
Blauwhoff Martjan, MALLINCKRODT Deutschland, Radiopharmaka, 53761 Hennet, D
Bodei Lisa, Centro Regionale di Medicina Nucleare, Via Roma 67, 56100 Pisa, I
Bohuslavizki Karl H., Dr., Nuklearmedizinische Klinik, Christian-Albrechts-Universität, Arnold-Heller-Straße 9, 24105 Kiel, D
Bourguignon Michel, Prof. Dr., CEA/SHFJ Orsay France, 4 Place du Général Leclerc, 91401 Orsay, F
Braun Erika, Dr., LKH Salzburg, Nukl. Med., Müllner Hauptstr. 48, 5020 Salzburg, A
Bremer Per Oscar, Prof., Institutt for Energiteknikk, Post Box 40, 02007 Kjeller, N

Britton K. E., Prof., St. Bartholomew's Hospital, West Smithfield, EC1A73E London, UK
Brunnöder Wolfgang, RZ PV-Ang., Vogelsangweg, 7431 Bad Tatzmannsdorf, A
Bucher C., DU PONT Pharma, Du-Pont-Str. 1, 61343 Bad Homburg, D
Buchinger Wolfgang, OA Dr., KH Graz-Eggenberg, Bergstr. 27, 8020 Graz, A
Burroni Luca, Dr., Policlinico "Le Scotte", Dept. of Nuclear Medicine, University of Siena, Viale Bracci, 53100 Siena, I
Busemann-Sokole Ellinor, Dr., Academic Medical Centre, Meibergdreef 9, 1105 AZ Amsterdam, NL

Chbicheb Abdelkrim, Prof., Hopital Avicenne Rabat, 08031 Rabat, Nations-Unies, Morocco, BP
Chinol Marco, Dr., European Institut of Oncology, Via Ripamonti 435, 20141 Milano, I
Chiti Arturo, Dr., National Cancer Institute, Via Venezian 1, 20133 Milano, I
Clausen M., Prof. Dr., Institut f. Nuklearmedizin, Arnold-Heller-Str. 9, 24105 Kiel, D
Cokragan Ahmet, IBA, Chemin du Cyclotron 2, 1348 Louvain-la-Neuve, B
Coli Antonio, Dr., Nuclear Medicine Service, Town Hospital ASL 5 La Spezia, Via dei Colli 9, 19121 La Spezia, I
Czernin Johannes, Prof. Dr., UCLA School of Medicine, Nuclear Medicine & Biophysics Dept., 10833 Le Conte Av., Los Angeles, USA

Dahlström Jan Anders, Dr., Fysiologiska Audelningen, Helsingborgs Lasarett, 25654 Helsingborg, S
De Geeter Frank, Dr., AZ Sint. Jan Brugge, Klumedreef 10, 08020 Oostkamp, B
De Roo Michel, Prof., Dept. of Nuclear Medicine, University Hospitals Leuven, Merendreef 26, 03001 Heverlee, B
Deckart Harald F., Prof. Dr.med.habil., Nuklearmedizinische Klinik, Klinikum Berlin-Buch, Wiltbergstraße 50, 13122 Berlin, D
Deckart Eva, Dr., 13187 Berlin, D
Decristoforo Clemens, Mag., Univ.-Klinik für Nuklearmedizin, Anichstraße 35, 6020 Innsbruck, A
Denk Eva, BIOCIS HandelsgesmbH, Divischg. 4, 1210 Vienna, A
Doepp Manfred, Dr., Ord. f. Nuklearmedizin, Faberstr. 2, 5020 Salzburg, A
Donaldson John, Dr., British Army, 52, West Court, Prince Imperial Rd., London SE18 4JW, UK
Donnemiller Eveline, Univ.-Klinik f. Nuklearmedizin, Anichstr. 35, 6020 Innsbruck, A
Dorner Elke, ZRI Leoben, Johann-Straußg. 10/5/17, 8010 Graz, A
Douglas Tibor, Dr., RZ PV-Ang., Vogelsangweg 113, 7431 Bad Tatzmannsdorf, A
Dwelshauvers Jean, Dr., CHR "La Tourelle" Verviers, Rue du Bief, 24, 04652 Xhendelesse, B
Dziuk Eugeniusz, Prof. Dr., Department of Nuclear Medicine, Central Clinical Hospital WAM, ul. Szaserow 128, 00909 Warsaw, PL

Edelmann Kurt, SIEMENS AG, Bereich Med. Technik, Henkestr. 127, 91052 Erlangen, D
Eghbalian Farzad, PV-Ang. RZ Hochegg, Friedrich-Hillegeist-Str. 2, 2840 Grimmenstein, A
Eisenkolb Gerlinde, Dept. of Nuclear Medicine, Röntgenweg 13, 72076 Tübingen, D
Ell P. J., Prof. Dr., Middlesex Hospital, Institute of Nuclear Medicine, Mortimer Street, London W1N 8AA, UK
Epple Brigitte, Rad. Klinik, Nuklearmedizin. Abt., Röntgenweg 13, 72076 Tübingen, D

Falk C., Dipl.-Ing., ELIMPEX-Medizintechnik GesmbH, Spechtgasse 32, 2340 Mödling, A
Feichtinger Helmut, Dr., KH Barmh. Schwestern, Seilerstätte 4, 4020 Linz, A

Feine Ulrich, Prof. Dr., Abt. für Nuklearmedizin, Röntgenweg 13, 72076 Tübingen, D
Fettich Jure, Dr., Nuclear Medicine Dept., University Medical Center Ljubljana, Zaloska 7, 61000 Ljubljana, SLO
Fischer Sibylle, Department of Nuclear Medicine, LMU Munich, Ziemssenstr. 1, 80336 Munich, D
Flores Juan, Dr., Department of Nuclear Medicine, Vienna University Hospital AKH, Währinger Gürtel 18-20, 1090 Vienna, A
Franceschini Rodolfo, SORIN BIOMEDICA Diagnostics S.p.A., Radiopharmaceutical Business Unit, 13040 Saluggia (UC), I
Franken Philippe, Dr., Academic Hospital AZ VUB, 101 Laarbeeklaan, 01090 Brussels, B
Frassine Harald S., Department of Nuclear Medicine, Vienna University Hospital AKH, Währinger Gürtel 18-20, 1090 Vienna, A
Fridrich Leo, Prim. Doz. Dr., Institut f. Nuklearmedizin, LKH, 4400 Steyr, A
Fritzsche Heinz, Prim. Doz. Dr., Nuklearmedizinische Abteilung, LKH Feldkirch, Carinagasse 47, 6800 Feldkirch, A
Frohn Jürgen, Dr., Südharz-Krankenhaus, Dr.-Robert-Koch-Straße 39, 99734 Nordhausen, D
Furlan Werner, Dr., Nukl. Med., Runastr. 38, 6800 Feldkirch, A

Galvan Günther, Prof. Dr., Institut für Nuklearmedizin u. Endokrinologie, LKH Salzburg, 5020 Salzburg, A
Gane Smaranda Mihaela, Dr., Université Catholique Louvain (U.C.L.), 12 Rue du Gruyer, Boite 3, 1170 Bruxelles, B
Gasparini Massimo, Dr., National Cancer Institute, Via Venezian 1, 20133 Milano, I
Gattinger Arno, Dr., Institut f. Nuklearmedizin, Müllner Hauptstr. 48, 5020 Salzburg, A
Giorgetti Gianluigi, Dr., Bufalini Hospital, Health Physics Dept., Vle. Ghirotti 286, 47023 Cesena (FO), I
Glatz Steffen, Dr., Abt. für Nuklearmedizin, Klinikum der Universität Ulm, Robert-Koch-Straße 8, 89070 Ulm, D
Goldschmidt Klaus, Medical Consulting, Rohrwiesenstr. 22, 63654 Büdingen, D
Goodwin David A., Prof., VA Palo Alto Health Care System, 3801 Miranda Ave. (115), Palo Alto, CA 94304, U.S.A.
Gottschild Dietmar, Prof. Dr., Friedrich-Schiller-Universität Jena, Bachstraße 18, 07740 Jena, D
Granowska Marie, Dr., St. Bartholomew's Hospital, West Smithfield, London EC1A 73E, UK
Grillenberger Kurt, Dr., Universitätsklinik Ulm, Nuklearmedizin, Robert-Koch-Straße 8, 89081 Ulm, D
Grossegger Carmen, Dr., Institut für Nuklearmedizin, KA Rudolfstiftung, Juchgasse 25, 1030 Vienna, A
Guhlmann Carl Albrecht, Dr., Abt. für Nuklearmedizin, Klinikum der Universität Ulm, Robert-Koch-Straße 8, 89081 Ulm, D
Günnewig Bernd, SIEMENS AG, Bereich Med. Technik, Henkestr. 127, 91052 Erlangen, D

Haas Christian, DI, Department of Medical Physics, LKH Feldkirch, Carinagasse 47, 6800 Feldkirch, A
Hahn Klaus, Prof. Dr., University of Munich, Ziemssenstr. 1, 80336 Munich, D
Hammer Johann, Dr., Univ.-Klinik für Innere Med. IV, AKH, Währinger Gürtel 18-20, 1090 Vienna, A
Handgriff Daphne, Dr., Kaiserin-Elisabeth-Spital, Huglgasse 1-3, 1150 Vienna, A
Hanner Christian, PV-Ang, Vogelsangweg 113, 7431 Bad Tatzmannsdorf, A
Hantelle Marie-Claude, CIS bio international, BP 32, 91192 Gif-sur-Yvette Cédex, F

Hartmann Tamara, Dr., KH St. Pölten, Ringelnatzstr. 5/C1, 3100 St. Pölten, A

Hatzl Margit, Dr., Starhembergstr. 66, 4020 Linz, A

Havlik Ernst, Doz. Dr., Department of Biomedical Engineering and Physics, Vienna University Hospital AKH, Währinger Gürtel 18-20/4L, 1090 Vienna, A

Haydl Hannes, Prim. Dr., A. Ö. Kardinal Schwarzenberg´sches Krankenhaus, 5620 Schwarzach, A

Heckenberg Andrea, Mag., Department of Biomedical Engineering and Physics, Vienna University Hospital AKH, Währinger Gürtel 18-20/4L, 1090 Vienna, A

Heidenreich Peter, Prof. Dr., Klinik für Nuklearmedizin, Zentralklinikum Augsburg, Stenglinstraße 2, 86156 Augsburg, D

Heinisch Martin, Dr., Nuklearmed. KH Melk, Krankenhausstr. 11, 3390 Melk, A

Henze E., Prof. Dr., Klinik für Nuklearmedizin, Christian-Albrechts-Universität zu Kiel, Arnold-Heller-Str. 9, 24105 Kiel, D

Hěrmanska Jindriska, Doc. Ing., CSc., Clinic of Nuclear Medicine, Faculty Hospital Motol, v. Úvalu 84, 15018 Prague 5, CZ

Höfer R., Prof. Dr., Ungargasse 39, 1030 Vienna, A

Hofmann Andrea, Dr., Institut f. Nuklearmedizin u. Endokrinologie, Müllner Hauptstr. 48, 5020 Salzburg, A

Höfs Renate, Dr., Am Marstall, 30165 Hannover, D

Hojker Sergej, Dr., Nuclear Medicine Dept., University Medical Center Ljubljana, Zaloska 7, 61000 Ljubljana, SLO

Holley Andy, CTI Europe, 15 Knowles Avenue, Crowthorne, Berkshire RG45 6DU, GB

Jacobs Axel, Dr., Department of Nuclear Medicine, Virga Jesse Hospital, Stadsomvaart 11, 03500 Hasselt, B

Jaracz Jan, Dr., Dept. of Psychiatry, University of Medical Sciences, ul. Szpitalna 27/33, 60572 Poznan, PL

John-Scheder Alexander, Ing., ELSCINT Medical Technology, Am Föhrenhang 1, 2551 Enzesfeld, A

Jörg Lutz, Dr., KH d. Barmherzigen Schwestern, Seilerstätte 4, 4010 Linz, A

Kampf Gudrun, Dr. rer. nat. habil., Klinik für Nuklearmedizin, Technische Universität Dresden, Fetscherstraße 74, 01307 Dresden, D

Karanikas Georg, Dr., Department of Nuclear Medicine, Vienna University Hospital AKH, Währinger Gürtel 18-20, 1090 Vienna, A

Kelly Duncan, Amersham, White Lion RD, HP79AX Amersham, UK

Kenda Rajko, Dr., Pediatric Hospital, University Medical Center Ljubljana, Stare pravde 4, 61000 Ljubljana, SLO

Kletter Kurt, Doz. DDr., Department of Nuclear Medicine, Vienna University Hospital AKH, Währinger Gürtel 18-20, 1090 Vienna, A

Kluge Regine, Dr., Klinik u. Poliklinik für Nuklearmedizin, Liebigstraße 20a, 04103 Leipzig, D

Knapp W. H., Prof. Dr., Klinik f. Nuklearmedizin, Liebigstr. 20a, 04103 Leipzig, D

Knierim Andreas, Dr., Praxis für Nuklearmedizin, Spitalmühlenstraße 3, 74523 Schwäbisch Hall, D

Knoll Peter, Mag., Wilhelminenspital, Montleartstr. 37, 1171 Vienna, A

Köhn Horst, Prof. Dr., Abt. für Nuklearmedizin, Wilhelminenspital, Montleartstraße 37, 1171 Vienna, A

König Beatrix, Prim. Dr., Hanusch-KH, H.-Collin-Str. 30, 1140 Vienna, A

Könne Werner, Wieselpfad 1, 30635 Hannover, D

Meyer Gabriele, Dept. of Nuclear Medicine, Ludwig-Maximilians-Universität, Ziemssenstraße 1, 80336 München, D

Mikosch Peter, Ass. Dr., LKH Klagenfurt, St.-Veiter-Straße 47, 09020 Klagenfurt, A

Milcinski Metka, Dr., Nuclear Medicine Dept., University Medical Centre Ljubljana, Zaloska 7, 61000 Ljubljana, SLO

Minear Gregory, Department of Biomedical Engineering and Physics, Vienna University Hospital AKH, Währinger Gürtel 18-20/4L, 1090 Vienna, A

Moka Detlef, Dr., Klinik für Nuklearmedizin, Josef-Stelzmann-Straße 9, 50924 Köln, D

Moldrich Waltraud, Dr., Nuklearmedizinisches Institut, Wilhelminenspital, Montleartstraße 37, 1171 Vienna, A

Muehllehner G., PhD, Hosp. of the Univ. of Penn., Nuclear Med./Radiology Dept., 300 Spruce St., Philadelphia PA 19104, USA

Müller Jörg, Dr., Städtisches Klinikum Osnabruck, Nuklearmedizin, Memetesstr. 44, 30657 Hannover, D

Nagel Bernd, Dr., St.-Marien-Hospital, Altstadtstr. 23, 44534 Lünen, D

Nieder Birgit, LKH Graz, Kalvariengürtel 48c, 8010 Graz, A

Niemi Risto Sydanryhma, Central Hosp. of Vaasa, Hietalahderk 2-4, 65100 Vaasa, FIN

Norrgren Kristina, Dr., Dept. of Radiation Physics, Universitetssjukhuset Mas, 20502 Malmö, S

Novak-Hofer Ilse, Dr., Labor für Radiopharmazie, Paul Scherrer Institut, 05232 Villigen, CH

Oberladstätter M., Dr., Klinik f. Nuklearmedizin, Anichstr. 35, 6020 Innsbruck, A

Oehme Liane, Dipl.-Phys., Klinik für Nuklearmedizin, Uni-Klinikum Carl Gustrav Carus, Fetscherstraße 74, 01307 Dresden, D

Ogris E., Prof. Dr., Abt. f. Nuklearmedizin, Donauspital-SMZO, Langobardenstr. 122, 1220 Vienna, A

Oliver T. Barry, Dr., Royal Infirmary, Edinburgh, 6, Craighall Terrace, Edinburgh EH6 4RF, Scotland, UK

Onder Brigitte, KH Barmh. Brüder, Große Mohreng. 9, 1020 Vienna, A

Otto Lothar, Dr., Nuklearmedizinische Klinik, Universität Leipzig, Liebigstraße 20a, 04103 Leipzig, D

Palumbo Renato, Prof. Dr., Medicina Nucleare, Università di Perugia, 06121 Perugia, I

Palumbo Barbara, Dr., Medicina Nucleare, Università di Perugia, 06121 Perugia, I

Panholzer Peter Josef, Dr., Seilerstätte 4, 4020 Linz, A

Pappo Itzhak, Prof. Dr., Assrf-Harojeh Medical Center, Dept. of Nuclear Medicine, Horne Tifha Dr., 70300 Zerifin, Israel,

Pinkert Jörg, Klinik für Nuklearmedizin, Uni-Klinikum Carl Gustav Carus, Fetscherstraße 74, 01307 Dresden, D

Podreka Ivo, Prim. Prof. Dr., Neurolog. Abteilung KH Rudolfsstiftung, Juchg. 25, 1030 Vienna, A

Pozenel H., Prim. Dr., Herz-Kreislauf-Zentrum, Parkstr. 12, 4540 Bad Hall, A

Predic Peter, Dr., Lab. Nuclear Medicine, Hospital Celje, Oblakova 5, 63000 Celje, SLO

Prohaska Rudolf, Dr., Nuklearmedizin, KH Melk, 3390 Melk, A

Rakiás Ferenc, Dr., National Institute of Pharmacy, P.O. Box 450, 01342 Budapest, H

Rees John, Dr., Department of Radiology, University Hospital of Wales, Cardiff, Heath Park, Cardiff, Wales, UK

Reske S.N., Prof. Dr., Klinikum der Universität Ulm, Robert-Koch-Str. 8, 89070 Ulm, D

Rettenbacher Lukas, Dr., LKH Salzburg, Nukl. Med., Müllner Hauptstr. 48, 5020 Salzburg, A
Riccabona Georg, Prof. Dr., Univ.-Klinik für Nuklearmedizin, Anichstraße 35, 06020 Innsbruck, A
Riedl Peter, Dr., MedPro - Vertrieb für med.-diagnost. Produkte Ges.m.b.H., Gersthofer Str. 9, 1180 Vienna, A
Rigo P., Prof., Service de Médecine Nucléaire, Centre Hospitalier Universitaire de Liège, 4000 Liège, B
Riva Pietro, Dr., Nuclear Medicine Department, M. Bufalini Hospital, Via Ghirotti 286, 47023 Cesena (FO), I
Rodrigues Margarida, Dr., Department of Nuclear Medicine, Vienna University Hospital AKH, Währinger Gürtel 18-20, 1090 Vienna, A
Ruckgaber Jochen, Abt. für Nuklearmedizin, Klinikum der Universität Ulm, Robert-Koch-Straße 8, 89070 Ulm, D

Šámal Martin, MD, DSc., Charles University Prague, Salmovská 3, 12000 Praha 2, CZ
Sauer Jürgen, Dr., Radiol. Klinik, Nuklearmedizin, ZKH St.-Jürgen-Str., 28205 Bremen, D
Schachner Liane, LKH Graz, Unterer Plattenweg 64, 8043 Graz, A
Schedlmayer F., BSM-Diagnostica GesmbH, Alser Str. 25, 1080 Vienna, A
Schenner Michael, Dr., KH d. Barmh. Brüder, Große Mohreng. 9, 1020 Vienna, A
Schmid Christine, Dr., Nuklearmedizinisches Institut, Kaiserin-Elisabeth-Spital, Heinrich-Collin-Straße 8-14/6/14, 1150 Wien, A
Schmidlin Peter, Dr., DKFZ, Im Neuenheimer Feld 280, 69120 Heidelberg, D
Schmidt Clemens, BIOCIS HandelsgesmbH, Divischg. 4, 1210 Vienna, A
Schmidt Matthias, AKH Hamburg-Barmbek, Walddörferstr. 279, 22047 Hamburg, D
Schmidt Ulrich, AKH Hamburg-Barmbek, Walddörferstr. 277, 22047 Hamburg, D
Schomäcker Klaus, Dr., Clinic of Nuclear Medicine, University of Cologne, Josef-Stelz-mann-Straße 9, 50924 Cologne, D
Schöppy H., PICKER International GmbH, Marienwerderstr. 2, 32339 Espelkamp, D
Shukla Shyama Kant, Prof. Dr., Servizio di Medicina Nucleare, Ospedale S. Eugenio, Piazzale Umanesimo 10, 00144 Roma, I
Sinzinger Helmut, Prof. Dr., Department of Nuclear Medicine, Vienna University Hospital AKH, Währinger Gürtel 18-20, 1090 Vienna, A
Skretting Arne, Prof., Department of Medical Physics and Technology, The Norwegian Radium Hospital, Montebello, 00310 Oslo, N
Sobal Grazyna, Mag., Dept. of Nuclear Medicine, Vienna University Hospital AKH, Währinger Gürtel 18-20, 1090 Vienna, A
Sochor Heinz, Prof. Dr., Dept. of Cardiology, Vienna University Hospital AKH, Währinger Gürtel 18-20, 1090 Vienna, A
Standke Rüdiger, Dr., i.c.t., Trazerbergg. 76, 1130 Vienna, A
Steinhardt Wolfgang, ELSCINT Medical Technology, Oskar-Helmer-Str., 2000 Stockerau, A
Sterba Sabine, ZRI Leoben, Grazerstr. 34g, 8045 Graz, A
Stockhammer M., Dr., KH Wels, Max-Mell-Str. 8, 4600 Wels, A
Strobl Eva, Dr., RZ Hochegg, 2840 Grimmenstein, A
Stubenrauch Doris, LKH Graz, Frauenklinik, Auenbruggerpl. 14, 8036 Graz, A
Šustarsic Janez, Institute of Oncology, Zaloska 2, 61000 Ljubljana, SLO
Synak Rastislav, Dr., MEDISO Medical Equipment Development & Service Ltd., Alsótörokvész u. 14, 1022 Budapest, H
Syslo H., SANABO GmbH, Brunner Str. 59, 1230 Wien, A
Szemethy G., DU PONT Pharma, Du-Pont-Str. 1, 61343 Bad Homburg, D

Szilvási Istvàn, Dr., Haynal Univ., P.O.Box 112, 1389 Budapest, H

Talbot Jean-Noel, Prof. Dr., Hopital Tenon, 4 Rue de Chine, 75970 Paris Cédex, F
Theissen Peter, Dr., Klinik für Nuklearmedizin, Universität Köln, Joseph-Stelzmann-Straße 9, 50924 Köln, D
Theurl Anton, Dr., Nukl. Med., BKH-Lienz, E.-v.-Hiblerstr. 5, 9900 Lienz, A
Thierfelder Hans, Gemeinschafts-KH Havelhöhe, Kladower Damm 221, 1000 Berlin, D
Thirion Bruno, CIS bio international, BP 32, 91192 Gif-sur-Yvette Cédex, F
Thomson William, City Hospital NHS Trust, Dept. of Physics and Nuclear Medicine, Dudley Road, Birmingham B18 7QH, UK
Tiling Reinhold, Dr., Dept. of Nuclear Medicine, University of Munich, Marchioninistraße 15, 81377 Munich, D
Todd-Pokropek Andrew, Prof., Medical Physics, University College London, Gower Street, London WC1 E6BT, UK
Torniainen Pentii, Dr., OYKS Isotooppilaboratorio, Oulu University Hospital, 90220 Oulu, FIN

Unterluggauer Paula, KH Barmh. Brüder, Große Mohreng. 8/67, 1020 Vienna, A

van Loon P., ADAC Laboratories Europe BV, P.O.Box 1419, 3600 BK Maarssen, NL
Veenstra Hinke, VEENSTRA Instrumenten BV, Joure, 8500, NL
Verbruggen Rudich, IBA, Av. J. Lenoir 6, 1348 Louvain-la-Neuve, B
Vidergar Barbara, Inst. of Oncology, Zaloska 2, 61000 Ljubljana, SLO
Visser Frans, Dr., Dept. of Cardiology, Free University Hospital, De Boelelaan 1117, 01081 HV Amsterdam, NL
Volterrani Duccio, Dr., Policlinico "Le Scotte", Dept. of Nuclear Medicine, University of Siena, Viale Bracci, 53100 Siena, I
von Gumppenberg Rolf M., Dr., Schweizer Paraplegiker-Zentrum, Radiologie, 06207 Nottwil, CH

Walamies Markku, M.D., North-Karelia Central Hospital, Männiköntie 17 as 1, 80100 Joensuu, FIN
Weber Andrea, LKH-Graz, Univ.-Frauenklinik, Hormonlabor, Auenbruggerpl. 14, 8036 Graz, A
Wegener Bernd, Dr., B.R.A.H.M.S. Diagnostica GmbH, Komturstr. 19-20, 12099 Berlin, D
Weingartmann P., BEHRING Institut GesmbH, Altmannsdorfer Str. 104, 1121 Vienna, A
Weiss Manfred, Dr., Schwanthalergasse 13, 4910 Ried, A
Weller Rolf, Dr., Dept. of Nuclear Medicine, University of Ulm, Robert-Koch-Straße 8, 89070 Ulm, D
Wiederin Herbert, Dr., Nuklearmedizin, LKH Feldkirch, Carinagasse 47, 06800 Feldkirch, A
Winderen Mette, Dr., Nuclear Medicine Department, The Norwegian Radium Hospital, Montebello, 00310 Oslo, N
Woloszczuk Wolfgang, Prof. Dr., LBI f. Exp. Endokrinologie, 1. Univ.-Frauenklinik, AKH-Wien, Währinger Gürtel 18-20, 1090 Vienna, A

Zakarias Herbert, BIOMEDICA HandelsgesmbH, Joseph-Marx-Straße 5, 8043 Graz, A
Zimmermann Rainer, Priv.-Doz. Dr., Dept. of Cardiology, Univ. of Heidelberg, Bergheimer Str. 58, 69115 Heidelberg, D
Zink Hannelore, Nukl. Med., KH Graz-Eggenberg, Bergstr. 28, 8020 Graz, A
Zolle Ilse, Dr., Department of Nuclear Medicine, Vienna University Hospital AKH, Währinger Gürtel 18-20, 1090 Vienna, A

22nd International Symposium

"Radioactive Isotopes in Clinical Medicine and Research"

International Scientific Committee

H. Bergmann (Vienna)
H.J. Biersack (Bonn)
A. Bischof-Delaloye (Lausanne)
U. Büll (Aachen)
H. Fritzsche (Feldkirch)
D.A. Goodwin (Palo Alto, CA)
H. Köhn (Vienna)

A. Kroiss (Vienna)
J. Martín-Comín (Barcelona)
R. Palumbo (Perugia)
G. Riccabona (Innsbruck)
H. Sinzinger (Vienna)
A.E. Todd-Pokropek (London)

Organizing Committee

Honorary President:

Prof. Dr. R. Höfer

Chairmen Organizing Committee:

Prof. Dr. H. Bergmann
Prim. Doz. Dr. A. Kroiss (President ÖNG)
Prof. Dr. H. Sinzinger

Staff Members of Congress Office:

Dr. A. Becherer
Dr. J. Flores
Susanne Granegger
Doz. Dr. E. Havlik
Mag. Andrea Heckenberg
Dr. G. Karanikas
DI P. Kopp

Adelheid Maringer
Dr. Susan Meghdadi
G. Minear, B.Sc.
K. Pogats
Eleonore Tinti
Gabriela Vida

List of exhibitors

ADAC Laboratories Europe B.V.
Zonnebaan 34
P.O.B. 1419
NL-3600 BK MAARSSEN

BEHRING Institut Ges.m.b.H.
Diagnostika
Altmannsdorfer Straße 104
A-1121 WIEN

BIOCIS Handelsges.m.b.H.
Divischgasse 4
A-1210 WIEN

BIOMEDICA Handelsges.m.b.H.
Divischgasse 4
A-1210 WIEN

BSM-DIAGNOSTICA Ges.m.b.H.
Alser Straße 25
A-1080 WIEN

COMTEC Laborgeräte GmbH
Alser Straße 25
A-1080 WIEN

DuPont Pharma, Abt. Radiopharmazeutika
Dupontstraße 1
D-61343 BAD HOMBURG

ELIMPEX-Medizintechnik GesmbH
Spechtgasse 32
A-2340 MÖDLING

GENERAL ELECTRIC MEDICAL
SYSTEMS
Praunheimer Landstraße 50
D-60488 FRANKFURT

HENNING Berlin GmbH
Zollergasse 2/18
A-1070 WIEN

i c t Chemikalien
VertriebsgesmbH
Trazerberggasse 76
A-1130 WIEN

IASON Labormedizin
Mag. Christoph Artner KEG
Rechbauerstraße 3/2
A-8010 GRAZ

MEDISO Medical Equipment
Development & Service Ltd.
Alsótötökvész u. 14
H-1022 BUDAPEST

MedPro
Vertrieb für med.-diagnost. Produkte
GesmbH
Gersthofer Str. 9
A-1180 WIEN

NUCLEAR SERVICES & SUPPLIES
ROST GmbH
Ortsstraße 18
Postfach 22
A-2331 VÖSENDORF

PICKER INTERNATIONAL GmbH
Robert-Bosch-Str. 11
D-65719 HOFHEIM -WALLAU

SIEMENS AG
Bereich Med. Technik
Med. GDW 5
Henkestraße 127
D-91052 ERLANGEN

TOSHIBA Medical Systems Europe
Zilverstraat 1
NL-2718 RP ZOETERMEER

VAN GAHLEN Nederland B.V.
Kelvinstraat 9
P.O.B. 25
NL-6940 BA DIDAM

VEENSTRA Instrumenten b.v.
Madame-Curie-Weg 1
P.O.B. 115
NL-8500 AC JOURE

The Badgastein Lecture

Radioactive Isotopes in
Clinical Medicine and Research XXII
ed. by H. Bergmann, A. Kroiss and H. Sinzinger
© 1997 Birkhäuser Verlag Basel/Switzerland

CLINICAL PET IN ONCOLOGY

P. Rigo, P. Paulus, T. Bury, G. Jerusalem, R. Hustinx, T. Benoit, M.P. Larock, J. Foidart.

University Hospital, Sart Tilman, Liege, Belgium

Summary : 18-FDG is accumulated in cancer cells. It has been proven useful to image a variety of tumors in conjunction with whole-body positron emission tomography. This review details some of the indications of PET at various stages of the cancerous process : differential diagnosis, preoperative staging, diagnosis of residual or recurrent disease as well as follow-up of therapy. Consideration of several potential improvements in clinical PET and of the need for careful patients selection conclude this review.

PET delivers high resolution images of different substrates and ligands' distribution or utilization in normal and pathological tissues. Initially focused on blood flow, metabolic and receptor studies of the brain and the heart, PET is now primarily used in Oncological indications. This development has resulted from the successful application of 18-FDG to a growing number of clinical indications at varying stages of diagnosis, staging and therapy follow-up in cancers of many types and origins.

It is therefore appropriate to review the advantages and limitations of FDG as a tumor seeking agent, its present and potential clinical role, the requirement for clinical improvement and widespread application of PET, as well as some research perspectives.

Biological characteristics of 18-FDG

Use of 18-FDG for in vivo cancer imaging results from the observation of an enhanced glycolysis in tumor cells. High rate of aerobic glycolysis (degradation of glucose to lactic acid in the presence of oxygen) in several types of cancer cells was first described by Warburg in 1930 (1). This phenomenon has been linked to both an increase in the amount of glucose membrane transporters and to an increase in the activity of the principal enzymes controlling the glycolytic pathways (2-7).

FDG following intracellular transport is a substrate for hexokinase, the first enzyme of glycolysis. It is phosphorylated to FDG-6-phosphate (8). The second enzyme however, glucose-6-phosphate isomerase, which transforms glucose-6-phosphate into fructose-6-phosphate does not react with FDG-6-phosphate. Further, as the concentration of glucose-6-phosphatase is very low (except in the hepatocyte), the reverse transformation is not possible and FDG-6-phosphate remains trapped. Accessory metabolic pathways to gluconate and glucuronate are very slow and can be considered negligible within the time frame of 18-F. The cellular concentration in 18-F is therefore closely representative of the accumulated FDG-6-phosphate and of the glycolytic activity of exogenous glucose (8,9).

Numerous studies have attempted to relate cellular FDG uptake to the biological properties of the tumor such as the histological grade, the proliferative activity, the doubling time, the number of viable tumor cells, etc. A positive correlation between 18-FDG uptake and the tumor grade has been reported in several tumor types including cerebral gliomas (10), liver tumors (11), non Hodgkin lymphomas (12) and some musculo-skeletal tumor types (13). The relationship between tumor grade and uptake is however less marked in pulmonary and other tumors (14).

It is important to stress that 18-FDG uptake by neoplasic tumors in vivo remains under the dependence of various physiological factors, such as tissue oxygenation, regional blood flow, peritumoral inflammatory reactions, etc. FDG-PET therefore although very sensitive, is a technique whose specificity is imperfect and must be compensated for by careful patients selection (patients with medium to high prevalence) and rigorous correlation with anatomical images (including image fusion, whenever possible).

Other tracers designed to evaluate amino acid uptake (11C-Methionine), protein synthesis (11C-Tyrosine) or DNA synthesis and cellular proliferation (11C-Thymidine and 18F-Fluorodeoxyuridine) have been proposed as tumor imaging agents (15, 16). Less experience has however been accumulated using these tracers. While theoretically attractive, they are more difficult to produce and usually do not provide the same image contrast that make FDG so impressive (with the notable exception of 11C-Methionine for brain tumor). Use of tracer modeling technique is required and in particular, labelled metabolites in blood and tissues have to be taken into account.

Clinical indications of 18-FDG in Oncology

As it is not possible in a short review to detail the clinical indications of FDG tumor by tumor, I have tried to group the indications along the course of the disease and will illustrate each of these indications by one or several examples.

Differential diagnosis of benign versus malignant disease

FDG-PET has proven useful in several differential diagnosis indications including the diagnosis of solitary pulmonary nodules, the differentiation of pancreatic carcinoma versus mass forming pancreatitis and the diagnosis of breast carcinoma in selected cases of mammography and/or biopsy failure (in particular in dense breasts and in implants). Other potentially valuable indications such as diagnosis of thyroid cancer in patients with cold nules may not be cost effective.

Considerable experience is currently available on solitary pulmonary nodule (17,18). Despite the progress of imaging, few criteria can reliably differentiate benign from malignant nodules. By instance, central calcifications are not always present in benign nodules. The clinician must therefore choose between expectation, potentially dangerous in malignant lesion and invasive diagnostic or therapeutic measures carrying high morbidity and also some mortality risk for a benign lesion.

We have prospectively studied 50 patients with an undetermined solitary pulmonary nodule (19,20). Results of the whole-body PET (neck to mid abdomen) were correlated to the surgical or needle-biopsy of the lesion. Thirty-four pulmonary cancers were correctly identified while 14 of 16 benign nodules were recognized. There were 2 false positives (1 active tuberculosis and 1 case of pseudotumoral anthracosilicosis with partial necrosis and peri-necrotic inflammation). Our results confirm the experience of other authors reporting high sensitivity of the technique in solitary pulmonary nodules. The rate of false positives although usually low shows however some regional variations depending on the local prevalence of pulmonary granulomatous diseases (table 1).

TABLE 1 : FDG IN SOLITARY PULMONARY NODULES

Author	Year	Pts #	Sensitivity (%)	Specificity (%)	PPV	NPV
Dewan	93	30	95	80	90	89
Slosman	93	36	93	-	-	-
Gupta	94	61	93	85	-	-
Lowe	94	88	97	89	95	92
Scott	94	62	93	80	-	-
Dewan	95	26	100	78	93	100
Bury	96	50	100	88	94	100
Total		317	96			
Multicenter	94	237	96	90		

Application of quantitative technique to lung cancer has been evaluated (17,21). It appears effective and certainly increases the objectivity of analysis but it does not appear to significantly improve the diagnosis as compared to visual analysis. Reproducibility is maximum for SUV (SUV related to lean-body mass and corrected for blood glucose concentration) and for Ki (slope of the graphical analysis as defined by Patlak). Parameters of the standard three compartments model were less reproducible (21). Use of FDG-PET for differentiation of solitary pulmonary nodules could lead to significant savings in addition to reducing the number of complications during management (22).

Several groups predominantly from Japan and Germany have evaluated the role of FDG-PET for differentiation of pancreatic cancer from benign chronic pancreatitis and mass forming pancreatitis (23-26). Results indicate a sensitivity of ± 94% with a specificity varying from 78 to 90%. The optimal SUV cut off varies between studies but is rather low (± 2) as glucose uptake in the normal pancreas is also low. On rare occasions, uptake in a pancreatitis site is markedly elevated. Here again visual analysis provided results comparable to those obtained with quantitation. Bares et al (23) first commented on the importance of adequate blood glucose control for optimal FDG uptake by the tumor. Patients with insulin dependent diabetes had lower uptake.

Initial (preoperative) staging of cancer

The importance of initial staging for optimal cancer management cannot be overemphasized. The success of therapy indeed depends on adequate staging. The role of diagnostic techniques in this staging is variable depending on the efficacy of screening methods for that cancer, on the propensity of the tumor for early metastases and on the role of surgery itself in staging. Initial staging by FDG has been proven useful for lung cancer, for melanoma, for sarcoma. Initial staging in lymphoma is probably indicated as a baseline for therapy follow-up. FDG-PET staging is also probably indicated in selected cases of other tumor types, specially when the tumor is at an advanced stage or when metastatic lesions are suspected by conventional imaging. Indeed in these cases, FDG-PET can provide sensitive whole-body screening. This is certainly the case for ovarian, head and neck and pancreatic carcinomas. Initial screening in colorectal cancer has been suggested but results today are not conclusive. Initial staging in breast carcinoma has been the subject of several studies (table 2) (27,28). Although initial results were optimistic, recent reports in larger non selected groups of patients have suggested that the sensitivity to detect axillary nodes metastases is around 75% (29). FDG-PET can however depict internal mammary nodes metastases that are not routinely explored by the surgeon. At this stage, the role of PET in staging and prognostic evaluation of breast carcinoma remain to be clarified.

TABLE 2 : BREAST CARCINOMA - NODAL EXTENT

Author	Pts. #	Sensitivity (%)	Specificity (%)	Acquisition technique
WAHL	7	100	-	Attenuation corrected
TSE	10	57	100	Whole-body
ADLER	20	90	100	Attenuation corrected
HOH	14	67	100	Whole-body
AVRIL	18	72	96	Attenuation corrected
NIEWEG	5	100	-	Attenuation corrected
MULTICENTER STUDY	49	96	96	Various

Several studies have evaluated the role of FDG-PET for staging of lung carcinoma. These studies must be separated in 2 groups. Some investigators have used focal techniques and have concentrated on hilar and mediastinal lymph nodes staging, while others have used whole-body techniques and have evaluated extrathoracic metastases as well (table 3). The reported sensitivity for lymph nodes staging in lung cancer varies from 82 to 100% and the specificity from 73 to 100%. In a prospective study of 30 patients studied prior to thoracotomy, we obtained values of 87% (sensitivity) and 79% (specificity) with 82% PPV and 83% NPV, compared to CT 64% and 56% respectively (table 4). It is interesting to note that CT both underestimated and overestimated the extent of disease so that in comparison PET would have contributed both to cancel and to confirm surgery as a therapeutic modality. Whole-body FDG-PET also contributes to significant management changes as first assessed by Lewis (30). In this study, unsuspected malignant metastatic lesions were recognized in 10 patients (12 extrathoracic sites and 8 thoracic sites). Management changes were noted in 14 patients. 6 (+2) patients were classified as unsuitable for surgery while 8 patients with equivocal finding were found to have single PET lesions. A frequent location of suspected metastasis are the surrenals where CT detects many non specific abnormalities. PET can confirm or infirm these effectively. Our own results confirm the data of Lewis (31).

TABLE 3 : STAGING OF LUNG CANCER BY FDG-PET

Author	Year	Pts. #	Sensitivity (%)	Specificity (%)	Comments
Berlangieri	94	22	90	100	Med. lymph node
Sasaki	94	9	86	100	Med. lymph node
Patz	94	21	100	73	Med. lymph node
Wahl	94	19	82	81	Med. lymph node
Buchpiguel	94	26	93	83	W.B.
Lewis	94	34	199	97	W.B.
Valk	95	62	85	93	W.B.
Bury	96	61	100	95	W.B.

TABLE 4 : STAGING OF NON SMALL CELL LUNG CARCINOMA BY
WHOLE-BODY FDG-PET
Prospective study in 30 patients with thoracotomy

	Positive nodes (16)	Negative nodes (14)	PPV	NPV
PET +	14	3		
			82	83
PET -	2	11		
CT +	9	5		
			64	56
CT -	7	9		

**Differentiation of scar and residual or recurrent disease** is a frequent indication of PET and one of the first to be documented. In 1982, Di Chiro showed the value of FDG-PET to distinguish radiation necrosis from recurrent tumor in the brain (10,32). A similar differentiation has been reported to be useful in lung and in head and neck tumors. Undeterminate pelvic masses on CT are frequent in the follow-up of colorectal cancer and require biopsic evaluation. Strauss et al described in 1989 the value of PET for distinguishing scar from recurrence (33). The use of an iterative reconstruction technique to avoid bladder artefacts was essential in their success. FDG has also proven useful in the evaluation of residual masses after therapy for lymphoma. Gallium has been previously found useful in this indication but FDG unlike Gallium does not require a baseline examination to verify that the tumor indeed accumulates the tracer.

Other cases of suspected recurrences occur when tumor markers increase or when the patient presents general or local clinical signs suggestive of tumor recurrences.Tumor markers are used routinely to follow patients with colorectal, ovarian, breast, thyroid, pancreatic cancers, etc and in many cases, conventional imaging fails to detect the recurrence because of its small size or of its occurrence at a distance from the initial site.

Several studies have concentrated on the value of PET to detect early recurrences in these cases based on its high sensitivity and on its whole-body capability. Indeed, whenever a recurrence is confirmed the extent of recurrence becomes the next question as the clinician pounders the therapeutic options. Data from Beets and Schiepers from Leuven (34), Wahl (35), Gupta (36) as well as our own have stressed the value of whole-body PET for staging recurrent disease in colorectal carcinoma (table 5). Data from the same groups have also demonstrated the value of PET to detect or confirm liver metastases. Overall, as demonstrated by Beets in a study of 35 patients, PET changed the therapeutic regimen in 7 of 16 cases with known metastatic lesions; it detected distant metastases in 2 patients suspected of local recurrences and it detected pelvic recurrence in 2 of 3 patients with an isolated CEA elevation (34).

TABLE 5 : PET IN COLORECTAL CARCINOMA
Staging recurrent disease after initial therapy

Author	Year	n (pts, sites)	Sensitivity(%)	Specificity(%)
Gupta	1991	18	100	86
Multicenter	1994	59	93	78
Schiepers	1995	76	94	98
Valk	1995	57, 78	95	87
Daenen	1995	19, 29	95	67

The impact of PET on management, avoiding unnecessary surgery, allowing more complete surgery or allowing surgery when it had seemed contra-indicated form the basis of its cost-effectiveness (37).

Follow-up of therapy

FDG-PET has been shown useful to evaluate early therapeutic response. FDG uptake can be markedly diminished or even completely suppressed after one or two cycles of chemotherapy, well before tumor mass can be shown to decrease by conventional imaging. With the use of quantification, this technique has wide indications and is of interest for most cancers submitted to chemotherapy or radiotherapy (lymphoma, breast, sarcoma, ovarian tumor, germ cell tumor, head and neck carcinomas, lung cancer, colorectal cancer, hepatic metastases, etc. Early determination of therapeutic resistance is also important to avoid the toxicity of an ineffective therapy and to allow selection of a new therapeutic regimen.

In our study of patients with non Hodgkin lymphoma, patients with negative scans after 2 or 3 chemotherapy cycles had good prognosis (1 recurrence in 8 patients 6-12 months after end of therapy) while patients with persistent disease had poor prognosis (4 deaths in 10 patients). Results of Hoekstra (38) and of Okada (39) are similar.

The prognostic value of FDG uptake has also been stressed by Alavi (40) in cerebral tumors and by Reisser (41) in head and neck tumors.

How to improve clinical PET

Improvement in clinical PET already results from increased sensitivity. The use of 3D-imaging techniques and of large field of view detectors have considerably increased system sensitivity and reduced statistical noise.

Reduction in image artefact can be obtained through transmission correction, iterative reconstruction and better patient preparation. Transmission correction up to now impractical for whole-body imaging (due to excessive time duration of acquisition), will become possible with the use of a single photon emitter (Cs-137). Further the use of transmission image segmentation has been shown to decrease statistical noise and improve the quality of image reconstruction. Maximum likelihood iterative reconstruction also decrease artefacts, specially in areas of high heterogeneous count activity and can facilitate image interpretation. Improved speed of computing and better algorhythms make it easier to use in clinical practise.

Finally better patient preparation, adequate fasting, glucose level verification, adequate relaxation or use of diazepan as a muscle relaxant and use of forced diuresis (furisemide) for pelvic examination can also contribute to the quality of the examination.

Interpretation can also be improved by anatomical correlation in particular through the use of image fusion of FDG-PET with morphological images. Accurate quantification could also significantly contribute to interpretation. Most important however is patient selection. As FDG is a non specific tracer, its accuracy depends on proper patient selection. Inclusion of patients with low disease probability indeed favor the occurrence of false positives and the technique is not suited to unselected screening or even to detect occasional cancers as by instance in studying patients with possible paraneoplasic syndrome. In adequately selected groups with proper diagnosis verification, the technique has shown considerable impact.

REFERENCES

1. Warburg O, Wind F, Neglers E. On the metabolism of tumors in the body. In : Metabolism of tumors. Warburg O, ed. Constable, London 1930, 254- 270.
2. Hiraki Y, Rosen OM, Birnbaum MJ. Growth factors rapidly induce expression of the glucose transporter gene. J Biol Chem 1988; 27 13655-13662.
3. Shawver LK, Olson SA, White MK, Weber MH. Degradation and biosynthesis of the glucose transporter protein in chicken embryo fibroblasts transformed by the src oncogene. Mol Cell Biol 1987; 7: 2112-2118.
4. Birnbaum MJ, Haspel HC, Rosen OM. Transformation of rat fibroblasts by FSV rapidly increases glucose transporter gene transcription. Science 1987; 235: 1495-1498.
5. Flier JS, Mueckler MM, Usher P, Lodish H. Elevated levels of glucose transport and trasporter messenger RNA are induced by ras or src oncogenes. Science 1987; 235: 1492-1495.
6. Yamamoto T, Seino Y, Fukumoto H et al. Overexpression of facilitated glucose transporter genes in human cancer. Biochem Biophys Res Commun 1990; 170: 223-230.
7. Nishioka T, Oda Y, Seino Y et al. Distribution of the glucose transporters in human brain tumors. Cancer Res 1992; 52: 3972-3979.
8. Gallagher BM, Fowler JS, Gutterson NI et al. Metabolic trapping as a principle of radiopharmaceutical design : Some factors responsible for the biodistribution of F-18-2-deoxy-2-fluoro-D-glucose. J Nucl Med 1989; 19: 1154-1161.
9. Sokoloff L, Reivich M, Kennedy C et al. The (^{14}C)deoxyglucose method for the measurement of local cerebral glucose utilization : theory, procedure, and normal values in the conscious and anesthetized albino rat. J Neurochem 1977; 28: 897-916.
10. Di Chiro G, de la Paz RL, Brooks Ra et al. Glucose utilization of cerebral gliomas measured by F-18-fluorodeoxyglucose and positron emission tomography. Neurology 1982; 32: 1323-1329.
11. Okazumi S, Isono K, Enomoto K et al. evaluation of liver tumors using flurorine-18-fluorodeoxyglucose PET : characterization of tumor and assessment of effect of treatment. J Nucl Med 1992; 33: 333-339.
12. Okada J, Yoshikawa K, Itami M et al. Positron emission tomography using fluorine-18-fluorodeoxyglucose in malignant lymphoma : a comparison with proliferative activity. J Nucl Med 1992; 33: 325-329.
13. Adler LP, Blair HF, Williams RP et al. Grading liposarcomas with PET using 18F-FDG. J Comput Assist Tomogr 1990; 14: 960-962.
14. Strauss LG, Conti PS. The applications of PET in clinical oncology. J Nucl Med 1991; 32: 623-648.

15.Higashi K, Clavo AC, Wahl RL. Does FDG uptake measure proliferative activity of human cancer cells ? In vitro comparison with DNA flow cytometry and tritiated thymidine uptake. J Nucl Med 1993; 34: 414-419.

16.Kubota K, Ishiwata K, Kubota R et al. Tracer feasibility for monitoring tumor radiotherapy : a quadruple tracer study with fluorine-18-fluorodeoxyglucose or fluorine-18-fluorodeoxyuridine, L-{methyl-14C}methionine, {6-3H}thymidine, and gallium-67. J Nucl Med 1991; 32: 2118-2123.

17.Lowe VJ, Hoffman JM, DeLong DM et al. Semiquantitative and visual analysis of FDG-PET images in pulmonary abnormalities. J Nucl Med 1994; 35: 1771-1776.

18.Dewan NA, Reeb SD, Gupta NC et al. PET-FDG imaging and transthoracic needle lung aspiration biopsy in evaluation of pulmonary lesions. A comparative risk-benefit analysis. Chest 1995; 108: 441-446.

19.Bury T, Paulus P, Corhay JL et al. Apport diagnostique de la tomographie à émission de positons dans l'évaluation d'une opacité pulmonaire unique : étude préliminaire chez 30 patients. Médecine Nucléaire - Imagerie fonctionnelle et métabolique 1996; 20: 77-82.

20.Bury T, Dowlati A, Paulus P et al. Evaluation of the solitary pulmonary nodule by positron emission tomography imaging. Eur Resp J 1996: in press.

21.Minn H, Zasadny KR, Quint LE et al. Lung cancer : reproducibility of quantitative measurements for evaluating 2-[F-18]-fluoro-2-deoxy-D-glucose uptake at PET. Radiology 1995; 196: 167-173.

22.Coleman RE, Cascade E, Gupta NC et al. Clinical application and economic implications of PET in the assessment of solitary pulmonary nodules. A retrospective study. Proceedings, Sixth International PET Conference, ICP, Fairfax, Virginia, U.S.A., 1994.

23.Bares R, Klever P, Hauptmann S et al. F-18 Fluorodeoxyglucose PET in vivo evaluation of pancreatic glucose metabolism for detection of pancreatic cancer. Radiology 1994, 192, 79-83.

24.Friess H, Langhans J, Ebert M et al. Diagnosis of pancreatic cancer by 2[18F]-fluoro-2-deoxy-D-glucose positron emission tomography. Gut 1995, 36: 771-777.

25.Hawkins R. Pancreatic tumors : imaging with PET. Radiology 1995, 95, 320-322

26.Inokuma T, Tamaki N, Torizuka T et al. Value of fluorine-18-fluorodeoxyglucose and thallium-201 in the detection of pancreatic cancer. J Nucl Med 1995; 36: 229-235.

27.Wahl RL, Cody R, Hutchins G et al. Positron emission tomographic scanning of primary and metastatic breast with the radiolabeled glucose analogue 2-deoxy-2(18F)fluoro-D-glucose. N. Engl J Med 1991; 324: 200.

28.Adler LP, Crowe JP, Al-Kaisi NK, Sunshine JL. Evaluation of breast masses and axillary lymph nodes with (F-18)2-deoxy-2-fluoro-D-glucose PET. Radiology 1993; 187: 743-750.

29.Avril N, Janicke F, Dose J et al. FDG-PET evaluation of pelvic masses suspicious for primary or recurrent ovarian cancer. J Nucl Med 1994; 35: 231P.

30.Lewis P., Griffin S., Marsden P. et al. Whole-body 18F-fluorodeoxyglucose positron emission tomography in preoperative evaluation of lung cancer. Lancet 1994; 344: 1265-1266.

31.Bury T, Dowlati A, Paulus P et al. Staging of non small cell lung cancer by whole-body 18FDG-PET. Eur J Nucl Med 1996; 23: 204-206.

32.Patronas NJ, Di Chiro GD, Kufta C et al. Prediction of survival in glioma patients by PET. J Neurosurg 1986; 62: 816-822.

33.Strauss LG, Clorius JH, Schlag et al. Recurrence of colorectal tumor : PET evaluation. Radiology 1989; 170: 329-332.

34.Beets G, Penninckx F, Schiepers C et al. Clinical value of whole-body positron emission tomography with [18F]fluorodeoxyglucose in recurrent colorectal cancer. Br J Surg 1994; 81: 1666-1670.

35.Wahl Rl, Zasadny K, Helvie M et al. Metabolic monitoring of breast cancer chemohormonotherapy using positron emission tomography. Initial evaluation. J Clin Oncol 1993; 11: 2101-2111.

36.Gupta NC, Bowman BM, Frank AL et al. PET-FDG imaging for follow-up evaluation of treated colorectal cancer. Radiology 1991; 199: 181P.

37.Institute for Clinical PET Colorectal Cancer Task Force. Clinical application and economic implications of PET in the assessment of colorectal cancer recurrence : a retrospective study. Abstract from the 1994 ICP Meeting.

38.Hoekstra OS, Ossenkoppele GJ, Golding R et al. Early treatment response in malignant lymphoma as determined by planar fluorine-18-fluorodeoxyglucose scintigraphy. J Nucl Med 1993; 34: 1706-1710.

39.Okada J, Oonishi H, Yoshikawa K et al. FDG-PET for predicting the prognosis of malignant lymphoma. Ann Nucl Med 1994, 8: 187-191.

40.Alavi JB, Alavi A, Chawluk J et al. Positron emission tomography in patients with glioma : A predictor of prognosis. Cancer 1988; 62: 1074-1078.

41.Reisser C, Haberkorn U, Dimitrakopoulou-Strauss A et al. Chemotherapeutic management of head and neck malignancies with positron emission tomography. Arch Otolaryngol Head Neck Surg 1995; 121: 272-276.

Oncology

Radioactive Isotopes in
Clinical Medicine and Research XXII
ed. by H. Bergmann, A. Kroiss and H. Sinzinger
© 1997 Birkhäuser Verlag Basel/Switzerland

PRETARGETING: IMPROVED PHARMACOKINETICS AND THERAPEUTIC RATIO

D.A. Goodwin, C.F. Meares, N. Watanabe, M. McTigue, W. Chaovapong, C. Ransone, O. Renn, D.P. Greiner.

Nuclear Medicine Service, Veterans Affairs Health Sciences Center; Stanford University School of Medicine, Palo Alto, CA 94304 and Department of Chemistry, University of California, Davis, CA.

SUMMARY: Pre-clinical studies of three step pretargeting of an anti-hapten mAb were done in BALB/c mice with KHJJ mouse adenocarcinoma. An 80% reduction in whole body radiation burden and a 10 fold increase in Therapeutic Ratio was achieved, compared to directly labeled mAb in this model.

INTRODUCTION

Directly labeled mAb circulates for days after i.v. injection giving a high blood and normal organ background concentration (Fig. 1). This reduces the contrast in tumor imaging and increases the radiation dose to normal tissues in radioimmunotherapy. Pretargeting is one way to improve these vital parameters.

Pretargeting involves the administration of a long circulating *targeting* macromolecule (mAb) having a high affinity non-covalent binding site for a small rapidly excreted *effector* molecule (step 1). After the mAb has reached a maximum concentration in the target tumor (T), i.v. radiolabeled hapten will bind to circulating mAb (Fig. 2) unless it is rapidly removed from the circulation with a polyvalent *chase* macromolecule (step 2). After the chase, the *effector* molecule (radio-labeled hapten-chelate conjugate) is given i.v. (step 3). With 3 step pretargeting the radiolabel is quickly taken up by the tumor and the excess is rapidly excreted by the kidneys within one hour (Fig. 3)

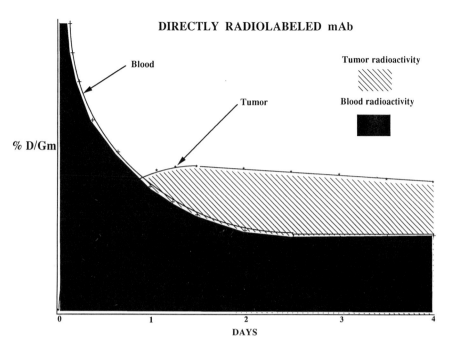

FIGURE 1. The time/concentration curves in tumor mice of covalent conjugates of directly labeled mAb in blood and tumor. The high tumor concentration is offset by high blood levels giving a TR ≈ 3/1 compared to ≈ 24/1 for pretargeting.

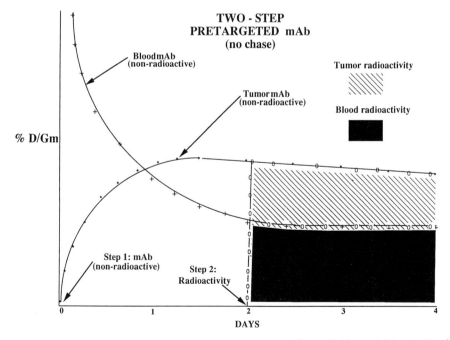

FIGURE 2. Pharmacokinetics of 2 step pretargeting. A long waiting period is needed for the blood mAb levels to fall. There is no radioactivity present during the mAb localization phase.

MATERIALS AND METHODS

Three step pretargeting for radioimmunotherapy in BALB/c, KHJJ tumor mice was done with mAb 2D12.5, which is specific for yttrium-DOTA, but nonspecific for the tumor. Tumor uptake was by passive diffusion of mAb through leaky neovasculature in the tumor. The 3 steps were: 1) anti-hapten mAb 2D12.5 (0 h), 2) polyvalent hapten-protein conjugate chase (20 h), 3) ^{88}Y-labeled monovalent DOTA, or bivalent Janus-DOTA haptens (21 h) and organ & tumor bioassay (24 h).

RESULTS AND DISCUSSION

With therapeutic radionuclides like ^{90}Y, the long biological half-life of directly labeled mAb imposes a high radiation burden on sensitive normal tissues from the large amount of retained radioactivity. Normal tissue toxicity, especially to the bone marrow, has been the major limiting factor in the application of radioimmunotherapy to solid tumors. Pretargeting techniques provide an alternate way to get high selective tumor uptake of ^{90}Y with simultaneous minimization of non-target tissue background.

Rapid tumor (T) uptake and high tumor to blood ratio (T/BL) was seen 3 h after injection of radioactivity (Fig. 3).

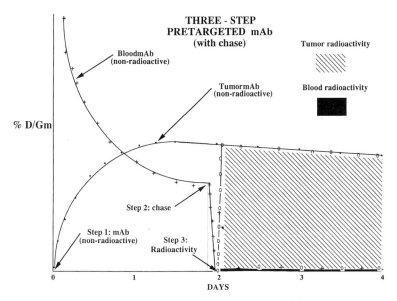

FIGURE 3. Pharmacokinetics of 3 step pretargeting. Rapid uptake at 3 h and slow release of hapten from the tumor is shown over 4 days with pretargeted mAb. Note the large difference between the rates of diffusion into and out of the tumor: very rapid uptake (hours) compared to very slow loss (days) from the tumor. Blood levels are low at all times.

For monovalent ^{88}Y- DOTA, T = *1.7 %/g and T/BL = 16/1; for bivalent ^{88}Y-Janus-DOTA, T = *4.41 %/g and T/BL = 21/1 at 3 h (*p< 0.001). Blood, and bone + marrow were << 1%/g and liver was < 1%/g. The 24 h whole body retention was ≈ 5% ID; 1% in T (20% of total remaining at 24 h), 1.8% in other organs and 2.2% in carcass. Compared to this, the 24 h whole body retention of covalent nonspecific antibody conjugates was > 80% ID. The biological half-life in the tumor of 0.9 µCi ^{88}Y-Janus-DOTA ≈ 24 h , measured daily for 5 days. The activity in µCi/g T and BL for ^{90}Y *equimolar* to ^{88}Y injected (0.9 0 µCi ^{88}Y = 0.744 pmoles = 36.47 µCi ^{90}Y) was used for calculating the area under the curve (AUC) of T & BL in µCi-h/g of ^{90}Y. The ^{90}Y radiation absorbed dose (RAD) from multiplying µCi-h/g x the ^{90}Y absorbed dose constant, 1.99 RAD-g/ µCi-h, gave: T = 89 RADS and BL = 3.7 RADS. The therapeutic ratio (TR) from; RAD T / RAD BL = 24/1 (14).

Thus pretargeting combines the pharmacokinetics of long circulating mAb with rapidly excreted small effector molecules to give *both* high tumor concentration and high tumor/normal tissue ratios. Non-specific localization at this stage in liver, spleen and bone marrow due to Fc receptor binding or phagocytosis of damaged or heavily labeled molecules and aggregates, does not contribute to normal tissue radiation since radioactivity injected later does not access these sites. Previous attempts to overcome non specific binding have required the administration of large amounts of "cold" mAb along with directly labeled mAb to saturate these non-specific binding sites. Two-step pretargeting requires a long waiting period for the blood concentration to fall, since any mAb still circulating must be saturated before any activity can reach the tumor (Fig. 2).

The aggregated mAb produced by cross-linking with the chase in the circulation, is rapidly endocytosed by reticuloendothelial cells (Kupfer cells), mostly in the liver (1). The intracellular location of the endocytosed mAb prevents the access and binding of charged hydrophilic effector molecules, so liver uptake of radioactivity remains low. The rapid entry of radiolabel into the tumor and its slow exit may be explained by cross linking of MAb by the bivalent JANUS hapten, forming ring dimers and trimers of high molecular weight (> 300 kd, Fig. 4), with greatly retarded diffusion out of the tumor extracellular fluid (Fig. 3).

Strategies to reduce the circulating half-time by decreasing the molecular size [F(Ab), F(v) fragments, peptides] also improve the tumor/blood ratio. But this also decreases the time integral in the blood (blood concentration x time), shortening the period of high concentration between the blood and the tumor, thus lowering the diffusion gradient and the final concentration in the tumor. In addition high concentration in non-target normal organs like the kidney [Fab] (11), and lung [VIP] (12) can be a problem with labeled fragments and peptides (13). Thus with directly labeled low molecular weight fragments or peptides, low blood concentration giving high T/Bl ratio is achieved only at the cost of a lower tumor uptake.

Several targeting macromolecule-conjugate/effector small molecule pairs have been proposed (Fig. 4). Examples are; mAb/hapten (2, 3, 4, 5), mAb-avidin/biotin (6), mAb-biotin/avidin (7), mAb-enzyme/prodrug (8, 9), and mAb-oligonucleotide/ antisense oligonucleotide (10) . All these systems give higher target to normal tissue ratios with less toxicity than covalent conjugates of mAbs and effector molecules.

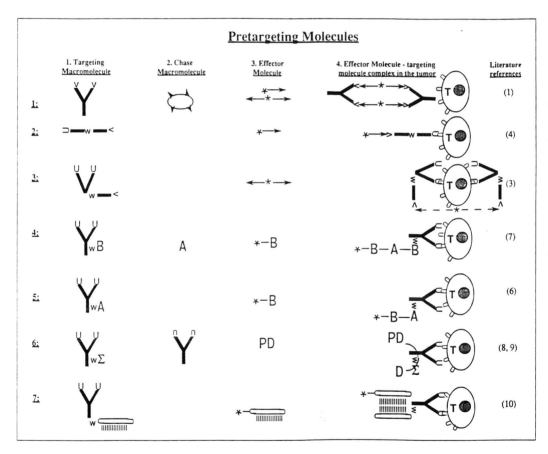

FIGURE 4. Pretargeting molecules based on MAbs. Seven pairs are shown: three hapten/anti hapten, two biotin/avidin, one enzyme/prodrug ADEPT (antibody dependent prodrug therapy) and one antibody-oligonucleotide/antisense. Three include a chase step. The targeting molecule is large and long-circulating, whereas the effector molecule is small, rapidly diffusable, short-circulating and quantitatively excreted by the kidneys without concentrating in any normal organs other than the kidney. ←→ is hapten radiolabeled, bivalent; ←•→ is hapten radiolabeled, monovalent; w is chemical linker; < is Anti-hapten CDR; ⊃ is Anti-tumor CDR; ≺ is whole antibody (MAb); < is F(ab')$_2$, MAb; — is Fab, MAb; A is avidin (streptavidin); •−B is biotin radiolabeled conjugate; Σ is enzyme (MAb conjugate); PD is prodrug; D is drug; •−▥▥ is radiolabeled antisense DNA; ⊂⊃ is polyvalent hapten (protein conjugate).

The essence of pretargeted tumor localization or therapy deals not only with the absolute concentration but also with the rate of clearance of radiolabel from the body (which should be fast) relative to the rate of clearance from the tumor (which should be as slow as possible). As a result of the chase, the therapeutic ratio (TR): area under curve tumor (AUC T)/ area under curve blood(AUC Bl)] is > 20/1, compared to 2/1 with conventional labeling, which is highly desirable for radioimmunotherapy.

The pharmacokinetics illustrated in figures 1-3 shows three key features of the effector molecules (biotin, hapten). They must be: 1) small, hydrophilic and rapidly diffusable, 2) quickly excreted, and 3) have little or no concentration in any normal tissues.

These results indicate that 3 step pretargeting ^{90}Y- hapten specific mAb for radioimmunotherapy has considerable promise.

ACKNOWLEDGMENTS

These studies were supported in part by a grant from the Veterans Administration (DAG) and PHS grants number CA 28343 and CA 48282 (DAG) and CA16861(CFM). Figures 1-4 were reprinted by permission from *Goodwin DA: Pretargeting: Almost the bottom line. J Nucl Med 36: 876-879, 1995.*

REFERENCES

1. Goodwin DA, Meares CF, McCall MJ, McTigue M, Chaovapong W. Pre-targeted immunoscintigraphy of murine tumors with indium-111 labeled bifunctional haptens. *J Nucl Med* 1988; 29: 226-234.

2. Reardon DT, Meares CF, Goodwin DA, et al: Antibodies against metal chelates. *Nature* 1985; 316:265-268.

3. Le Doussal J-M, Martin M, Gautherot E, Delaage M, and Barbet J. In vitro and in-vivo targeting of radiolabeled monovalent and divalent haptens with dual specificity monoclonal antibody conjugates: enhanced divalent hapten affinity for cell-bound antibody conjugate. *J Nucl Med* 1989; 30:1358-1366.

4. Stickney, D.R., Anderson, L.D., Slater, J.B., Ahlem, C.N., Kirk, G.A., Schweighardt, S.A., and Frincke, J.M. Bifunctional antibody: a binary radiopharmaceutical delivery system for imaging colorectal carcinoma. Cancer Res 1991;*51:*6650-6655.

5. Schuhmacher J, Klivényi G, Matys R et al. Multistep tumor targeting in nude mice using bispecific antibodies and a gallium chelate suitable for imminoscintigraphy with positron emission tomography. Cancer Res 1995; 55: 115-123.

6. Hnatowitch DJ, Virzi F, Rusckowski M: Investigations of avidin and biotin for imaging applications. J Nucl Med 28: 1294-1302, 1987

7. Paganelli G, Magnani P, Zito F, et al. Three-step monoclonal antibody tumor targeting in carcinoembryonic antigen-positive patients. *Ca Res* 1991; 51: 5960-5966.

8. Bagshawe KD. The First Bagshawe lecture. Towards generating cytotoxic agents at cancer sites. British Journal of Cancer 1989; 60:275-81.

9. Senter PD. Activation of prodrugs by antibody-enzyme conjugates: a new approach to cancer therapy. *The FASEB J* 1990; 4: 188-193.

10. Bos ES, Kuijpers WHA, Meesters-Winters M, et al. *In vitro* evaluation of DNA-DNA hybridization as a two-step approach in radioimmunotherapy of cancer. *Cancer Res* 1994; 54: 3479-3486.

11. Pimm MV, and Gribben SJ. Prevention of renal tubule re-absorption of radiometal (indium-111) labeled Fab fragment of a monoclonal antibody in mice by systemic administration of lysine. Eur J of Nucl Med 1994; 21: 663-664.

12. Virgolini I, Raderer M, Kurtaran A, et al. Vasoactive intestinal peptide-receptor imaging for the localization of intestinal adenocarcinomas and endocrine tumors. N Engl J Med 1994; 331: 1116-1121.

13. Fischman AJ, Babich JW and Strauss HW. A ticket to ride: peptide radiopharmaceuticals. J Nucl Med 1993; 34: 2253-2263.

14. DA Goodwin, CF Meares, N Watanabe et al. Pharmacokinetics of pretargeted MAb 2D12.5 and Y-88-JANUS-DOTA in BALB/c mice with KHJJ mouse acenocarcinoma: a model for Y-90 radioimmunotherapy. Cancer Research 1994; 54: 5937-5946.

Radioactive Isotopes in
Clinical Medicine and Research XXII
ed. by H. Bergmann, A. Kroiss and H. Sinzinger
© 1997 Birkhäuser Verlag Basel/Switzerland

BRAIN TUMORS - EFFECT OF RADIATION THERAPY ON AMINO ACID TRANSPORT

L. Otto, C. Dannenberg, P. Feyer, K. Papsdorf, A. Seese, I. Kämpfer, F.H. Kamprad, W.H. Knapp

Departments of Nuclear Medicine and Radiotherapy, University of Leipzig, Liebigstraße, D-04103 Leipzig, Germany

SUMMARY: Labeled amino acids have been successfully used to image brain tumors with PET and SPET. This study deals with the question whether percutaneous irradiation produces changes in 3-[^{123}I]iodo-L-α-methyltyrosine (IMT) uptake. 32 patients were investigated before, during, after radiotherapy and 4 weeks later using IMT-SPET. In high-grade tumors there was a significant decrease of the tumor-to-non-tumor activity ratio (T/N) after irradiation, whereas T/N remained unchanged in low-grade astrocytomas. It is concluded that IMT uptake by brain tumors could be used to identify responders from non-responders to radiotherapy.

INTRODUCTION

Individual therapy response of brain tumors following percutaneous irradiation cannot be reliably predicted on the basis of pathohistomorphology. CT and MRI are appropriate techniques for discovering brain tumors, but fail to identify or differentiate tumor response or recurrence immediately after irradiation.

Compared with brain tissue, many tumors have increased protein synthesis rates of amino acids corresponding with increased amino acid transport, according to data obtained with positron emission tomography (PET) using Carbon-11 labeled methionine (1,2). Tumor extent defined with [^{11}C]-methionine was larger than that defined with CT. The selective uptake of [^{11}C]methionine correlated with the degree of malignancy (3,4).

Labeled methyl tyrosine with iodine-123 offers the possibility of imaging brain tumors using the widely available SPET technique (5).

This study deals with the question, whether percutaneous irradiation produces changes in amino acid uptake, and if so, when these changes occur and whether there are differences in the degree of reactions as to different grades of malignancy.

MATERIALS AND METHODS

Patients: We investigated 32 patients (25 male, 7 female), aged between 25 and 75 years (mean 47.8 years). 27 patients underwent surgery with tumor resection, the remainder were classified inoperable. Tumor histology showed in 6 cases low-grade astrocytomas (grade II) and in 26 patients high-grade astrocytomas or glioblastomas (grade III to IV). In patients with astrocytoma grade II 60 Gy were admistered with single doses of 1.8 Gy per day. High-grade tumors underwent hyperfractionated therapy (2 irradiations with a total dose of 3 Gy per day and a total dose per irradiation course of 54 Gy to the hemisphere involved).

SPET studies: Patients unterwent scintigraphy with 250 MBq 3-[^{123}I]Iodo-L-α-methyltyrosine (IMT)
- before (A),
- after 50 - 60 % of the total dose (B),
- immediately after termination of irradiation course (C), and
- after a further interval of 4 weeks (D).

Acquisition was begun 10 min p.i. using a dual-head SPET camera system with LEHR-collimators (35 sec per view, 64 detector positions and 64 x 64 matrix).

For reconstruction Gaussian filter and attenuation correction (attenuation coefficient of 0.12) were used. Quantitation of tumor activity was obtained using irregular ROIs. The transverse slice showing a maximum in count density within the tumor area was selected to delineate the tumor. The so defined ROI was mirrored at the interhemispheric line into the normal brain. The ratio of the respective counts yielded the tumor-to-non-tumor ratio (T/N ratio). The same ROIs were repositioned for the next 3 examinations of each patient.

RESULTS AND DISCUSSION

On average, the T/N ratio decreased from 1.80 to 1.59 during irradiation (Table 1).

Table 1. Mean values of the tumor-to-non-tumor activity (T/N ratio; n = 32; p-values refer to A, paired Student's t-test)

(A)	1.80 ± 0.34 (range 1.00 - 2.59)	
(B)	1.72 ± 0.30	n.s.
(C)	1.64 ± 0.28	$p < 0.01$
(D)	1.61 ± 0.33	$p < 0.01$

The wide range of the initial values of the T/N ratio (before irradiation) seem to reflect rather the individually different active tumor volume after or without surgical resection than different grades of malignancy. The individual time course of the T/N ratios was independent of the initial value.

A typical course of the T/N ratio after irradiation is shown in Fig. 1. The T/N values of the 50 years old patient with an inoperable glioblastoma grade IV in the left hemisphere frontal decreased from 2.59 (A) to 1.68 (D).

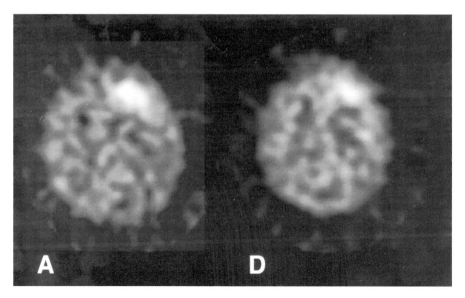

Figure 1. Transverse slice using IMT-SPET before (A) and 4 weeks after termination of the irradiation course (D). Note decrease in tumor activity uptake.

Out of the 26 patients with high-grade malignancies there was only one with an increase of the T/N ratio between A (before irradiation) and C (immediately after the irradiation course). It was a 75 years old patient with a partly resected glioblastoma grade IV of the left hemisphere temporobasal. Six weeks post operative tumor resection irradiation course was begun. Immediately before irradiation (A) the T/N ratio was 1.48, at the end of the irradiation course (C) the T/N ratio had increased to 1.71 with subsequent letal tumor progression.

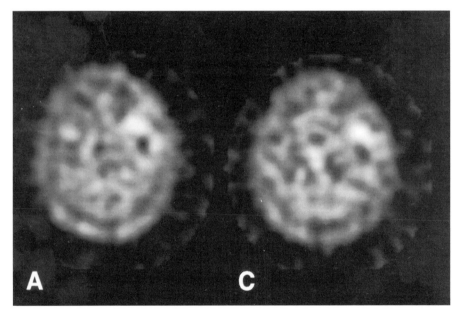

Figure 2. Transverse slice using IMT-SPET before (A) and at the end of irradiation course (C) of a patient with rapid letal tumor progression. Note increase in tumor activity uptake.

The mean values of the T/N ratio for the patients with high-grade brain tumors (Tab.1) did not change significantly between A and B. Only when data at A and C were compared the difference reached statistical significance. It suggests that the cytocidal effect of radiation therapy may be monitored by the T/N ratio (6). Between C and D there was considerable interindividual variability regarding the development of T/N ratios.

Table 2. Mean values of the T/N ratios of high-grade brain tumors ($n = 26$; p-values refer to A, paired Student's t-test)

(A)	1.83 ± 0.31	(range 1.00 - 2.59)
(B)	1.71 ± 0.31	n.s.
(C)	1.61 ± 0.27	$p < 0.01$
(D)	1.60 ± 0.23	$p < 0.01$

In contrast to patients with high-grade malignancies no decrease in T/N ratios was observed in low-grade astrocytomas, on average. Four out of six low-grade astrocytomas showed increased T/N ratios when therapy was terminated (Table 3). These tumors are known to be relatively radioresistant.

Table 3. Mean values of the T/N ratios of the low-grade astrocytomas ($n = 6$; p-values refer to A, paired Student's t-test)

(A)	1.63 ± 0.19	(range 1.44 - 1.90)
(B)	1.71 ± 0.23	n.s.
(C)	1.73 ± 0.40	n.s.
(D)	1.68 ± 0.48	n.s.

CONCLUSIONS

Percutaneous radiation therapy reduces the global amino acid uptake in the residual mass of high-grade astrocytomas and glioblastomas. There is no effect of radiation therapy on amino acid transport in low-grade astrocytomas. The data suggest that IMT uptake by brain tumors could be used to identify responders from non-responders to radiotherapy.

ACKNOWLEDGEMENT

This work was supported by a grant from Bundesministerium für Bildung, Wissenschaft und Forschung to W.H.K. (FKZ 01 ZZ 9103/2.4).

REFERENCES

1. Bergström M, Collins VP, Ehrin E, Ericson K, Eriksson L, Greitz T, Halldin C, Holst Hv, Langström B, Lilja A, Lundquist H, Nagren K. Discrepancies in brain tumor extent as shown by computed tomography and positron tomography using [^{68}Ga]EDTA, [^{11}C]glucose, and [^{11}C]methionine. J Comput Assist Tomogr 1983; 7:1062-6.

2. Ericson K, Lilja A, Bergström M, Collins VP, Eriksson L, Ehrin E, Holst Hv, Lundqvist H, Langström B, Mosskin M. Positron emission tomography with ([^{11}C]methyl)-L-methionine, [^{11}C]D-glucose, and [^{68}Ga]EDTA in supratentorial tumors. J Comput Assist Tomogr 1985; 9:683-9.

3. Schober O, Meyer GJ, Duden C, Lauenstein L, Niggemann J, Müller JA, Gaab MR, Becker H, Dietz H, Hundeshagen H. Die Aufnahme von Aminosäuren in Hirntumoren mit der Positronen-Emissionstomographie als Indikator für die Beurteilung von Stoffwechselaktivität und Malignität. Fortschr Röntgenstr 1987; 5:503-9.

4. Derlon JM, Bourdet C, Chatel M, Théron J, Darcel F, Bustany P, Syrota A. Study of [^{11}C]-L-methionine uptake in glial tumors by positron emission tomography: Metabolic grading and effect of radiotherapy and intraarterial chemotherapy. J Cereb Blood Flow Metab 1987; 7(Suppl 1): S476.

5. Biersack HJ, Coenen HH, Stöcklin G, Reichmann K, Bockisch A, Oehr P, Kashab M, Rollmann O. Imaging of brain tumors with L-3-[^{123}I]Iodo-α-methyl tyrosine and SPECT. J Nucl Med 1989; 30:110-2.

6. Kubota K, Matsuzawa T, Takahashi TTF. Rapid and sensitive response of carbon-11-L-methionine tumor uptake to irradiation. J Nucl Med 1989; 30:2012-6.

Radioactive Isotopes in
Clinical Medicine and Research XXII
ed. by H. Bergmann, A. Kroiss and H. Sinzinger
© 1997 Birkhäuser Verlag Basel/Switzerland

SCINTIMAMMOGRAPHY WITH TECHNETIUM-99M-SESTAMIBI: PLANAR SCANNING VS SPECT

A. Becherer, Th. Helbich, A. Staudenherz, and Th. Leitha

Departments of Nuclear Medicine and Radiology, Vienna General Hospital, Austria

SUMMARY: To determine the accuracy of planar scintimammography versus SPECT scintimammography 18 patients with 21 fibroadenomas and 21 patients with 24 breast cancer sites were investigated. The sensitivity and specificity reached 79% and 95% with the planar technique and 96% and 76% with SPECT scintimammography, respectively. Metastatic axillary lymph nodes were found in one of 4 cases in planar scans but in 3 of 4 by SPECT. Whereas 5 of 17 fibroadenomas were false positive in SPECT in patients under 40 years there were no false positives above 40 years. We conclude that particularly in the higher age group SPECT scintimammography is the method with the best diagnostic accuracy.

INTRODUCTION

Planar scintimammography has proved to be a method of good diagnostic values in a number of studies [1-5], yet those are hampered by lacking information about the tumour stages of their patient samples. SPECT should be a useful tool in the further classification of T1 and T2 lesions, which are found at increasing numbers through modern mammography devices with resolution capabilities down to 1 millimetre. Despite the weaker spatial resolution of planar scanning at present hardly data on SPECT scintimammography exist.

The purpose of the following investigation is to compare the sensitivity and specificity of planar and tomographic scintimammography in patients with node positive mammograms.

MATERIALS AND METHODS

We investigated 39 female patients with pathologic findings on palpation or node positive mammograms and ultrasound investigations, makes necessary subsequent histologic workup. After scintimammography they underwent diagnostic biopsy or surgery.

The patients were positioned supine, arms overhead. Dynamic and planar imaging was performed until 20 minutes after injection of 740 MBq Tc-99m-Sestamibi in a cubital vein contralateral to the lesion on a gamma camera with a wide FOV LEGAP collimator, 256x256 pixel matrix. One frame with a marker over the lesion was obtained for exact localisation of the lesion, further right and left lateral images were obtained.

For SPECT we investigated the patients also supine with arms overhead on a triple headed gamma camera equipped with LEUHR collimators, 128x128 pixel matrix.

Images were assessed by two observers, every focal tracer uptake in the breast was classified as positive scan and considered as malignant.

RESULTS

Of the breast cancers 9 patients were staged as pT1, 9 as pT2 stage, 2 as pT3 cancers and only one was in the pT4 stage, respectively. In 4 patients involvement of axillary lymph nodes was documented. Planar scanning detected 19 of the 24 cancers correctly and was false positive in one out of 21 fibroadenomas. These results represent a sensitivity of 79% and a specificity of 96%. Of 4 metastatic axillary lymphatic involvements only one was imaged clearly.

With SPECT 23 cancers were true positive but also 5 fibroadenomas showed focal tracer uptake, increasing the sensitivity to 96% at reduced specificity to 76%. Axillary metastases were true positive in 3 cases with no false positive SPECT in this region.

Confining the results to patients over 40 years, none of the 4 fibroadenomas was false positive in SPECT.

In one patient investigated for two small nodes in her breast a diffuse faint uptake in the cervicothoracal and right apical thoracal region on planar scintimammography was clearly shown by SPECT as focal uptake with central cold spot. Surgery confirmed a pancoast tumour of a low differentiated bronchial carcinoma. In the patient with the pT4 stage carcinoma, which presented already clinically as large tumour mass, the contribution of SPECT was the finding that also deeper structures like the thoracic wall muscles were involved. Planar scanning in this two special cases, particularly when performed only in prone position, probably would have missed the lung tumour and the extension of the breast cancer, respectively because of the different field of view.

DISCUSSION

In summary of our results, SPECT has following advantages:

- The patient can be investigated supine without need of a special positioning device.
- The sensitivity is increased by SPECT from 79% to 96%.

In two cases SPECT provided additional information, which might influence other therapeutic procedures like the decision about chemotherapy before surgery, particularly suggested by the correctly as T4 staged breast cancer. Also in the other patient with a pancoast tumour the finding of an apical lung uptake was markedly better visible and interpretable on the tomographic images.

A very important finding was the increased specificity in patients over 40 years. In their age group not only the breast cancer incidence rises but also the probability of accidentally breast node detection of radiologically unclear dignity [6, 7] by screening investigations. A similar age dependent phenomenon has been described for Gadolinium-DTPA enhancement in MRI-studies [8]. A possible explanation is a reduction of fibroadenoma vascularisation in elderly patients since there exists a correlation between Tc-99m-Sestamibi uptake with neoangiogenesis [9].

CONCLUSION

If the tendency of a high specificity of SPECT scintimammography in patients over 40 years of age can be confirmed in a larger patient sample, SPECT could become the method of choice for elderly women. In younger patients the advantage of increased sensitivity by SPECT is diminished through the loss of specificity. However, SPECT seems to be superior in tumour staging of the primary tumour and axillary involvement as well so that we recommend its performance at present.

REFERENCES

1. Khalkhali I, Mena I, Jouanne E, et al: Prone scintimammography in patients with suspicion of carcinoma of the breast. J Am Coll Surg 1994; 178: 491-497

2. Kao CH, Wang SJ, Liu TJ: The use of technetium-99m-methoxyisobutylnitrile breast scintigraphy to evaluate palpable breast masses. Eur J Nucl Med 1994; 21: 432-436

3. Burak Z, Argon M, Memis A, et al: Evaluation of palpable breast masses with Tc-99m-MIBI: A comparative study with mammography and ultrasonography. Nucl Med Commun 1994; 15: 604-612

4. Khalkhali I, Cutrone J, Mena I, et al: Scintimammography: The complementary role of Tc-99m sestamibi prone breast imaging for the diagnosis of breast carcinoma. Radiology 1995; 196: 421-426

5. Taillefer R, Robidoux, A, Lambert R, Turpin S, Laperrière J: Technetium-99m-sestamibi prone scintimammography to detect primary breast cancer and axillary lymph node involvement. J Nucl Med 1995; 36: 1758-1765

6. Bassett LW, Liu T-H, Giuliano AE, Gold RH: The prevalence of carcinoma in palpable vs impalpable, mammographically detected lesions. AJR 1991; 157: 21-24

7. Thurfjell EL, Lindgren JAA: Population-based mammography screening in Swedish clinical practice: prevalence and incidence screening in Uppsala county. Radiology 1994; 193: 351-357

8. Gilles R, Garnier C, Meingan P, et al: Fibroadenomas of the breast: histopathological/dynamic contrast-enhanced MR correlation. Eur Radiol 1995; 5, 511-517

9. Scopinaro F, Schillaci O, Scarpini M et al: Technetium-99m-MIBI: An indicator of breast cancer invasiveness. Eur J Nucl Med 1994; 21: 984-987

Radioactive Isotopes in
Clinical Medicine and Research XXII
ed. by H. Bergmann, A. Kroiss and H. Sinzinger
© 1997 Birkhäuser Verlag Basel/Switzerland

HOW TO FURTHER EVALUATE INDETERMINATE MAMMOGRAMS? A COMPARISON BETWEEN SEMIQUANTITATIVE TC-99m SESTAMIBI SCINTIMAMMOGRAPHY AND DYNAMIC MRI

R. Tiling, H. Sommer, R. Moser, M. Pechmann, G. Meyer, Th. Pfluger, K. Tatsch and K. Hahn

Departments of Nuclear Medicine, Radiology and Gynecology
Ludwig-Maximilians-University of Munich, Germany

SUMMARY: The clinical impact of semiquantitative scintimammography with Tc-99m sestamibi and contrast enhanced MRI was evaluated in 66 patients with indeterminate results of previous mammography. Scintimammography provided a sensitivity of 86% and a specificity of 82%; Gd-enhanced MRI revealed a higher sensitivity of 93%, but a considerable lower specificity of 47%. The data indicate, that scintimammography is the preferable method in the further diagnostic work up of these patients. In contrast, MRI seems not be able to reduce the number of biopsies yielding benign results mainly due to Gd-enhancement of different benign lesions.

INTRODUCTION

Recent publications (1-3) attribute to scintimammography with Tc-99m sestamibi very promising results in the diagnostic work up of breast masses. Evaluating the purpose of these data in the clinical routine, one has to note, that patients with palpable or mammographically detected suspicious or definitively abnormal lesions were included in these examinations. But the impact of new diagnostic modalities in routine breast assessment will be determined by their results in patients with indeterminate preliminary diagnosis. If physical examination, ultrasound and mammography are highly suspicious for carcinoma or if the mentioned methods are diagnostic in excluding malignancy, no further diagnostic work up is necessary and will be performed. Only in patients with indeterminate results there are major problems in deciding the further therapeutic proceedings. Thus up to now many patients with benign lesions undergo surgery in order to exclude malignancy. In consideration of these facts the aim of our study was to determine the results of scintimammography in patients with unclear preliminary diagnosis and to compare scintimammography with the results of contrast enhanced MRI.

MATERIALS AND METHODS

In order to obtain the above mentioned information, we examined a total of 62 patients, for whom indeterminate results of clinical examination, mammography and ultrasound warranted breast biopsy. All patients underwent scintimammography with Tc-99m sestamibi as well as contrast enhanced MRI. The reasons for the radiologists and gynecologists not being able to make a certain diagnosis are listed below:

- homogeneous dense breast tissue (n=7)
- severe fibrocystic mastopathy (n=6)
- unclear microcalcifications (n=19)
- unclear opacities or asymmetries (n=28)
- unclear differentiation between scar and recurrence (n=2)

Breast scintigraphy was done in prone position using a double headed camera system. Planar lateral and anterior views (acquisition times 600 sec) were acquired 5 - 30 min. p.i. Each patient received 740 MBq Tc-sestamibi intravenously in the arm contralateral to the breast with the suspected abnormality.

The MR images were obtained before, immediately and 5 minutes after the administration of Gd-DTPA using a 3D gradient echo sequence (TR=40 msec, TE=14 msec, Flipangle=50°). 24 continuous slices were acquired.

In scintigrams we determined the presence of any breast abnormality without knowledge of the findings in MRI and mammography. To assess visual sestamibi accumulation we used a score system (normal/equivocal , focal with low intensity, focal with medium intensity, focal with high intensity). Studies were considered positive, if a focal sestamibi accumulation was observed.

Regions of Interest were drawn on focal and equivocal sestamibi uptake sites and normal breast tissue, respectively. Thus a target/non target ratio for semiquantitative evaluation was obtained. The contrast behaviour in MR images was scored visually by independent observers also blinded for the suspected diagnosis. In a first step every focal contrast enhancement was considered as suspicious. To optimize the method we differentiated MR-diagnoses in benign, indeterminate and suspicious by rating the amount and dynamics of Gd uptake as well as the shape of the enhancing lesion. The uptake of sestamibi was compared with the signal increase in MRI after application of Gd-DTPA representing the major criterion for malignancy. After determination of the optimal threshold for judging a scintigraphic study as suspicious, diagnoses obtained by semiquantitative scintimammography were correlated with the findings in optimized MRI and with the final histopathologic results.

RESULTS

24 out of 28 carcinomas visually showed positive focal sestamibi accumulation (Fig. 1). 4 carcinomas (2 lobular invasive, one ductal invasive and one subepidermal spread) could not be detected scintigraphically. 7 cases with different benign lesions showing also focal uptake were diagnosed false positive (Table 1).

Table 1. Scintimammography: sestamibi uptake versus histology

	sestamibi uptake			
	normal/equivocal	focal low	focal medium	focal high
carcinoma	4	5	10	9
fibroadenoma	4	2	-	-
mastopathy	19	1	1	-
papillomatosis	2	1	-	-
chron. inflammation	-	-	2	-
scar	2	-	-	-

In MRI 26 of 28 carcinomas showed contrast enhancement after application of paramagnetic Gd-DTPA, so diagnoses were true positive (Fig. 1). 2 of 4 non sestamibi accumulating carcinomas showed no Gd-enhancement. On the other hand many of the benign lesions had a low, medium or even high signal increase after administration of Gd-DTPA and could therefore not be differentiated from carcinomas by assessment of Gd-uptake only (Table 2).

Table 2. MRI: contrast enhancement versus histology

	contrast enhancement			
	none	low	intermediate	high
carcinoma	2	2	8	16
fibroadenoma	1	-	2	3
mastopathy	2	3	8	8
papillomatosis	-	1	2	-
chron. inflammation	-	-	-	2
scar	1	1	-	-

After calculation of the target/non target ratio in lateral scintigrams an overlap of benign and malignant cases was established between values of 1.0 and 1.5. The maximal ratio seen in our study was 3.4 (invasive ductal carcinoma), the mean ratio of all carcinomas was 1.7. The maximal target/non target ratio in benign lesions (1.5) was calculated in a chronic inflammation. A ROC analysis was performed to optimize the threshold between benign and suspicious diagnoses. The optimal threshold for judging a sestamibi study as suspicious was a ratio of 1.3.

Compared to the results of visual analysis semiquantitative evaluation didn't change the sensitivity of 86% but improved the specificity of scintimammography from 79% (visual evaluation) moderately up to 82%.

Considering any contrast enhancement as criterion for malignancy, sensitivity of MRI was 93% and higher compared to scintimammography. In consequence of the high number of benign lesions with a low, medium or even a high signal increase after application of Gd-DTPA, malignancy could be excluded by MRI only in 4 out of 34 patients with benign lesions. After modification of MRI readings taking into account amount and dynamics of Gd- enhancement as well as the shape of the enhancing lesion, specificity increased up to 47%, sensitivity remained unchanged. The positive and negative predictive value representing important parameters in further evaluation of indeterminate preliminary diagnoses were 80% resp. 87% in scintimammography and 59% resp. 89% in modified MRI readings.

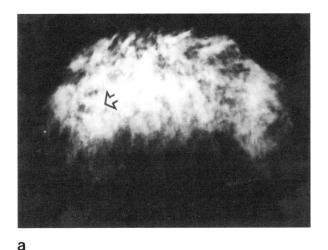

a

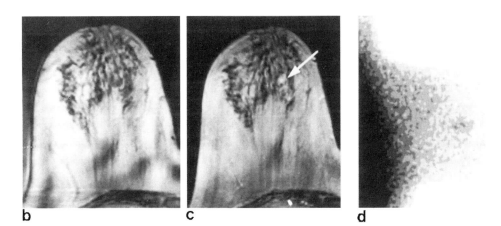

b   c   d

Figure 1. Mammography (a), plain and Gd-enhanced MRI (b,c) and scintimammography (d) in a 52 years old patient with severe fibrocystic mastopathy. Mammography detected unclear microcalcifications (short arrow), diagnosis was indeterminate. In MRI a very small and irregular enhancing lesion was observed (long arrow), so MRI reading was suspicious. Scintigraphically a small focal area with a low sestamibi uptake could be seen more clearly. Biopsy proved an invasive ductal carcinoma with a diameter of 0.6 cm.

DISCUSSION

Our data indicate, that a target / non target ratio of 1.3 is the optimal threshold for separating benign from suspicious lesions. Using the ratio seems to provide a little higher specificity and may increase the diagnostic certainty especially in cases of an indeterminate sestamibi uptake.

In the selected patient group with indeterminate findings of palpation and mammography semiquantitative evaluation of sestamibi uptake provided a sensitivity of 86% and a specificity of 82% for the detection of breast carcinoma. The previous reported values over 90 % (1-3) could not be reached in the subpopulation with unclear preliminary diagnosis. Nevertheless, the further role of scintimammography will be determined by the results in this patient group. In contrast to Gd-enhanced MRI, scintimammography using Tc-99m sestamibi provides a comparable higher specificity and may be able to reduce the number of biopsies which yield benign results.

Optimized MRI readings show a higher sensitivity but a considerable lower specificity due to intense contrast enhancement of different benign lesions. Thus, breast scintigraphy may be suggested as the preferable method for further evaluation of indeterminate mammographic findings, especially in patients with dense breast tissue, unclear microcalcifications or severe mastopathy.

REFERENCES

1. Khalkhali I, Cutrone J, Mena I, et al. Scintimammography: The complementary role of Tc-99m sestamibi prone breast imaging for the diagnosis of breast carcinoma. Radiology 1995; 196:421-426.
2. Khalkhali I, Cutrone J, Mena I, et al. Technetium-99m-sestamibi scintimammography of breast lesions: clinical and pathological follow-up. J Nucl Med 1995; 36:1784-1789.
3. Taillefer R, Robidoux A, Lambert R, Turpin S, Laperriere J. Technetium-99m-sestamibi prone scintimammography to detect primary breast cancer and axillary lymph node involvement. J Nucl Med 1995; 36:1758-1765.

Radioactive Isotopes in
Clinical Medicine and Research XXII
ed. by H. Bergmann, A. Kroiss and H. Sinzinger
© 1997 Birkhäuser Verlag Basel/Switzerland

THE USE OF TECHNETIUM-99m METHOXYISOBUTYLISONITRILE (Tc^{99}m-MIBI) BREAST SCINTIGRAPHY FOR EARLY DETECTION OF BREAST CANCER

T. Horne[1], I. Pappo[2], R. Reif[3], V. Kent[4], and R. Orda[2]

Departments of [1]Nuclear Medicine, [2]Surgery "A", [3]Pathology, and [4]Radiology, Assaf Harofeh Medical Center, Sackler Faculty of Medicine, Tel Aviv University, Israel.

SUMMARY: We evaluated the feasibility of Tc^{99}m-MIBI scintigraphy as a method for early detection of breast cancer in 142 patients. In 101 consecutive patients there was a suspicious lesion on physical examination or on mammography. In 41 high risk patients the scintigraphy was performed only as a screening test. **RESULTS:** The results demonstrated that in 101 patients who underwent biopsies, there were positive scans in 48 patients (29 of them were true positive), and 53 negative scans (51 of them were true negative). The sensitivity, specificity, positive predictive value and negative predictive value were 94%, 73%, 60%, and 96% respectively. Two false-negative results were in lesions 0.6 and 0.7 cm. in size. Among 19 false positive results 5 were in patients with active mastitis. **CONCLUSIONS:** Tc^{99}m-MIBI breast scintigraphy is a sensitive method for early detection of breast malignancies.

INTRODUCTION

Breast cancer is the leading cause of cancer related death among women in the western world (1). In spite of great advances in breast cancer research and therapy, the most efficient way for reducing morbidity and mortality of this disease remains early detection (2).

However, standard mammography has serious limitations. Given the fact that among an estimated 700,000 breast biopsies which are done yearly in the United States only in 1 out of 4 cases cancer has been found, it is obvious that a better tool is urgently needed in order to reduce this high number of useless invasive procedures.

Recent publications have demonstrated that an imaging agent used usually for cardiac imaging, Tc99m- methoxyisobutylisonitrile (Tc^{99}m-MIBI), was shown to demonstrate positive results in the imaging of tumors such as recurrent brain gliomas, bone and thyroid tumors, parathyroid adenomas (3-5). Recent data suggested that using Tc^{99}m-MIBI scintimammography may be a highly effective method for early breast cancer detection, with high rates of sensitivity and specificity (6-9).

The aim of the present study is to determine the sensitivity and specificity of Tc^{99}m-MIBI in a series of consecutive patients

MATERIALS AND METHODS

Patients: One hundred and one consecutive women who were found to have suspicious breast lesions, either on physical examination or on mammogram, were subjected to open biopsy or to fine needle aspiration of their lesions. Prior to their biopsies they were referred to perform Tc^{99}m-MIBI scintigraphy. An additional forty one patients with no definite breast lesions but with a history which may put them in higher risk for breast cancer (family history of cancer, previous malignant lesions of the breast or florid fibrocystic disease), also underwent breast scintigraphy. The average age of the patients was 48.6 years old (range: 17-83 years).

Seven patients had suspicious lesions on mammogram with no palpable lesions. These patients had mammography guided open biopsies. The Tc^{99}m-MIBI scintigraphy results were evaluated using histopathological or cytological examinations as gold standards.

Technetium-99m-MIBI Scintimammography: Technetium-99m methoxyisobutylisonitrile (Tc^{99}m-MIBI) is a commercial preparation ("Cardiolite") and was obtained from the DuPont Company through the Nahal Sorek atomic plant in Israel. The labeling and quality control procedures were carried out according to the manufacturer's instructions.

All patients received an intravenous injection of 20 mCi (740 Mbq) Tc^{99}m-MIBI, in the antecubital vein of the arm contralateral to the breast with the known lesion, to avoid any false-positive uptake in the axillary lymph nodes. Five minutes following the injection, 5 minutes planar images were obtained using a large field of view gamma camera (Elscint Apex SP-4) fitted with a low energy all purpose collimator. Five images were obtained: anterior, two posterior oblique and two lateral views.

The lateral and oblique images were obtained while the patient lay prone on a special table with semilunar aperture in each side, which enables the breast to be pending, and minimized the distance between the breast and the detector. The anterior view was obtained with the patient supine with arms raised and the hands placed behind the head to visualize the axilla.

All images were interpreted by two physicians. They were classified as positive when a focal abnormal accumulation was identified, and negative when no such focus of activity was found (Fig. 1).

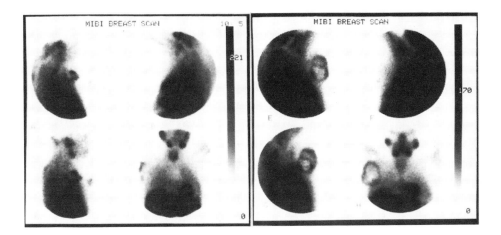

Figure 1. Scintigraphic study of two different patients. The four views (A,B,C,D) (first patient) show primary tumor in the right breast and metastatic axillary lymph node involvement on the same side. The four views (E,F,G,H) (second patient) show in the right breast (images E,G,H) increased tracer uptake in the edge of a palpable inflammatory mass, with focal area of increased uptake in the lower medial region seen in the anterior view (image H). There is also a focal area of increased uptake in the left breast (image F) which has been proven to be cancer.

RESULTS

Among 142 patients who were scanned we obtained pathological results in 101 cases following either open biopsy or fine needle aspiration (Table 1). Among them we found 31 breast malignancies and 70 benign lesions (Table 2).

While evaluating patients who had underwent biopsies, we demonstrated 48 positive MIBI scans (29 true-positive and 19 false-positive), and 53 negative scans (51 true-negative and 2 false-negative). We excluded 3 patients with active mastitis who were added in order to study specifically the behavior of Tc[99]m-MIIBI scan in active infection and obtained the following results: Sensitivity of the MIBI scan was: 94%, its specificity was 76%, positive predictive value: 64.5% and the negative predictive value was found to be 96%. (Including the cases of mastitis, specificity and positive predictive values were 73% and 60%, respectively)

In six patients the scintigraphy was performed during known active mastitis, in five the scan demonstrated false positive results. Another case of false positive result was a woman on Coumadin treatment who bled and suffered from focal hematoma in her left breast.

Two cases had false-negative results: The first woman who was post neo-adjuvant therapy for stage 3 breast cancer, had a complete disappearance of her lesion on both physical examination and on mammogram. Only in the mastectomy specimen a 0.7 cm. breast cancer focus was found. The second woman with false negative result had a 0.6 cm breast cancer mass in a large fibrocystic lesion.

Comparison of Tc[99]m-MIBI scintigraphy to mammography: In 109 of the scanned patients a mammography was available for comparison. In 68 of these patients, both mammography and Tc[99]m-MIBI scan were negative for malignant lesions. In two of these patients a malignant breast lesion was diagnosed. In 17 patients both examinations were positive for malignancy. Pathological examinations demonstrated malignant lesions in all 17 cases. Ten patients had suspicious mammographies while their corresponding Tc[99]m-MIBI scan was negative, no one of these women suffered a malignant tumor. On the other hand, in 14 patients only the Tc[99]m-MIBI scan was positive, while mammograms were negative for malignancy. Three patients out of the 14 patients were diagnosed as having malignant breast lesions.

Table 1. Tc[99]m-MIBI scintimammography for breast imaging
Results of patients who had biopsies (including 3 cases with mastitis)

Pathology/scan	Malignant	Benign
Positive	29	19
Negative	2	51
TOTAL	31	70

Sensitivity: 94%; Specificity 73%

Positive predictive value: 60%

Negative predictive value: 96%

Table 2. Tc^{99}m-MIBI scintimammography for breast imaging

Pathological results of patients with positive scans

Lobular/ductal carcinoma	27
Squamous cell carcinoma	1
Malignant phylloides tumor	1
Hematoma - post anticoagulation	1
Mastitis	5
Florid fibrocystic disease/fibroadenoma	13
TOTAL POSITIVE SCANS	48

DISCUSSION

Several radionuclide imaging techniques have been examined for tumor imaging and four of these approaches have been more extensively studied in humans (8,10).

Because of the better emission characteristics of Tc^{99}m-MIBI, and its biodistribution as shown in the myocardium, compared to ^{201}Tc-chloride, it was found to be a superior candidate for breast tumor imaging (11).

Although the exact mechanism of Tc^{99}m-MIBI concentration in breast cancer cells is not completely understood, it is known that in the heart it accumulates in viable myocardium proportional to regional blood flow. Crane and colleagues demonstrated, using c-neu OncoMouse, transgenic mice which develop spontaneously mammary tumors, that Tc^{99}m-MIBI concentrates in the periphery of the tumor (12). The center of the tumor which is acellular and often necrotic shows less retention. These results support the theory that Tc^{99}m-MIBI demonstrates viable cells.

The results obtained in the present study confirm the findings of previous studies using Tc^{99}m-MIBI for early detection of breast cancer (8,9). Among the patients in the present study, there was a false-negative rate of 2% with a negative predictive rate of 96%, demonstrating the very high sensitivity of this examination. However, the specificity and positive predictive value of the present study were lower, 73% and 60%, respectively (with exclusions of the cases with mastitis 76% and 64.5%). Possible explanations for these lower rates were the high rate of patients with active mastitis, and the fact that we studied 142 consecutive patients without any selection.

Multiple views, especially the lateral and the oblique prone images, improved the sensitivity of the examination and the rate of detection breast malignancy.

The smallest breast tumor that was diagnosed by Tc^{99}m-MIBI scintigraphy was 1 centimeter. This confirms the findings of others who also mentioned 1 cm as being the lower limit of detection.

Among 31 cases of malignancy, two were not detected by the scintigraphy and gave false-negative results. Their sizes were 0.6 and 0.7 cm. The latter was in a patient following neo-adjuvant radiochemotherapy with no evidence of disease on physical examination or mammogram and the focus of cancer was found in the mastectomy specimen.

Comparing scintimammography to mammography demonstrated that among 22 patients with cancer who underwent mammogram prior to the scan, only 17 were correctly diagnosed, while Tc^{99}m-MIBI demonstrated malignancy in 20 patients. This demonstrates the higher sensitivity of scintimammography over mammography. Among 87 patients with benign breast lesion, Tc^{99}m-MIBI scintigraphy correctly identified 76 patients while mammography was negative in 77 patients, demonstrating similar rates of specificity.

In conclusion we believe that MIBI scintigraphy cannot replace mammography but may provide additional information about suspicious breast lesions. The high negative predictive value of this examination, as demonstrated in this study, may reduce negative breast biopsies especially in the high risk population of patients.

REFERENCES

1. Harris JR, Morrow M, Bonadonna G. Cancer of the breast in: De Vita VT, Hellman S, Rosenberg S,.eds: Cancer, Principles & Practice of Oncology, J.B. Lippincott 1993;pp:1264-1332.

2. Taba L, Fagerberg GJG, Gad A, et al. Reduction in mortality from breast cancer after mass screening with mammography: randomized trial from the Breast Screening Working Group of the Swedish National Board of Health and Welfare. Lancet 1985;1:829-32.

3. Caner B, Kitapel M, Unlu M, et al. Technetium-99m-MIBI uptake in benign and malignant bone lesions: A comparative study with Technetium-99m-MDP. J Nucl Med 1992;33:319-24.

4. Balon HR, Fink-Bennet DM, Stoffer SS. Technetium-99m uptake by recurrent Hurtle cell carcinoma of the thyroid. J Nucl Med 1992;33:1393-1395.

5. Taillefer R, Boucher Y, Potvin C, et al. Detection and localization of parathyroid adenomas in patients with hyperparathyroidism using a single radionuclide imaging procedure with Technetium-99m-sestamibi (double-phase study). J Nucl Med 1992;33:1801-7.

6. Kao CH, Wang SJ, Lui TJ. The use of technetium-99m methoxyisobutyl isonitrile breast scintigraphy to evaluate palpable breast masses. Eur J Nucl Med 1994;21:432-6.

7. Burak Z, Argon M, Memis A, et al. Evaluation of palpable breast masses with mammography and ultrasonography. Nucl Med Comm 1994;15:604-12.

8. Taillefer R, Robidoux A, Lambert R, et al. Technetium-99m-sestamibi prone scintimammography to detect primary breast cancer and axillary lymph node involvement. J Nucl Med 1995;36:1758-65.

9. Khalkhali I, Cutrone J, Mena I, et al. Technetium-99m-sestamibi scintimammography of breast lesions: clinical and pathological follow-up. J Nucl Med 1995;36:1784-9.

10. Launder JP, Lowe J, Baker JR, et al. Gallium-67 citrate scanning in neoplastic and inflammatory lesions. Br J Radiol 1971;44:361.

11. Aktolum C, Bayhan H, Kir M. Clinical experience with Tc-99m MIBI imaging in patients with malignant tumors. Preliminary results and comparison with TI-201. Clin Nucl Med 1992;17:171-6.

12. Crane P, Onthank D, Retos C, et al. Technetium-99m sestamibi retention in the c-neu oncomouse: an in-vivo model for breast tumor imaging (Abstract). J Nucl Med 1994;35:21P.

Radioactive Isotopes in
Clinical Medicine and Research XXII
ed. by H. Bergmann, A. Kroiss and H. Sinzinger
© 1997 Birkhäuser Verlag Basel/Switzerland

FDG SPECT TO MONITOR LUNG CANCER CHEMOTHERAPY

RA Lengauer*, CD Colder°, A van Lingen°, OS Hoekstra°, PE Postmus°, GJJ Teule°

*Elisabethinen's Hospital, Fadingerstr. 1, A-4020 Linz, Austria
°Free University Hospital, De Boelelaan 1117, 1007 MB Amsterdam, The Netherlands

SUMMARY: Resectability after neoadjuvant chemotherapy for locally advanced non small cell lung cancer (NSCLC) is difficult to predict due to incomplete or delayed CT response. We found residual masses in > 90% of our patients in whom resection was attempted. FDG SPECT provided independent information above the detection limit, which was found to be ≥ 2cm. In more than 60%, the perhaps prognostically relevant FDG detected response rate can be followed throughout chemotherapy. Absent or faint FDG uptake suggested resectability, avid uptake was associated with viable tumor and mediastinal uptake with inoperability. Preliminary data suggest that rapid responders have a better prognosis. Such metabolic imaging may therefore help to individualize patient management in neoadjuvant schedules.

INTRODUCTION

Each year 8000 new cases of lung cancer are detected in the Netherlands, 6300 of the non small cell type. At presentation 25-33% of non small lung cancer (NSCLC) is locally advanced and inoperable. In recent years, favorable results were reported with preoperative chemotherapy (1), attempting to "downstage" the malignant process to the extent that resection becomes feasible. The clinical response is variable, however: No viable tumor is left in 10%, no volume reduction is seen in < 50%. Volume response as defined with radiological techniques does not predict surgical success and at present there is no way to predict or monitor the impact of the treatment prior to operation. So only if progression is evident, chemotherapy is stopped. This results in a high number of unnecessary thoracotomies. The problem with volume response relates to the lack of tissue specifity of radiological techniques: true tumor size may not be measurable due to concurrent atelectasis or necrosis and delayed or incomplete response may occur.

[18]Fluoro-2-deoxyglycose (FDG) has shown promising results in malignant disease, and in lung cancer in particular. Most (PET) studies deal with preoperative staging, usually attempting to avoid unnecessary surgery for spreaded desease. Only few used the opportunity offered by short-lived tracers to define the prognostically relevant response rate during treatment (2,3,4). This concept is especially attractive if volume response is delayed or incomplete. Since we, as many others, have access to FDG but not to PET, we are evaluating the applicability of gamma-cameras and FDG (5,6,7) in various malignancies, focusing on response monitoring.

In the present study we first established the detection limit of FDG SPECT in NSCLC, then the potential of FDG SPECT in chemotherapeutically treated patients, and finally performed in vitro and patient studies to assess the feasibility and limits of the technique in monitoring the impact of chemotherapy as indicated by FDG.

MATERIALS AND METHODS

Aiming at detection limit we performed SPECT studies in 18 untreated NSCLC patients (group A), and compared with CT and clinical data. Lesions were analyzed visually and semiquantitatively, using regions of interest (ROI's) over tumor and a contralateral mirror ROI (expressed as T-NT ratio).

Group B consisted of 15 patients treated with chemotherapy (cisplatin, etoposide). In 8/15 multiple scans were done during chemotherapy. Treatment was continued unless progression was evident from CT, and all patients with non progressive disease were operated. CT volume response was classified according to standard techniques, lymph nodes > 1 cm were considered abnormal. The protocol required CT and FDG scans prior to treatment, after 2 and 4 courses, and an additional FDG study after first course. We obtained 17/30 possible comparisons between FDG studies. Missing data result from stopped treatment (upstaging n=1, therapy related death n=1, progressive disease n=2 and of bad [patient or doctor] compliance). The FDG acquisition started with a 10 min whole body scan (30 min pi), ca. 15 min. (53±11min.) later followed by SPECT. SPECT studies were later analyzed by 2 observers (RL, OSH). SPECT data were compared to CT, surgical and histological findings. Serum glucose was measured in all patients.

Quantitative analysis (in vitro and patient studies)/sources of error:

a. Whole body scan (to account for potential changes of FDG biodistribution): geometric mean of counts in brain, liver, contralateral chest, tumor and leg muscle, normalized for ROI size and whole body counts. Whole body scans were used to check for stable biodistribution of FDG in consecutive studies, which proved to be the case (pooled coefficients of variation: contralateral chest: 2.6%, brain 2.5%, liver 3.2%, lower extremity 1.9%). One study was discarded because of severely altered biodistribution during newly developed steroid-diabetes (readily recognized because of reduced cerebral uptake). In the other patients serum glucose was normal.

b. SPECT: in vitro studies (AvL) had shown that quantitation of FDG changes in longitudinal studies is feasible in tumors >2cm and T-NT > 1.1 (corresponding with actual concentration ratios of at least 2.4), since recovery losses are minor in such lesions. In cases where CT cannot estimate tumor size, the ROI size of SPECT may be used (in operated patients we found an acceptable correlation between actual and calculated diameter, r=.93, FDG size=1.7+0.8 [true size]). In the patient studies, regions of interest were drawn in axial 15mm slices around tumor and a reference region (background subtraction ≤10%, saturation unchanged). Three approaches were studied: ratio of counts in tumor vs contralateral mirror ROI, in tumor vs the average of the contralateral hemithorax, in tumor vs the decay corrected injected dose, using the mean of 2 observer data (the latter 2 correlated best; r^2=0.8, p>0.05). In the analysis of SPECT data (ROI's) the interobserver variation was 2.5%. As either method has pros and cons we used their mean values. Data are presented as means ± SD unless specified otherwise.

RESULTS

Group A (untreated NSCLC)

All malignant lung lesions > 2cm were readily recognized with SPECT, at tumor-nontumor ratios of 3.1±0.8. All tumors ≤2cm were not recognized (n=3). CT could separate tumor, atelectasis and necrosis in 10/18 patients, maximal tumor diameter in the others was 5.2 ±3.4cm. SPECT clearly delineated viable tumor and non malignant tissue in all patients.

Group B (treated NSCLC)

13 patients were operated, 2 had progressive disease (on CT as well as SPECT); 9 had resectable disease. One had a complete CT response, the rest partial response or stable disease, with residual masses measuring 3.6±1.9cm (pathology data or, if not available, CT). The volume response did not predict resectability (table 1). Patients with absent or faint FDG uptake were always resectable, and midline FDG foci reflected inoperable disease.

table 1

CT criteria	CT	operable - FDG	operable +	inoperable - FDG	inoperable +
complete response	1	1	0	0	0
partial response	7	2	2	0	3[*]
stable disease	5	2[**]	2	0	1
progression	2	0	0	0	2

[*] mediastinal foci (2/3)

[**] 1 proved to have carcinoid rather than NSCLC

FDG uptake reflected viable tumor (10/10). The relative tracer uptake was not related to the CT response. Histological examination revealed nodal (N2) metastases in 6 patients, in 4 these were missed by CT and SPECT (nodes < 1cm). The preliminary patient data suggest that rapid

responders have a better
prognosis and seem to
confirm the clinical
impression that
intraindividual responses
can be heterogeneous
(figure 1). One patient
initially had a clear
response, but delay
occurred between the last
cycle of chemotherapy
and surgery: his
preoperative scan
showed progression and
mediastinal involvement,
which was confirmed at
surgery.

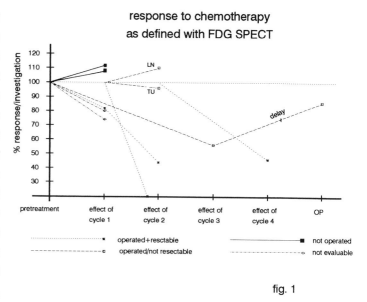

fig. 1

DISCUSSION

Neoadjuvant chemotherapy is increasingly used as part of multimodality approach in oncology. In lung cancer, the aim is to get the tumor process resectable. It would be very helpful to have better tools than CT to assess the impact of preoperative chemotherapy: too often, failure is only detected during the operation. Anatomically orientated, ie. radiological techniques may fail to reflect tumor kill in case of delayed or incomplete volume response. As shown in group A, it can even be difficult to determine the initial (ie. reference) tumor size because of atelectasis or necrosis. Earlier stratification would prevent non responders to receive therapy from which they derive no benefit and, on the other extreme, may lead to more intense/prolonged treatment in others.

Theoretically, longitudinal studies comparing FDG accumulation during chemotherapy may suffer from many confounding factors, mostly concerning the specificity of the "FDG signal". Some of the unsolved issues are: to what extent are we looking at tumor or macrophages (8), is FDG uptake related to the number of tumor cells or is it rather a function of hypoxia or variable proliferative activity (9) ? How about reversible cell damage, what is the impact of perfusion changes, initiated by the tumor itself or by the therapy? And, above all, do these complex matters preclude response monitoring? The conflicting results of sophisticated animal studies appear not to be able to solve these issues. Others tend to use a rather phenomenological approach, observing change during therapy and relating this to outcome (10). Such studies have confirmed and extended the notion that metabolic precede anatomic changes during chemotherapy.

Diagnostic procedures like FDG PET or SPECT (11,12) could be helpful in initial staging, during therapy and prior to attempted resection. Staging should be improved because today too many patients, as in our study, have in fact (undiagnosed) macroscopically disseminated rather than locally advanced disease. It is unlikely that FDG imaged with gamma-cameras will have major impact in this respect, taking into account, that in the lung, where low background levels allow for good contrast, the detection limit for SPECT is already 2cm. Our data suggest that besides PET, SPECT may play a role in preoperative restaging of such patients: irrespective of the CT resonse, absent FDG suggests resectability, avid uptake means tumor viability and if mediastinal, inoperability. For the subset with persistent noncentral FDG uptake, the response rate could be of help. Our data show that in >60% of these patients this, at least in other tumors prognostically relevant, criterium can be assessed with SPECT, provided that larger masses are studied. This is different from the situation with lymphoma and SCLC where the detection limit, in our experience, for SPECT is usually reached half-way during chemotherapy.

We conclude that FDG SPECT and CT provide independent information. SPECT allows tumor visualisation to the extent that the early response to chemotherapy can be monitored and may help to individualize treatment schedules. Our preliminary data suggest that non responders can be identified, and that rapid responders do better.

REFERENCES

1. Rosell R, Gomez-Codina J, Camps C, Maestre J, Padille J, Canto A, Mate JL, Canela M, Ariza A, Skacel Z, Morera-Prat J, Abad A. A randomized trial comparing preoperative chemotherapy plus surgery with surgery alone in patients with non-small-cell-lung cancer. N Engl J Med 1994; 330: 153-8

2. Hoekstra OS, Ossenkoppele GJ, Golding R, van Lingen A, Visser GWM, Teule GJJ, Huijgens PC. Early treatment response in malignant Lymphoma, as determined by planar Fluorine-18-Fluorodeoxyglucose scintigraphy. J Nucl Med 1993; 34:1706-1710

3. Wahl RL, Zasadny K, Helvie M, Hutchins GD, Weber B, Cody R. Metabolic monitoring of breast cancer chemotherapy using positron emission tomography: initial evaluation. J Clin Onkol 1993, 11: 2101-2111

4. Hoekstra OS, van Lingen A, Ossenkoppele GJ, Golding R. Early response monitoring in malignant lymphoma using fluorine-18 fluorodeoxyglucose single-photon emission tomography. Eur J Nucl Med 1993; 20: 1214-1217

5. van Lingen A, Huijgens PC, Visser FC, Ossenkoppele GJ, Hoekstra OS, Teule GJJ. Performance characteristics of a 511-keV collimator for imaging positron emitters with a standard gamma-camera. Eur J Nucl Med 1992; 19:315-321

6. Macfarlane DJ; Cotton L; Ackermann RJ; Minn H; Ficaro EP; Shreve PD; Wahl RLTriple-head SPECT with 2-[fluorine-18]fluoro-2-deoxy-D-glucose (FDG): initial evaluation in oncology and comparison with FDG PET. Radiology 1995 ; 194(2): 425-429

7. Drane WE, Abbott FD, Nicole MW, Mastin ST, Kuperus JH. Technology for FDG SPECT with a relatively inexpensive gamma camera. Work in progress. Radiology 1994; 191(2): 461-465

8. Kubota R; Kubota K; Yamada S; Tada M; Ido T; Tamahashi N. Microautoradiographic study for the differentiation of intratumoral macrophages, granulation tissues and cancer cells by the dynamics of fluorine-18-fluorodeoxyglucose uptake.   J-Nucl-Med. 1994 Jan; 35(1): 104-12

9. Kubota R, Kubota K, Yamada S, Tada M, Ido T, Tamahashi N. Active and passive mechanisms of [Fluorine-18] Fluorodeoxyglucose uptake by proliferating and prenecrotic cancer cells in vivo: a microautoradiographic study.   J-Nucl-Med. 1994; 35: 1067-1075

10. Ichiya Y, Kuwabara Y, Otsuka M, Tahara T, Yoshikai T, Fukumura T,Jingo K, Masuda K. Assessment of response to cancer therapy using fluorine-18-fluorodeoxyglucose and positron emission tomography J Nucl Med 1991; 32:1655-1660

11. Martin WH, Delbeke D, Patton JA, Hendrix B, Weinfeld Z, Ohana I, Kessler RM, Sandler MP. FDG-SPECT: Correlation with FDG-PET. J Nucl Med 1995; 36: 988-995

12. Trampert L, Holle LH, Berberich R, Alexander C, Ukena D, Ruth Th, Sybrecht GW, Oberhausen E. [18]FDG beim primären staging von Lungentumoren. [18]FDG in the primary staging of lung tumors. Results with a gamma camera and a 511 keV Collimator. Nucl.-Med. 1995; 34:79-86

Radioactive Isotopes in
Clinical Medicine and Research XXII
ed. by H. Bergmann, A. Kroiss and H. Sinzinger
© 1997 Birkhäuser Verlag Basel/Switzerland

DIAGNOSIS AND THERAPY CONTROL OF OCULAR MELANOMA WITH [18]FDG-PET

A PILOT STUDY

U. Feine[1], A. Stanowsky[2], R. Lietzenmayer[1], J. Held[1], I. Kreissig[2]
Department of Nuclear Medicine[1], Department of Ophthalmology[2],
Eberhard-Karls-Universität Tübingen,Germany

Summary: 12 patients suspected for choroidal melanoma of the eye were examined in a pilot study with [18]FDG-PET. A well visible tumor uptake with significantly elevated Standardized Uptake Values (SUV) for tumors with a prominence > 5 mm was demonstrated. In one patient a non-malignant choroidal lesion (choroidal hemorrhage) could be differentiated. In two patients the simultaneously performed [18]FDG-WB-PET showed unknown extraocular metastases, influencing further therapy procedures. In two patients treated with brachytherapy (Iodine-125, Ruthenium-106) a clear response to the radiation was observed. Further studies are needed to clarify the diagnostic value of this method and radiation-dose-effects on [18]FDG uptake. As far as we know [18]FDG-PET is at the moment the only non-invasive method that provides clinical data concerning the vitality of melanoma cells after radiotherapy. Therefore this method might serve as an important parameter for the effectiveness of therapy and for optimizing radiation protocols.

Introduction

The ophthalmologic diagnostics of malignant choroidal melanoma with fundoscopy, ultrasonography, fluourescein angiography or scanning laser ophthalmoscopy together with the radiological examinations of CT and MRI has reached a high standard (1,2,3). But in few cases of about 2% there are difficulties in differentiating malignant melanoma from benign alterations as e.g. hemorrage, pseudomelanoma etc. (4,5). Therefore the Ophthalmologic Clinic in Tübingen asked for a method to confirm the malignancy of a suspected eye melanoma. Out of this reasons we performed the presented pilot study with [18]FDG based upon the positive results with [18]FDG-PET examinations in cutaneous melanomas and their metastases (6-7).

The other aim of the study was to determine the tumor vitality following an eye brachytherapy to optimize radiation protocols for treatment of eye melanomas.

Patients and Methods

12 patients with presumed choroidal melanoma (maximal base diameter 8,5 - 16,5 mm, highest prominence 2,6 - 12,4 mm) were examined with a PET-scanner (General Electric ADVANCE) with 15 cm axial Field of View (FOV), high sensitivity mode allowing total body scanning and transmission correction to obtain a quantitive ^{18}FDG uptake of the tumor with determination of Standardized Uptake Values (SUV).

All patients, after informed consent, were examined at least 12 hours after their last meal in order to keep the glucose level as low as possible. Each patient received 5 MBq of ^{18}FDG per kilogram body weight 45 minutes prior to the PET-scan. A transmission scan over 10 to 15 minutes was performed only for the ocular field. The patients were asked not to move the eyes and to fixate a point during the running emission scan of the eye region..The whole body scans with 5-7 bed positions were performed without transmission correction. For evaluation of the orbital region tomograms were performed in axial, sagittal and coronary sections. Quantitative uptake data were calculated from four different regions of interest (ROI´s) in transaxial slices of the ocular melanoma and for comparison over the corresponding area of the fellow eye. Reference ROI´s were obtained in the area of one of the ocular muscles and in the cortical region of the brain.

Standardized Uptake Values corrected for body weight (SUV_{bw}) and for recovery effect were calculated. For the calculations the formulas of Kim (8) respectively Zasadny et al (9) were slightly modified: For best approximation of the activity concentration within a structure smaller than 15 mm the maximum values in the ROIs were used for calculation.To correct for the recovery-effect it was necessary to multiply the activity concentration values with correction values which were experimentally determined for the Tübingen PET-scanner by measuring phantoms with known activity and different sizes. These measurements demonstrated that correction of activity concentration values is necessary, if the measured structure is smaller than 18 mm (for Hanning-filter[10]).

Results

12 patients with the clinical diagnosis of a choroidal melanoma were subjected to 15 examinations with ^{18} FDG PET-scan. In two of these patients, two respectively three examinations were performed 4 - 32 weeks following brachytherapy with Iodine-125 irradiation of the melanoma. In 8 patients a significant ^{18}FDG-uptake in the PET-scan was found in three different tomogram-directions (fig 1). The SUV_{bw} ranged from 4.0 to 10.8 in the tumor and from 1.4 to 2.8 in the control region of the healthy eye.

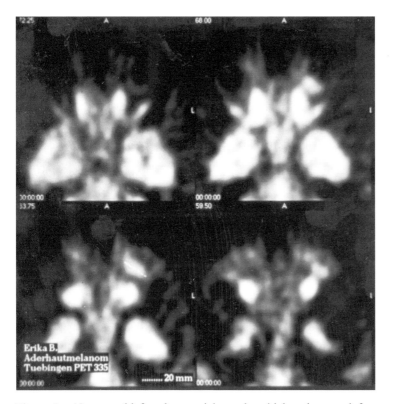

Figure 1   45-years-old female, suspicious choroidal melanoma left eye, nasocaudal. Base diameter: 18x16 mm, prominence: 7 mm. ^{18}FDG-PET: 4 axial tomograms in 3 sections: the melanoma is clearly outlined, largest diameter about 20 mm(-----).The outer eye muscles demonstrate a high ^{18}FDG-trapping too.

Of the 4 [18] FDG negative patients one turned out to suffer from a subchoroidal hemorrhage. In the 3 other patients the maximal tumor prominence was < 4.8 mm. One of these patients had had a laser treatment prior to the PET-scan, another a questionable recurrence 2 years following Ruthenium-106 plaque treatment. In one patient the choroidal lesion clinically proved to be a metastasis of a cutaneous melanoma. Therefore it was demonstrated, that choroidal melanomas with a minimal prominence of about 5 mm are suitable to be detected with [18]FDG in a PET-scan with high resolution capacity.

The treated melanomas (brachytherapy with Iodine-125/Ruthenium-106 applicators, sclera contact dose 350 - 400 Gy, at the apex 80 - 90 Gy) in one patient demonstrated an increased uptake 4 weeks after the first brachytherapy, ressembling to a flare effect. In this patient an increase of the exsudative detachment was present at the time of PET-scan examination. Even eight months after radiation therapy this tumor demonstrated a significant difference in uptake in comparison to the fellow eye, clinically an inhomogeneous tumor regression was observed The other patient showed a decrease of the SUV's after 4 weeks .

Discussion

This pilot study demonstrates that choroidal melanomas can be displayed by the[18]FDG-PET-scan depending on the tumor prominence (in our series > 4.8 mm) and the resolution of the scanner and can be differentiated from non-malignant tumors (e.g. hematoma). The high [18]FDG-uptake of the choroidal melanoma of the eye corresponds to the reports of others (5,6), that undifferentiated carcinomas and to a high degree melanomas have an elevated glucose metabolism and therefore an increased [18]FDG-uptake in comparison to non-malignant tumors. The visual evaluation controlled by the determination of the SUV's in the eye tumor compared to the control region in the healthy eye demonstrated significant differences in [18]FDG-uptake for malignant melanomas with a prominence > 5 mm.

In two patients control PET was performed 4 weeks after brachytherapy and in one of these 32 weeks after radiation too. The SUV_{bw} of these patients demonstrated, that the radiation effects after brachytherapy may be controlled by [18]FDG-PET. The increased SUV in one patient 4 weeks after brachytherapy (tumor dose 400 Gy at the base, 80 Gy at the top) can be interpreted as a flare effect following therapy. This phenomen corresponds well to the clinical observation of an increased exsudative retinal detachment. Performing a total body [18]FDG-PET-scan, unknown metastases were detected in three patients, inducing an alteration in treatment. The total body PET-scan did not subject the patients to additional radiation exposure, however, the total examination time was extended for another 30 to 40 minutes.

Conclusion: Whenever there is doubt in the diagnosis of an ocular malignancy we therefore suggest to perform a PET-scan prior to enucleation or brachytherapy. However larger series of patients are needed to obtain more data concerning [18]FDG PET-scan examinations in diagnosis and therapy of malignant melanomas of the eye.

References

(1) Mafee MF, Peyman GA, Grisolano JE, Fletcher ME, Spigos DG, Wehrli FW, Rasouli F, Capek V.: Malignant uveal melanoma and simulating lesions: MR imaging evaluation. Radiology. 1986; 160(3): 773-80

(2) Mafee MF, Peyman GA, Peace JH, Cohen SB, Mitchell MW: Magnetic resonance imaging in the evaluation and differentiation of uveal melanoma.Ophthalmology1987; 94(4): 341-8

(3) Ossoinig KC, Bigar F, Kaefring SL: Malignant melanoma of the choroid and ciliary body (A differential diagnosis in clinical echography). Bibl. Ophthalmol. S. Karger, Basel 1988, 83:141-154

(4) Shields JA, Augsburger JJ, Brown GC, ,Stephens RF: The differential diagnosis of posterior uveal melanoma: Ophthalmology 1980; 87 (6): 518-22

(5) Chang M, Zimmermann LE, McLean I: The persisting pseudomelanoma problem. Arch Ophthalmol. 1984;102(5):726-7

(6) Strauss LG, Conti PS: The Applications of PET in Clinical Oncology. J. Nucl. Med. 1991 (32): 623-648

(7) Steinert HC, Huch Böni RA, Buck A, Böni R, Berthold T, Marincek B, Burg G, v. Schulthess GK: Malignant Melanoma: Staging with Whole-Body Positron Emission Tomography and 2-[18-F]-Fluoro-2-Deoxy-D-Glucose. Radiology 1995; 195: 705-709

(8) Kim CK, Gupta NC, Chandramouli B., Alavi A: Standardized uptake values of FDG: Body Surface Area Correction is preferable to Body Weight Correction. J. Nucl. Med. 1994; 35 (1): 164-167

(9) Zasadny KR, Wahl RL: Standardized Uptake Values of normal tissues at PET with 2[Fluorine-18]-Fluoro-2-deoxy-D-glucose: Variations with Body Weight and a method for correction. Radiology 1993; 189: 847-850

(10) Bilger H; Keller;KD,. Nüsslin F.. Feine U: Einflüsse der Objektgröße und der Ortsabhängigkeit des Auflösungsvermögens auf die quantitative Bildauswertung mit einem Positronen Emissions Tomographen. Diplomarbeit. 1995, Depart.Nuclearmed., Med.Physik Universität Tübingen.

Radioactive Isotopes in
Clinical Medicine and Research XXII
ed. by H. Bergmann, A. Kroiss and H. Sinzinger
© 1997 Birkhäuser Verlag Basel/Switzerland

FDG-PET, I-131 and MIBI SCINTIGRAPHY IN THE FOLLOW-UP OF DIFFERENTIATED THYROID CANCER

F. Grünwald, H.-J. Biersack, E. Klemm, C. Menzel, H. Bender, T. Bultmann, A. Schomburg, J. Ruhlmann, H. Palmedo

Department of Nuclear Medicine, University of Bonn, Germany

INTRODUCTION

Serum thyroglobulin (Tg) measurement and whole-body-scintigraphy with [131]I (WBS) are widely used for detection of local recurrence, lymph node and distant metastases in the follow-up of differentiated thyroid cancer (1,2). The "myocardial tracers" thallium and ^{99m}Tc-MIBI have been proven to be useful besides [131]I. [18]FDG is known to be retained in malignant tissue, depending on the grade of malignancy. Some reports have been published dealing with FDG uptake in thyroid cancer, partly using a regional-body positron-emission tomography (PET) scanner and partly using a conventional gamma camera (3-6). Recently, Feine et al. (3) published first results obtained with a whole-body PET scanner. The aim of the present study was to evaluate the use of whole-body FDG-PET imaging in the follow-up of patients who have been treated with ^{131}I and to compare the results with other imaging modalities, particularly with MIBI-scintigraphy since this radiopharmaceutical has been proven to be useful in the follow-up of (also ^{131}I-negative) thyroid carcinomas (7).

MATERIALS AND METHODS

33 patients with differentiated thyroid cancer were included in the study. There were 26 cases with papillary and 7 cases with follicular carcinomas. Tumor stage was pT1 in 6

cases, pT2 in 8 cases, pT3 in 3 cases pT4 in 14 cases and pTx in 2 cases, respectively. Histological grading of the primary tumor was obtained in 10 cases (5 G1 and 5 G2 each). Tumors were classified according to the suggestions of the International Union Against Cancer/Union Internationale Contre le Cancer (UICC) (8). The FDG-PET studies were performed when no major benign remnant tissue was expected. Nearly all PET scans were done under thyroxine replacement therapy. PET imaging was performed using a Siemens/CTI ECAT Exact 921/47 PET scanner. 220-380 MBq (about 6-10 mCi) FDG were administered intravenously 45 minutes before the start of static emission images in multiple (4-5) bed positions, starting from the base of the skull. A MIBI scintigraphy (740 MBq) including whole-body imaging and a SPECT study of head and neck was done in 20 cases. Tg was measured prior to ^{131}I treatment in all patients.

RESULTS

FDG-PET was normal in 18 cases. In 3 patients an only slightly increased glucose metabolism was observed in the thyroid bed, supposed to be related to remnant tissue. In 1 case local recurrence, in 10 cases lymph node metastases (one false-positive) and in 3 cases distant metastases were found with FDG-PET. Among the patients with pathological PET results, there was one patient with local recurrence as well as lung metastases and one patient with lymph node and lung metastases. In 3 cases the glucose metabolism was only moderately increased and the result could not be confirmed either by other imaging techniques or surgically. 8 out of 18 PET-normal cases showed a clear normal ^{131}I scan without any tracer uptake in the thyroid bed. In 5 of these patients a MIBI scan was available, showing a normal result in all cases. In 6 patients remnant tissue could be visualized with ^{131}I, but not with FDG, in one case the ^{131}I scan showed a mediastinal tracer uptake which was diagnosed as unspecific since magnetic resonance imaging (MRI) and Tg values were normal. MIBI scintigraphy, performed in 5 out of these 7 patients, corresponded in 3 cases with the PET scan, but only in one case with the ^{131}I scan and suggested local recurrence in one case as the only functional imaging technique. Two out of the 3 cases with suspected remnant tissue/local inflammation (PET) showed a congruent [131]I- and MIBI-result, in one case [131]I- and [201]Thallium-scintigraphy were completely normal. For further evaluation, scans showing only remnant tissue/unspecific tracer uptake were summarized with the complete normal results and addressed as "normal". The table gives an overall comparison of FDG-PET and ^{131}I scintigraphy.

Comparison of FDG-PET and ^{131}I whole-body scintigraphy in the follow-up of differentiated thyroid cancer (sites reported in all positive cases)

| | FDG-PET | | | |
	normal	local recurrence	lymph node mets.	distant mets.
^{131}I scan				
normal	18	1	5*	2
local rec.	0	0	0	0
lymph node mets.	2	0	4	0
distant mets.	3	0	0	1
not done	0	0	1	0

* one false-positive (sarcoidosis)

Comparison of FDG-PET and MIBI scintigraphy in the follow-up of differentiated thyroid cancer (sites reported in all positive cases)

| | FDG-PET | | | |
	normal	local recurrence	lymph node mets.	distant mets.
MIBI				
normal	11	0	3	2
local rec.	1	1	0	1
lymph node mets.	0	0	3	0
distant mets.	0	0	0	0
not done	9	0	4*	0

* one false-positive (sarcoidosis)

Corresponding results (FDG-PET/^{131}I scan) were obtained in 23 cases. It is noted that most discrepancies exist regarding lymph node metastases since in 5 patients these were observed with PET (one false-positive), but not with ^{131}I. MIBI scintigraphy was positive in 2 of these cases, negative in another 2 patients and not done in the false-positive case. In the latter case, the FDG-PET scan showed an increased tracer uptake in mediastinal lymph nodes, but a sarcoidosis was surgically proven lateron. Remarkable is that in only one of 6 cases distant metastases were correctly diagnosed by both techniques. Unfortunately, MIBI-scintigraphy was available in only 3 cases with distant metastases. In none of these patients the metastases were detectable with MIBI. In no case of concordant pathological "staging" (PET and ^{131}I, 5 patients), completely identical results were obtained as to exact lesion localization. There were ^{131}I-positive/PET-negative and ^{131}I-negative/PET-positive sites coexisting with ^{131}I-positive/PET-positive lesions in all these patients.

DISCUSSION

Concerning differentiated thyroid cancer, FDG-PET has to compete not only with the tumor-seeking agents ^{201}Thallium and MIBI, but also with the "physiological" marker of thyroid tissue, ^{131}I, which has the advantage of very high uptake values in most types of highly-differentiated thyroid cancer. Since there were 3 cases with normal FDG-PET scan and proven distant metastases (^{131}I-positive) in our patient group and similar results have been reported by other investigators, a replacement of WBS by FDG-PET cannot be recommended. For the differentiation of remnant tissue from residual tumor or recurrence, PET (and also MIBI) seems to be superior, since there were 2 cases with a completely normal PET scan but ^{131}I uptake in the thyroid bed. For the detection of lymph node metastases, PET showed a higher sensitivity than WBS, correlating closer to MIBI scintigraphy. Two out of the 5 cases with lymph node metastases, which were detectable only with PET (but not with ^{131}I), 2 were MIBI-positive. Since ^{131}I-uptake is known to be correlated positively and FDG-uptake is known to be correlated negatively to the grade of tumor differentiation, discrepancies between the imaging results were expected. The phenomenon of highly diverging uptake behaviour has been addressed as "flipflop" by Feine et al. (3). Our results suggest that the detectability with both tracers depends on the grade of malignancy. In 2 cases with high differentiation (G1), ^{131}I-uptake was observed in distant metastases, whereas FDG-PET was completely normal. Additionally, ^{131}I-positive and FDG-negative lymph node metastases existed in one of these patients. In contrast, in one patient with a G2-tumor, FDG-PET (and also MIBI) were able to detect local recurrence in spite of a negative ^{131}I scan. A significantly higher rate for positive FDG-PET results is obvious in patients with higher pT-stage. Whereas in only 2 out of 14 cases with a pT1/pT2 tumor stage a pathological PET scan was obtained, 8 out of 17 patients (47%) suffering from pT3/pT4 carcinoma were PET-positive. This is not surprising since higher tumor stages are known to be associated with a higher rate of recurrence and lymph node as well as distant metastases, but it suggests, that the clinical use of FDG-PET should be recommended mainly in higher pT-stages.

CONCLUSION

From the results of the present study it can be concluded that in the routine follow-up of differentiated thyroid cancer serum Tg measurement and WBS seem to be primarily sufficient. Nevertheless, if metastases are proven, e.g. with ^{131}I, a PET scan should be performed in addition to localize coexisting ^{131}I-negative metastases, particularly in low-differentiated tumors. This is especially important for the mediastinum, which cannot be evaluated sonographically. FDG-PET is particularly useful during follow-up of thyroid cancer, when elevated Tg levels combined with normal WBS occur.

REFERENCES

1.   Goolden AWG. The indication for ablating normal thyroid tissue with ^{131}I in differentiated thyroid cancer. Clin Endocrinol 1985; 23: 81-86

2.   Dadparvar S, Krishna L, Brady LW, et al. The role of [131]Iodine-Na and [201]Thallium imaging and serum thyroglobulin in the management of differentiated carcinoma. Cancer 1993; 71: 3767-3773

3.   Feine U, Lietzenmayer R, Hanke JP, Wöhrle H, Müller-Schauenburg W. [18]FDG whole-body PET in differentiated thyroid carcinoma. Nucl Med 1995; 34: 127-134.

4.   Joensuu H, Ahonen A. Imaging of metastases of thyroid carcinoma with fluorine-18 fluorodeoxyglucose. J Nucl Med 1987; 28: 910-914

5.   Sisson JC, Ackermann RJ, Meyer MA. Uptake of 18-fluoro-2-deoxy-D-glucose by thyroid cancer: implications for diagnosis and therapy. J Clin Endocrin Metabol 1993; 77: 1090-1094

6.   Baqai FH, Conti PS, Singer PA, et al. ^{18}F-FDG-PET scanning - a diagnostic tool for detection of recurrent and metastatic differentiated thyroid cancers. Abstract, 68th annual meeting of the American Thyroid Association, Chicago 1994, pp 9

7.   Briele B, Hotze AL, Kropp J, et al. A comparison of ^{201}Tl and ^{99m}Tc-MIBI in the follow-up of differentiated thyroid carcinoma. Nucl Med 1991; 30: 115-124

8.   Spiessl B, Beahrs OH, Hermanek P, et al. TNM-Atlas. Illustrierter Leitfaden zur TNM/pTNM-Klassifikation maligner Tumoren/International Union Against Cancer/Union Internationale Contre le Cancer (UICC). Springer-Verlag, Berlin-Heidelberg-New York, 1993, pp 58

Radioactive Isotopes in
Clinical Medicine and Research XXII
ed. by H. Bergmann, A. Kroiss and H. Sinzinger
© 1997 Birkhäuser Verlag Basel/Switzerland

[18]FDG/^{131}I-ALTERNATING UPTAKE IN DIFFERENTIATED THYROID CANCER - WHOLE BODY PET IN 41 PATIENTS

U. Feine, R. Lietzenmayer, J.P. Hanke, H. Wöhrle, J. Held and W. Müller-Schauenburg

Department of Nuclear Medicine,
Eberhard-Karls-University Tuebingen
Germany

Summary: In the follow up of 41 patients with thyroid cancer we found with the combined examination of [18]FDG-WB PET and ^{131}I-WB planar scans an alternating behavior of [131]I- and [18]FDG-uptake in the metastases like a Flipflop (Flipflop: Electronic device or a circuit, as in a computer, capable of assuming either of two stable states). The combination of [18]FDG and ^{131}I-Scanning has a high sensitivity of about 95%. This permits the detection of local recurrence or metastases in the WB-scan, which are often not shown by other imaging methods. Furthermore it seems to be possible to perform a biochemical grading of thyroid cancer with [18]FDG and [131]I. Low grade tumors have low glucose metabolism, high grade tumors show high glucose metabolism. [131]I uptake seems to be a sign for higher differentiation, [18]FDG uptake for higher malignancy. Such a grading may also be possible in other tumors.

INTRODUCTION

The determination of human thyroglobuline (hTg) for the detection of local tumor recurrence and metastases together with the ^{131}I-WB-scan are well established methods in the follow-up of patients with thyroid carcinoma (1). Other imaging procedures such as X-ray, Ultrasound, CT and MR offer additional control methods in the follow-up. Newer scintigraphic examinations with ^{201}Tl-Chloride, ^{99m}Tc-Sestamibi and ^{111}In-Octreotide, the latter for diagnosing C-cell carcinoma, are not yet completely evaluated (2).

After ^{131}I-elimination of remaining thyroid tissue increasing hTg-levels as a sign of tumor recurrence need to be followed up. With the conventional diagnostic procedures hTg producing tissue cannot always be localized. With 2-[^{18}F]-Fluorodeoxyglucose ([18]FDG) it is possible to mark malignant tumors with a high sensitivity of about 80-90% (3).

Only a few publications deal with [18]FDG-uptake of malignant thyroid tumors; most of the examinations were conducted with only one or two field PET examinations in the neck region. Some cases without [18]FDG-uptake in thyroid cancer were reported (4, 5,6).

This prospective study was designed to define the sensitivity of detecting thyroid cancer and metastases by means of [18]FDG-Whole-Body-Positron-Emission-Tomography (WB-PET) in combination with ^{131}I-WB-scanning in patients in the follow up.

Patients

41 patients with differentiated thyroid carcinoma after thyroidectomy and ^{131}I-elimination of the remaining thyroid were investigated in the follow-up with [18]FDG-WB-PET in 52 examinations in the period from December 1993 to August 1995. 12 of the 41 patients in this study had papillary carcinoma, 23 patients follicular carcinoma and 6 patients Hürthle-cell carcinoma. Three additional patients with C-cell carcinoma, all MEN II, and with elevated calcitonine levels had no uptake of [18]FDG, and are not further mentioned in this study. All patients were subjected to a ^{131}I-WB-gamma camera scan; ultrasound of the neck and abdomen; CT and a determination of the hTg level. All patients gave informed consent for their participation in the study.

Methods

The examinations with [18]FDG were performed with a *General-Electric ADVANCE*-PET Scanner with Whole-Body- and High Sensitivity Mode. The Field of View (FOV) was 15 cm; 5-7 FOV = 75-105 cm body-scan. Patients fasted 18 hours prior to injection of [18]FDG (5 MBq /kg body weight), and were scanned 45 min. after injection. The scan time for one FOV was 5-7 min. [18]FDG was commercially produced by the Nuclear Research Center in Karlsruhe (Germany). Transmission correction were performed for the quantitative evaluation of tumor uptake in 31 examinations. Standardized uptake values (SUV) were calculated and corrected for body weight (SUV_{bw}) and for body surface area (SUV_{bsa}), as described by Kim et al. (7). A correction for the finite resolution with recovery coefficients was not necessary because the metastases evaluated had sizes of > 18 mm and due to the high resolution of the *ADVANCE* PET (8). For ^{131}I-WB-scanning we used a body scanner (*Siemens*) with two opposite large field gamma camera detectors and high energy collimators. The dose of ^{131}I was between 100 MBq and 6 GBq (therapy doses), and patients were scanned 48 h to 5 days after application. All patients were examined for ^{131}I-uptake without hormone substitution at high TSH-levels. ^{18}FDG-PET was performed before or after ^{131}I-WB-scanning, some ^{18}FDG-WB-scans with thyroxin substitution. Four cases examined with ^{18}FDG without Thyroxin substitution were controlled later with Thyroxin substitution.

Results

We found an alternating behaviour of ^{131}I- and ^{18}FDG uptake in these tumor patients. Tumors and metastases showed either an ^{131}I or an ^{18}FDG uptake (figures 1; 2).

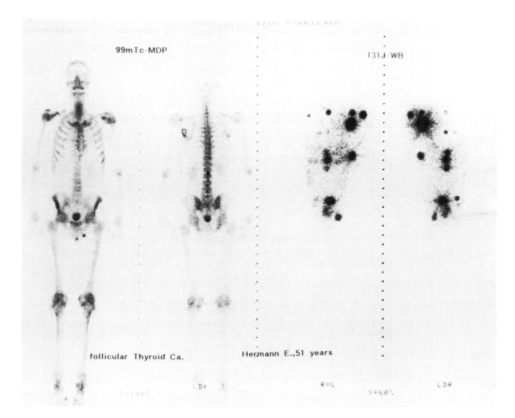

Fig. 1(a) and (b): 51 year old male with follicular thyroid carcinoma and bone metastases with **uptake-type II**:
(a) Left: WB bone scan (MDP): no sure bone metastases visible (only in the left scapula a pathologic fracture with ^{99m}Tc-MDP uptake). - Right: ^{131}I-WB-scan with multiple ^{131}I-trapping metastases.

A combined ^{131}I/ [18]FDG uptake could be clearly identified only in 4 patients in 5 metastases. There could be some more localisations with a combined uptake in a few additional patients, where the comparison between the different imaging modalities of whole-body iodine scans and [18]FDG tomograms was difficult, especially in cases with multiple metastases. Such an alternating uptake can be called like in the

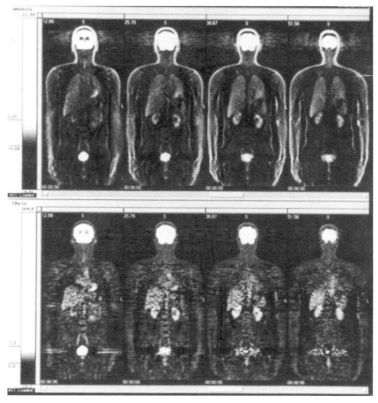

Fig.1 (b): [18]FDG-WB-PET: above: emission scan non corrected; below: transmission corrected scan: no metastases visible

electronic- and computer-technology a"flipflop",that means the logical connection between two states and describes an electronic device or a circuit (as in a computer), capable of assuming either of two stable states. It distinguishes between better differentiated thyroid carcinoma cells which still have iodine metabolism for hormone synthesis and normal glucose metabolism, and less differentiated carcinoma cells without iodine uptake and elevated glucose metabolism.

We classified the uptake pattern of the metastases of our 41 patients in five different uptake types. Table 1 shows the 5 uptake types according to their histological differentiation:

Table 1: 41 Patients with Differentiated Thyriod Cancer: ^{18}FDG/^{131}I-Uptake Types and Histological Classification

Uptake-Type	papillary Ca.	follicular Ca.	Hürthle Cell Ca	Total
I ^{18}FDG-positive/ ^{131}I-negative	7**	8	4	19
II ^{18}FDG-negative/ ^{131}I-positive	1	5	-	6
III mixed type*	1	4	-	5
IV ^{18}FDG- and ^{131}I-positive	1	3	-	4
V ^{18}FDG- and ^{131}I-negative	2***	3****	2*****	7
Total	12	23	6	41

*Type III: either ^{18}FDG-positive/^{131}I-negative or ^{18}FDG-negative/^{131}I-positive (mixed type)

**4 patients post-operative histologically confirmed, 2 of them hTG-negative prior to surgery!

***1 true negative (hTG < 1 ng/ml), 1 false negative (hTG < 10 ng/ml)

****2 true negative (hTG < 1 ng/ml), 1 false negative (hTG > 100 ng/ml) after radioiodine therapy

*****true negative (hTG < 1 ng/ml)

In 3 of 5 metastasesof autake typIV we found areas of different uptake levels of 131I and 18FDG within the same metastasis. Therefore it seems that this flipflop behaviour may be found within the same metastatic lesion. We suppose that for other lesions the resolution did not allow a further differentiation (spatial resolution for PET is about 6 mm, for the ^{131}I whole-body gamma camera above 20 mm).

Discussion

Based on our results we assume that there are two different types of cellular differentiation in papillary and follicular thyroid carcinoma. They
correspond to the uptake types
I, II, and III (figs 1 and 2).
The carcinoma cell seems to
de-differentiate from a functionally higher level to a lower
one. According to the uptake
pattern there is no continuous
reciprocal change from iodine
hormone metabolism to

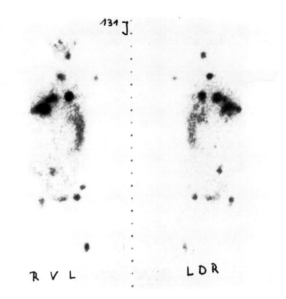

Fig. 2,(a) and (b): **Uptake Type III** 63 years old female
with variable differentiated papillary thyroid carcinoma and
multiple metastases.
(a): ^{131}I-WB scan with multiple trapping metastases

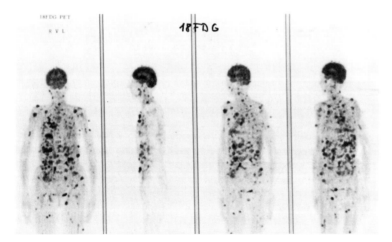

Fig.2(b): ^{18}FDG-WB-PET (sinogram projections): three times or more ^{18}FDG trapping
metasases, but at different localisations as the ^{131}I trapping metastases.

glucose metabolism, but there is rather a yes/no,no/yes alternative. We therefore characterized
the alternating uptake as a flip-flop logic according to the use of this term in electronics or
computer sciences for an alternating behaviour between two stable states(7). With the higher

glucose metabolism the thyroid carcinoma cells seem to change into a higher degree of malignancy and a higher level of aggression since the metastases with iodine uptake and normal glucose metabolism were all found in those patients which had been already in our follow-up and treatment for up to 30 years. On the other side the missing ^{18}FDG uptake in our group of patients correlates with thyroid carcinoma with a missing uptake of bone tracers in the imaging of bone metastases by phosphonates (^{99m}Tc-MDP). This behaviour corresponds to a lower level of aggression of the slowly growing differentiated thyroid carcinoma cells with iodine uptake. This type of behaviour is well-known in the literature(8).

The alternating uptake for the diagnosis of carcinoma metastases means, that a combination of ^{18}FDG and^{131}I gives a high sensitivity of about 95 % for the combined use of both tracers in papillary and follicular thyroid carcinoma according to our results in 41 patients. Especially this combined examination was useful in patients with elevated levels of thyroglobulin, the main tumor marker in thyroid carcinoma. The combined examination was even there successful when the combination of CT, MR, sonography and ^{201}Tl-scintigraphy failed to find the lesions.

Of special interest is the biochemical behaviour of the thyroid carcinoma cell that is loosing the ability of iodine metabolism, i.e. the cell is loosing its functional differentiation accompanied by a change to an elevated glucose metabolism. The phenomenon of switching to an elevated glucose metabolism in a process of de-differentiation of the cell seems not to be confined to follicular and papillary thyroid carcinoma. It may be a principle in oncology: 8 patients with neuroblastoma examined with ^{18}FDG-whole-body-PET showed a high ^{18}FDG-uptake in the tumor while two better differentiated ganglioneuroblastoma did not show ^{18}FDG-uptake. All ganglioneuroblastoma were $^{131/123}$I-MIBG-positive. Also two higher differentiated hepatocellular carcinoma of the fibrolamellar type were FDG-negative. DiChiro described 1987 the similar behaviour in brain tumors(9). Astrocytoma and glioma of grade I or II did not show an elevated ^{18}FDG uptake, while astrocytoma grade III and IV and glioblastoma had a high FDG-uptake. But the higher ^{18}FDG-uptake is not specific for malignancy: We found five benign thyroid adenomas with elevated ^{18}FDG uptake as described also by Bloom et al. 1993(10). Inflammatory foci as lymph nodes ect. have mostly an increased ^{18}FDG uptake too.

Conclusion: In the combined examination with ^{18}FDG and ^{131}I we could demonstrate in 41 patients with follicular and papillary thyroid carcinoma a diagnostic sensitivity of about 95%. The alternating uptake allows to detect local recurrence or metastases in the whole body, often not found by other imaging methods, and to bring them to surgery. It also seems to be possible that no [18]FDG- and good ^{131}I-uptake in thyroid cancer and its metastases represents a higher functional differentiation with a better prognosis. That means we could get a biochemical in vivo grading for thyroid carcinomas based on this alternating flipflop type uptake.

We finally could like to assume, that this switching to an elevated glucose metabolism in a process of de-differentiation of the tumor cell could be a general principle in oncology and needs further studies in a large spectrum of different tumors.

References

1. Ng Tang Fui,SC,Hoffenberg,R.,Maisey,MN,Black,E : Serum thyroglobulin concentrations and whole body radiodine scan in follow-up of differentiated thyroid cancer after thyroid ablation. Br.Med.J. 1979; 2: 298-300.
2. Lawson M., Dusick D, Bandy D et al. Comparison of [^{18}F]- FDG and Tl-201 for detection of recurrent metastatic differentiated thyroid cancer. J.Nucl.Med. 1995; 36: 203P.
3. Strauss L,Conti PS:The application of PET in clinical oncology.J.Nucl.Med.1991, 32: 623-648
4. Hawkins RA, Hoh C, Glapsy J, et al and Phelps ME: The role of positron emission tomography in oncology and other whole body application. Sem. Nucl. Med. 22(4) 1992: 268-284.
5. Hoh CK, Hawkins RA, Glaspy JA, Dahlborn M, Tse NY, et al: Cancer detection with whole body PET using[18]F-fluoro-deoxyclucose. J.Comput.assist.Tomography 1993; 17 (4): 582-589
6. Voth E., Börner AR., Theissen P., Schicha, H. Positron emission tomography (PET) in benign thyroid diseases.Exp. Clin.Endocronol. 1994; 102: 71-74
7. Feine U, Lietzenmayer R, Hanke J, Müller-Schauenburg W.1995: Ganzkörper-^{18}F-Fluordeoxyglucose- Positronen-Emmissions-Tomographie (GK-FDG-PET) bei differenzierten Schilddrüsen-Carcinomen - Flipflop im Speichermuster von [18]FDG und [131]J. NuklearMedizin 34:127-34.
8. Castillo, LA, Yeh, DJ, Leeper, LD, Benua, RS1980:Bone scans in bone metastases.Clin.Nucl.Med., 5: 200-8.
9. DiChiro G., Positron emission tomography using ^{18}F-fluorodeoxyglucose in brain tumors. A powerful diagnostic and prognostic tool. Invest. Radiol. 1987, 22: 360-371

Bloom AD, Adler LP, Shuck JM: Determination of malignancy of thyroid nodules with positron emission tomography. Surgery 1993; 114: 728-735

Correspondence adress :Prof.Dr.U.Feine MD, Department of Nuclear Medicine;
                                     D72076 Tuebingen, Roentgenweg 13 Germany

1.

Radioactive Isotopes in   77
Clinical Medicine and Research XXII
ed. by H. Bergmann, A. Kroiss and H. Sinzinger
© 1997 Birkhäuser Verlag Basel/Switzerland

Tc-99m-SESTAMIBI WHOLE BODY SCINTIGRAPHY: AN USEFUL TOOL IN THE
FOLLOW UP OF PATIENTS WITH DIFFERENTIATED THYROID CARCINOMA?

G. Meyer, U. Kleine, R. Tiling, K. Stein, K. Hahn

Department of Nuclear Medicine, Ludwig-Maximilians-University of Munich, Germany

SUMMARY: Purpose of this study was to assess the clinical value of sestamibi whole body
scintigraphy in detecting local recurrences and metastases in patients with differentiated thyroid
carcinoma and to compare these results with diagnostic 131-radioiodine scans and serum thyroglobulin determinations. 75 patients - following all total thyroidectomy and high dosed
radioiodine therapy - underwent sestamibi and diagnostic iodine scintigraphy. In addition,
serum thyroglobulin levels were determined. Only patients with elevated thyroglobulin levels
showed positive sestamibi and/or iodine uptake. In comparison with iodine scans sestamibi
scintigraphy revealed with a higher sensitivity recurrences and metastases especially in follicular
and Hürthle cell carcinoma.

INTRODUCTION

As a lipophilic cation Technetium-99m-methoxyisobutylisonitrile (Tc-99m-sestamibi) has been

successfully used in imaging iodine-negative thyroid carcinoma as well as other malignant

tumors especially lung and breast carcinoma (1-4). Previous studies predominantly compared

131- iodine scintigraphy and thallium-201 scintigraphy in patients with differentiated thyroid

carcinoma (4,6).

The purpose of this present study was to assess the clinical value of sestamibi whole body

scintigraphy in detecting local recurrences and metastases in patients with differentiated thyroid

carcinoma and to compare these results with diagnostic iodine-131 whole body scans. The

sensitivity and specificity of sestamibi and iodine planar scintigraphy was evaluated. In

addition, in all patients serum thyroglobulin was determined.

Table 1: Positive whole body scans in 49/75 patients with differentiated thyroid carcinoma and elevated serum thyroglobulin

n	histology	Iodine +	Sestamibi +	Iodine/Sestamibi +
21	follicular	8	8	5
15	papillary	15	-	-
9	Hürthle	2	6	1
4	follicular/ papillary	2	2	-

The results reveal that of 49 patients with positive whole body scans, twenty seven patients had only positive iodine uptake, 16 patients had increased Sestamibi accumulation and in six cases, both positive iodine and sestamibi uptake was detected.

In no case with papillary carcinoma positive sestamibi uptake was observed. Particularly in patients with follicular carcinoma and Hürthle cell carcinoma positive findings in the sestamibi scintigraphy could be detected.

In follicular carcinomas (n = 37), five patients had positive iodine and sestamibi scans. Eight patients showed a selective sestamibi accumulation in especially the lung parenchyma and in projection to the thyroid gland. Eight of the thirty seven cases had only increased iodine uptake in projection to the thyroid gland.

In the group of Hürthle cell carcinoma, six patients showed a selective sestamibi uptake, one patient had positive iodine and sestamibi uptake, two patients had only positive iodine accumulation and in one case no positive tracer uptake could be detected.

The positive tracer findings were insured by computertomography, MRI and in the most cases biopsy was taken. In thirteen patients local recurrences were confirmed. In 21 cases metastases especially of the lung and mediastinum could be diagnosed (fig 1a, fig 1b).

When we reviewed the results, in particular for follicular carcinoma, Hürthle cell carcinoma and papillary/follicular carcinoma, seventeen patients had a selective iodine accumulation and twenty two patients showed only positive sestamibi uptake.

Sestamibi scintigraphy detected metastases or local recurrences with a sensitivity of 63 % and a specificity of 96 %, whereas diagnostic iodine scintigraphy had a sensitivity of 58 % and a specificity of 100 %.

MATERIALS AND METHODS

75 patients with histopathologically confirmed carcinomas of the thyroid were included in this prospective study. The histopathologies studied were as followed: twenty papillary carcinoma, thirty seven follicular carcinoma, ten Hürthle cell carcinoma and eight papillary - follicular carcinoma. All patients underwent total thyroidectomy, radioiodine therapy (3700 - 7400 MBq I-131) and, in some cases, external radiation.

Planar sestamibi whole body scans were performed 10 min and 1 hour after intravenous administration of 700 MBq Tc-99m-Sestamibi. Additionally, SPECT images were obtained using a Picker Prism 2000 camera. Under optimal endogenous TSH-stimulation (TSH > 25 mU/ml), diagnostic raioiodine scans were performed 72 hours after oral application of 370 MBq I-131. In all patients serum thyroglobulin levels were measured after hormone discontinuation for at least two weeks. The range of normal values was 0.2 - 1.6 ng/ml.

Positive findings in the sestamibi and iodine scans were confirmed by computertomography, MRI and/or by biopsy. A finding was classified as true-positive if it showed an increased tracer uptake especially in projection to the thyroid gland and/or the lung parenchyma and if the findings could be confirmed by other diagnostic methods. A study was classified as false-positive if it showed an increased tracer uptake but no confirmation with CT, MRI or by biopsy was possible. True-negative findings had no positive uptake in the sestamibi and iodine scans or in other radiological methods. False-negative findings showed no abnormal tracer accumulation in the scintigraphy but positive findings were confirmed with CT,MRI and/or biopsy.

RESULTS

15/75 patients showed normal thyroglobulin levels and negative findings in the sestamibi as well as in the iodine scintigraphy. 60 of the investigated patients presented an increased thyroglobulin level (> 3 ng/ml), 11/60 cases had negative findings in both, sestamibi and iodine scans. 49 patients had elevated thyroglobulin levels and positive tracer accumulation in the iodine and/or sestamibi scintigraphy (table 1).

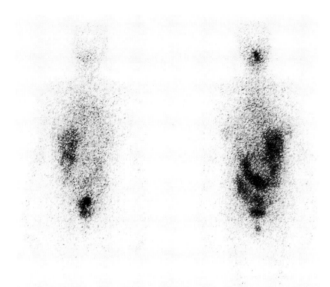

Fig. 1a: Follicular Ca, diagnostic iodine scintigraphy with normal iodine uptake in projection to the thyroid gland or to the lungs.

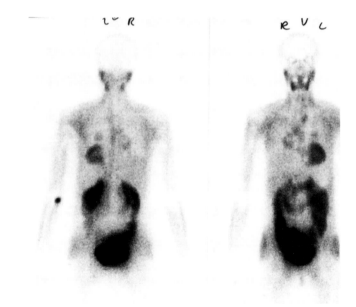

Fig 1b: The sestamibi scintigraphy shows multiple areas of increased uptake in the posterior and anterior lung fields. These findings were confirmed by CT as mestastases of the follicular carcinoma.

DISCUSSION

The gold standard for detecting recurrences and metastases in differentiated thyroid carcinoma is the use of 131-iodine. In the past, radiopharmaceuticals other than 131-iodine have been considered for the detection of metastastic lesions of thyroid carcinomas. Especially Tc-99m-pentavalent-dimercaptosuccinic acid has successfully been used to diagnose differentiated thyroid carcinoma and medullary thyroid carcinoma (6). Previous studies showed that thallium-201 scintigraphy has been used in the follow up in thyroid carcinoma while the patients are on hormonal suppression (4). In particular, in patients with Hürthle cell carcinoma following total thyroidectomy and presenting an elevated serum thyroglobulin thallium-201 has been successfully used for the detection of metastases and recurrences (2). Thallium -201 could give complementary information to iodine-131 especially in those cases of thyroid carcinoma with an increased serum thyroglobulin level and negative iodine scintigraphy (4,5).

Biochemical studies have suggested that Tc-99m-sestamibi as a lipophilic cation enters the tumor cells by passive diffusion and is retended in mitochondrial cells. The uptake of sestamibi is described in relationship to an increased blood perfusion and capillary permeability in tumor cells (1,8). In abundance of negatively charged mitochondria in tumor cells sestamibi is preferential accumulted within these mitochondria (9).

In this study all patients were investigated in an optimal endogenous stimulation, although other studies has been performed onder hormonal suppression. Caused to the increased blood perfusion in tumor cells, images were obtained 10 min and 1 hours after administration of sestamibi. Compared to iodine scintigraphy sestamibi has the advantage of imaging within the same day and better image resolution.

Among the diagnostic methods used in our study, iodine scintigraphy was the superior method for detecting recurrences and metastses in patients with papillary carcinoma. The use of iodine was limited in the value due to the poor uptake in Hürthle cell carcinoma and in different cases of follicular carcinoma. In these tumors sestamibi provided complementary information to iodine -131 imaging for the detection especially of lung metastases. Based on the results of our study, we conclude that iodine scintigraphy and the determination of serum thyroglobulin should be the primary diagnostic methods in the follow up of differentiated thyroid carcinoma, except in Hürthle cell carcinoma, where sestamibi scintigraphy should be the method of choice in detecting local recurrences and metastases.

In patients with follicular carcinoma, elevated serum thyroglobulin and negative iodine scans, sestamibi scintigraphy reveals recurrences and metastases with high sensitivity and specificity . Therefore, in follicular carcinoma sestamibi scintigraphy should be performed in addition to iodine scans.

REFERENCES

1. Aktolun C., Bayhan H.,Kir M. Clinical experience with 99m-Tc-MIBI imaging in patients with malignant tumors: preliminary results and comparison with 201-thallium. Clin Nucl Med 1992:17: 171-176

2. Balone HR. Fink-Benett D, Stoffer SS. 99mTechnetium-sestamibi uptake by recurrent Hürthle cell carcinoma of the thyroid. J Nucl Med 1992; 33: 1393-1395

3. Briele B., Hotze A., Kropp J. et al. A Comparison of 201-Tl and 99m-Tc-MIBI in the follow up of differentiated thyroid carcinoma. Nuklearmedizin 1991; 30: 115-124

4. Dadparvar S.,Kirshna L.,Brady LW, et al. The role of 131-iodine-Na and 201-thallium imaging and serum thyroglobulin in the management of differentiated thyroid carcinoma. Cancer 1993; 71:3767-3773

5. Dadparvar S, Chevres A, Tulchinsky M, Kirshna-Badrinath L, Khan a, Slizofski W.Clinical utility of Tc-99m methoxisobutylisonitrile imaging in differentiated thyroid carcinoma: comparison with thallium-201 and iodine-131 Na scintigraphy, and serum thyroglobulin quantitation. Eur J Nucl Med 1995; 22:1330-1338

6.Lastoria S, Vergara E, Varrella P, et al. Imaging of differentiated thyroid tumors with99m Tc (V) DMSA J Nucl Med 1993; 34:12p

7. Ramanna L, Waxman A, Braunstein G. 201 Thallium scintigraphy in differentiated thyroid cancer: comparison with radioiodine scintigraphy and serum determinations. J Nucl Med 1991; 32: 441-446

8. Wackers FJT, Berman DS, Maddahi J, et al. 99m Technetium hexakis 2 methoxyisobutyl isonitrile: human biodistribution, dosimetry, safety, and preliminary comparison to 201-thallium for myocardial perfusion imaging. J Nucl Med 1989; 30: 301-311

9. Waxman AD. Non-cardiac uses of 201-thallium and 99m-Tc-sestamibi. Clinical nuclear medicine. Harvard Medical School Annual Lectureship, 1994,p86-86

Radioactive Isotopes in
Clinical Medicine and Research XXII
ed. by H. Bergmann, A. Kroiss and H. Sinzinger
© 1997 Birkhäuser Verlag Basel/Switzerland

HÜRTHLE CELL TUMOR AND TECHNETIUM-99m-SESTAMIBI SCINTIGRAPHY
(SINGLE INJECTION DOUBLE-PHASE STUDY).

A. Vattimo, D. Volterrani, P. Bertelli, L. Burroni, A. Vella

Nuclear Medicine Unit at the University of Siena, Italy

SUMMARY: Single injection dual-phase MIBI thyroid scintigraphy was performed
on 49 pts with a cold nodule on a previous Tc99m scintigraphy. In 8 pts the
nodule displayed intense and persistent MIBI uptake (8 Hürthle cell tumors).
In 23 pts the nodule displayed early intense uptake with late fading activity
(9 benign and 14 malignant nodules). In 18 patients the nodule showed no MIBI
uptake (3 malignant and 15 benign nodules). This tecnique is able to identify
Hürthle cell tumors since they retain MIBI due to the presence of an abundant
granular acidophilic cytoplasm represented by crowded mitochondria.

INTRODUCTION

The Hürthle cell tumor is one of the most controversial in thyroid
oncology. Most authors believe in the existence of both benign (adenoma) and
malignant (carcinoma) forms and in the malignant transformation of the
adenoma (1). The carcinoma form is most invasive and has high morbidity and
mortality: therefore adequate identification is needed. As reported in the
literature, thyroid ultrasound (2) and double-phase scintigraphy with 201Tl
(3-6) can give useful results, with various degrees of sensitivity and
specificity, for the differential diagnosis between benign and malignant
nodules, although they cannot be conclusive; neither, however, in the
available literature has been mentioned as being able to differentiate among
the various malignant nodules. Experienced cytologists are able to correctly
diagnose malignant nodules by means of thyroid aspiration or biopsy while
also obtaining the histologic type. During the last decade, Technetium-99m-
Sestamibi (MIBI) has been introduced for perfusion myocardial imaging as an
alternative to 201Tl (7). In addition MIBI concentrates on thyroid (8) and

parathyroid adenomas (9). In the present paper we present the scintigraphic aspects of the Hürthle cell tumor in comparison with other thyroid tumors using early (15-30 min.) and a delayed (3-4 hrs) thyroid scintigraphy following i.v. injection of MIBI

PATIENTS & METHODS

The study was carried out on 49 patients who had displayed a cold thyroid nodule on a 99mTc scan. Thirty women, aged 27-70 yrs, and 16 men, aged 40-60 yrs, participated in the study. All underwent thyroid surgery.

MIBI scintigraphy. An early image at 15-30 min and a late image at 3-4 hr were acquired after tracer injection, using a small field-of-view gammacamera (20 cm in diameter) fitted with a pin-hole collimator encompassing an area of 10x10 cm. The images were fixed on 64x64 matrices and stored on hard disk for the further processing. The late image was not obtained for those patients with a cold nodule in the early MIBI image.

Scintigraphic data processing. A visual inspection of the images was performed using a score method for MIBI uptake   0= no uptake; 1= uptake in the nodule superior to the background and inferior to the thyroidal tissue, 2= uptake in the nodule equal to the thyroidal tissue; 3= uptake in the nodule superior to that of the thyroidal tissue. Squared regions of interest were drawn over the nodule, the normal thyroid tissue and the surrounding extrathyroidal tissue in the early and late images. After background subtraction, the counts in the nodule and extranodular tissue were normalized for the acquisition time and the decay of 99mTc. The nodular-to-extranodular normal thyroidal tissue (N/T) uptake ratio was calculated in the early and late images, and the washout rate from the nodule (WON) and from the extranodular normal thyroidal tissue (WOT) was also calculated and expressed as fraction of the tracer removed per hour ($\% \ h^{-1}$). Mann-Whitney (between groups) and Wilcoxon signed-rank (within groups) tests were used for statistical analysis.

Histopathologic data analysis. Since some patients were operated on in different hospitals, surgical specimens were collected and given to our pathologist for preparation and reading. The pathologist, unaware of the

scintigraphic data, was first asked to dignose the lesion and secondly to
score the percentage of oxyphilic cells as compared to the whole cellularity.

RESULTS

Scintigraphic data. Visual inspection identified 31 patients exhibiting a
clear uptake of MIBI in the nodule (score 1, 2, 3) in the early image: among
these in the late study 8 patients (Group A) showed a persistent uptake in
the nodule and a wash-out in the thyroid (score 3), whereas 23 patients
(Group B) showed a wash-out both in the nodule and in the thyroid tissue
(score 0). Eighteen patients (Group C) did not show any significant uptake of
MIBI in the nodule in the early study (score 0) and had no scintigraphic data
processing. In the early image the N/T ratio resulted higher than 1 for
patients in both group A and B, but the ratio increased in group A and
decreased in group B in the late image. The washout rate was found to be
lower in the nodule of group A patients than in group B and similar in normal
thyroid tissue in both groups. The following table summarizes the results and
shows the statistical analysis.

Table 1 - Scintigraphic data and statistical analysis

	Early score	Late score	
group A	2.63±0.48	3.00±0.00	NS
group B	1.85±0.78	0.00±0.00	p<.001
	p<.01	p<.001	

	Early N/T uptake	Late N/T uptake	
group A	1.67±0.42	3.26±1.47	p<.01
group B	1.54±0.45	0.94±0.32	p<.001
	NS	p<.0001	

	WON (% h-1)	WOT (% h-1)	
group A	17.6±6.8	25.7±7.6	p<.001
group B	32.6±7.8	24.8±7.8	p<.001
	p<.001	NS	

Figure 1 displays the pattern in each group.

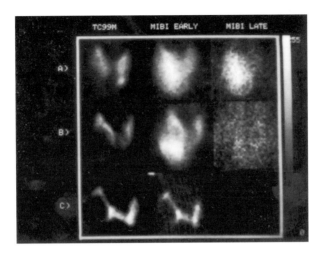

Figure.1. A): intense and persistent deposition of MIBI
in a cold nodule on 99mTc scan; B): intense uptake of
MIBI with fading activity in a cold nodule on 99mTc; C):
no uptake of MIBI in a cold nodule on 99mTc scan.

Histopathologic data. A Hürthle cell tumor was diagnosed in the group A
patients (3 carcinoma and 5 adenoma). The oxyphilic cellularity ranged from
50% to 100%. Hystopathology of the group B patients revealed colloid cysts
(n=1), adenomatous goiters (n=8), papillary carcinoma (n=6) and follicular
carcinoma (n=8). In patients from group C, colloid nodules (n=6), follicular
adenoma (n=9), papillary carcinoma (n=1) and follicular carcinoma (n=2) were
diagnosed. Oxyphilic cellularity was not observed in any patients from group
B or C.

DISCUSSION

Thyroid nodularity is a common finding but, fortunately, the rate of
malignancy is relatively low. Although a hypoechoic lesion was more likely to
be malignant than benign, malignancy was detected only in 63% of lesions,
whereas 4% of hyperechoic lesions, more likely to be benign, resulted
malignant (2). Thyroid aspiration and biopsy are widely performed in the
assessment of nodules and experienced centers are able to get adequate

specimens. Thyroid scintigraphy with 201Tl, potassium analog tracer has not lead to conclusive results. In a group of 76 patients who had undergone surgery, Ochi et al. (3) found intense uptake in the early image and retention in the late image in 35/37 malignant and in 4/39 benign nodules using a visual scoring method. This promising pattern for differentiating between benign and malignant nodules has not been confirmed by others (4,5). Since visual interpretation of 201Tl uptake may be inconclusive in detecting malignancy, recently Hardoff et al. (6) have suggested the early and late lesion-to-non-lesion ratio for this purpose: they have found a sensitivity of 100% and specificity of 62%. In is generally accepted that 201Tl cannot be the ideal tracer for diagnostic assessment of thyroid nodules: its suboptimal physical properties give images of poor quality leading to misinterpretation and its recirculation may continuously supply the nodule with tracer so as to mimic persistent uptake. For such purposes MIBI may be considered superior to 201Tl: the optimal physical properties of 99mTc and the lack of recirculation lead to a better delineation of nodules and to better differentiation between true and apparent uptake in late acquisition. Recently, in a series of 34 surgically diagnosed nodules, Földes et al. (10) found dual-phase MIBI scintigraphy to not be specific for thyroid malignancy: the late image in their series was performed 1 hr following the injection. Our findings partly support these results. In fact, in our group of patients, although limited, double-phase scintigraphy with MIBI correctly identified patients with a Hürthle cell tumor displaying persistent uptake of the tracer in the late image in contrast with other tumors, some of which showed an intense uptake with washout and others which did not show any uptake of the tracer. The cellular mechanisms of uptake and retention of MIBI is due to its lipophilic-cationic nature by means of which it can distribute across the biologic membranes and concentrate especially into the mitochondria, since they generate a large negative potential across the inner mitochondrial membrane; moreover, the number of mitochondria contributes to the overall accumulation of MIBI. The Hürthle cell tumor is a neoplasm composed esclusively or predominantly of follicular cells exhibiting oxyphilic features due to the presence of abundant granular acidophilic cytoplasm represented by crowded mitochondria and, therefore, responsible for high MIBI uptake. This tumor, also known as oxyphil tumor, oncocytomas or Askenazy cell tumor, is one of the most controversial in thyroid oncology. The debate arises from the view that all Hürthle cell tumors are malignant (carcinoma) or potentially malignant (adenoma), and therefore total thyroidectomy is suggested as the treatment of choice (11). This suggestion is supported by the fact that the adenoma has the property of undergoing malignant transformation, (1) the carcinoma may spread to the lymph nodes and metastatize in the lungs, because it has higher morbidity and mortality and usually does not concentrate radioiodine (12). Therefore it is important to correctly diagnose such a tumor and our data are promising in this regard; in fact, persistent MIBI uptake seems to be a particular characteristic of the Hürthle cell tumor.

REFERENCES
1. McDonald RJ, Wu S, Jensen JL, et al. Malignant trasformation of a Hürthle cell tumor: case report and survey of the literature. J Nucl Med 1991; 32:1266-1269.
2. Solbiati L, Volterrani L, Rizzato G, et al. The thyroid gland with low uptake lesions: evaluation by ultrasound. Radiology 1985; 155:187-191.
3. Ochi H, Sawa H, Fukuda T, et al. Thallium-201-chloride thyroid scintigraphy to evaluate benign and/or malignant nodules. Cancer 1982; 50:236-240.
4. Bleichrodt RP, Vermey A, Piers A, et al. Early and delayed thallium 201 imaging. Diagnosis of patients with cold thyroid nodules. Cancer 1987; 60:2621-2623.
5. Henze E, Roth J, Boerer H, et al. Diagnostic value of early and delayed Tl-201 thyroid scintigraphy in the evaluation of cold nodules for malignancy. Eur J Nucl Med 1986; 211:413-416.
6. Hardoff R, Baron E and Sheinfeld M. Early and late lesion-to-non-lesion ratio of thallium-201-chloride uptake in the evaluation of "cold" thyroid nodules. J Nucl Med 1991; 32:1873-1876.
7. Taillefer R, Lambert R, Dupras G, et al. Clinical comparison between thallium-201 and Tc99m-methoxy isobutyl isonitrile (hexamibi) myocardial perfusion imaging for detection for coronary artery disease. Eur J Nucl Med 1989; 15:280-286.
8. Vattimo A, Bertelli P and Burroni L. Effective visualization of suppressed thyroid tissue by means of baseline Methoxy-isobutyl-isonitrile in comparison with Tc99m pertechnetate scintigraphy after TSH stimulation. J Nucl Biol Med 1992; 36:315-318.
9. Taillefer R, Boucher Y, Potvin C, et al. Detection and localization of parathyroid adenomas in patients with hyperparathyroidism using a single radionuclide imaging procedure with technetium-99m-sestamibi (double-phase study). J Nucl Med 1992; 33:1801-1807.
10. Földes I, Lèvay A and Stotz G. Comparative scanning of thyroid nodules with technetium-99m pertecnetate and technetium-99m methoxyisobutylisonitrile. Eur J Nucl Med 1993; 20:330-333.
11. Gundry SR, Burney RE, Thompson NW, et al. Total thyroidectomy for Hurthle cell neoplasm of the thyroid. Arch Surg 1983; 118:529-532.
12. Yen T, Lin H, Lee C, et al. The role of technetium-99m sestamibi whole body scans in diagnosing metastatic Hürthle cell carcinoma of the thyroid gland after total thyroidectomy: a comparison with iodine-131 and thallium-201 whole body scans. Eur J Nucl Med 1994; 21:980-983.

Radioactive Isotopes in
Clinical Medicine and Research XXII
ed. by H. Bergmann, A. Kroiss and H. Sinzinger
© 1997 Birkhäuser Verlag Basel/Switzerland

GALLIUM AND MAGNETIC RESONANCE IMAGING IN THE FOLLOW-UP OF MEDIASTINAL LYMPHOMA

M. Gasparini, L. Maffioli, J.D. Tesoro Tess, A. Chiti, [1]M. Castellani and E. Bombardieri
Istituto Nazionale per lo Studio e la Cura dei Tumori, Via Venezian 1, Milano Italy
[1]Ospedale Maggiore di Milano, Via F. Sforza 35 Milano Italy

SUMMARY: A residual mediastinal mass after treatment represents a common diagnostic problem in the management of a lymphoma patient. Conventional radiology and computed tomography (CT) do not adequately reflect changes as fibrosis or necrosis. We compared the ability of gallium-67 scintigraphy and magnetic resonance imaging (MRI) to evaluate the mediastinal disease in the follow up of a lymphoma patient. This study included 247 previously treated patients (200 Hodgkins disease and 47 non-Hodgkin lymphoma) were investigated with gallium scan, MRI (372 examinations) and all other investigations to evaluate the mediastinal region. High values of sensitivity (90%) and specificity (96%) were found for both methods. We want to stress the complementary role of these two tests.

Introduction

Intrathoracic disease is present in 80% of newly diagnosed cases of Hodgkin disease (HD), compared with 30% to 40% in non-Hodgkin lymphoma (NHL) (1). The mediastinum is involved in almost all patients with HD with intrathoracic lymphoma, whereas in patients with NHL different sites such as other lymph-node groups, lung, pleura and pericardium are involved and often as an isolated finding. Especially in bulky mediastinal lymphoma, a residual mediastinal mass is a common pattern after treatment (2).

Conventional diagnostic radiology and computed tomography (CT) give information about tumor size and distribution of lesions, but do not adequately reflect changes such as fibrosis, necrosis and inflammation. A residual mediastinal mass does not necessarily indicate active disease (3,4) and this fact can represents a difficult diagnostic problem.

Gallium-67 (^{67}Ga) scintigraphy has been useful for evaluating neoplastic disease in the mediastinum (5,6) and the lack of accumulation of ^{67}Ga in fibrotic tissue makes it particularly attractive to study the follow up of lymphoma patients. Magnetic resonance imaging (MRI) can potentially differentiate between viable tumor and fibrosis (7,8) and for this reason in this study we compare the overall utility of this techniques and ^{67}Ga scintigraphy with regard to mediastinal disease activity in the follow-up of patients with lymphoma.

Materials and Methods

From January 1990 to June 1995 we tested in our Institute more than 300 patients with Hodgkin and non-Hodgkin lymphoma. Out of these we selected 247 previously treated patients (117 males and 130 females), ages 8-58 years (mean 28.4) which were submitted, during the same period (approximately 15 days), both the gallium scan or MRI. Considering the pathology of the patients, 200 were HD (respectively 146 nodular sclerosing, 39 mixed cellularity and 15 lymphocytic depletion) and 47 were NHL (31 were classified as G, 7 as I and 9 as H of the Working Formulation). Regarding the staging of this group we had 19 patients in stage I, 135 in stage II, 38 in stage III and 55 in stage IV. All patients entered the study during the follow up of the disease, having received some form of treatment as multidrug chemotherapy and radiation therapy if necessary. The range of follow up time was 12-85 months. One hundred and sixty-one patients were in restaging after treatment and 86 patients were investigated for suspected radiologic recurrences in the mediastinum. The group of patients studied were given a physical examination, chest radiography and all other necessary imaging procedures.

Scintigraphy was performed 48-72 hours after i.v. injection of 185-295 MBq of ^{67}Ga. A large field-of-view digital gamma camera (Toshiba GCA-901A) equipped with a medium energy general-purpose collimator and three energy peaks of 93, 184 and 296 keV (window 20%) was utilized. Total body images (scan speed 10 cm x min⁻1, with 512x128 matrix) were supplemented with an appropriate spot of view of the mediastinum. When SPET study was performed in order to better define the mediastinal region, also a triple headed gamma camera (Picker Prism 3000) was utilized. In this case the study was acquired on a 64 x 64 matrix, collecting 120 projections in a 360-degree circular orbit at a rate of 30 seconds per projection. In general images were prefiltered using a Wiener filter and successively transaxial tomograms were reconstructed using a Ramp filter.

MRI was performed with a 1.5 Tesla Superconductive Magnet (Siemens Magneton). Spin echo sequences with cardiac gating were used in all cases. T1 and T2 weighted images were acquired. TR depended on the heart frequency rate (TR = 600-900 msec for T1 W and 1200-2000 msec for T2 W) and TE ranged from 17 to 90 msec. The area of interest was studied in axial and coronal planes with 6-8 mm of thick, noncontiguos slices and 2 mm of separation volume.
Imaging studies were reviewed by specialists without knowledge of the results of the other tests.

The results of gallium scintigraphy and MRI were matched with clinical findings during the follow up. An imaging which was in agreement with the clinical status of the patient was considered either true positive or true negative.

Results

Three-hundred and seventy-two gallium scans and MRI examinations of the mediastinal region were performed in the population of 247 patients.

In Table 1° we compared the two examinations in term of positivity and negativity results. The gallium scan was positive in 99 cases and negative in 273 circustances, while MRI was considered significant for active disease in 116 cases and negative in 256 studies. The concordant positive results were 91, while in terms of negativity there was agreement in 248 cases.

Table 1° Gallium-67 imaging results compared with MRI in 247 patients with lymphoma

	Ga-67 results		
	Positive	Negative	Total
MRI results			
Positive	91	25	116
Negative	8	248	256
Total	99	273	372

Moreover we compared the results in term of true positive and true negative. This results are summarize in Table 2. We obtained similar results for both methods. The true positive were 90 for the gallium scan and 91 for MRI; 262 examinations for the scintigraphic method were considered true negative versus 241 for MRI; also the false negative results (11 vs 10) were equal. An important difference was demonstrated when we considered the false positive results. In 30 examinations the MRI interpretated the residual mediastinal mass as pathologic tissue but the subsequenty follow up showed the absence of the disease. Instead the gallium scan was erroneously positive in 9 cases.

Table 2° Gallium-67 scintigraphy versus MRI (372 examinations)

	Ga-67	MRI
True positive	90	91
True negative	262	241
False positive	9	30
False negative	11	10

In only 2 cases both examinatios resulted false positive for medistinal disease. In the first case there was a young patient with NHD. After treatment a SPET gallium scan showed an important uptake behind the sternum. This was confirmed by RMI. This examinations were repeated two months later with the same results. The successive surgical approach do not confirm the presence of lymphoma,

The gallium scan has been regarded by many as the gold standard for the detection of activity in the residual mediastinal masses, but unfortunately not all lymphomas take up gallium (11). MRI can be useful in solving this problem, because scarring or fibrosis are characterized by low signal intensity in all sequences, whereas high signal intensity on T2-weighted images suggests active tissue. However, necrosis or inflammation associated with disease responding to therapy can simulate viable tumor on T2-weighted images. Thus, when uniformly low signal intensity is observed, neoplastic activity can be reasonably excluded. Conversely, when there are areas of persistently high signal intensety, MRI can be inconclusive (12). In our preliminary report, in a limitated number of HD's patients (13), we suggested the high value and ability of the gallium scan and MRI to indicate whether a residual mass represents active neoplastic disease and the complementary role of the two tests. Also in this study we comfirm the ability of the two examinations. While the disappearance of gallium uptake in the mediastinal region after therapy may correspond to regression of tumor activity, a persistent uptake suggests the presence of active lymphoma. On 274 patients investigated we note only 9 (3.2%) cases of false positive results. MRI can be considered an alternative technique to conventional radiography and CT scan. In this experience the specificity resulted relatively low compared to the gallium scan tecnhique. In 30 cases MRI revealed a persistent mediastinal mass with a signal compatible with active lymphoma when only fibrotic tissue was present. Histopathological confirmation is the most effective method of establishing malignancy, but it would have been impractical for most of our patients. In this contest we utilized the patient's clinical status as a standard for comparison with imaging data.

We can conclude that gallium scintigraphy and MRI are accurate in assessing the activity of residual mediastinal mass after therapy, but however we want to point out the complementary role of the two tests. In our opinion the most appropriate way to utilize these techniques is to perform them currently if possible.

References

1) Musumeci R, Tesoro Tess JD. New imaging techniques in staging lymphomas. Current opinion in Oncology 1994; 6:464-469.

2) Jochelson MS, Mauch P, Balikian J et al. The significances of the residual mediastinal mass in treated Hodgkin's disease. J Clin Oncol 1985; 3:634-640.

3) Israel O, Front D, Epelbaum R et al. Residual mass and negative gallium scintigraphy in treated lymphoma. J Nucl Med 1990; 31:365-368.

4) Wylie BR, Southee AE, Joshua DE. gallium scanning in the management of mediastinal Hodgkin's disease. Eur J Haematol 1989;42:344-347.

5) Drossman SR, Schiff RG, Kronfeld GD et al. Lymphoma of the mediastinum and neck: evaluation with gallium-67 imaging and CT correlation. Radiology 1990;174: 171-175.

6) McLaughlin AF, Magee MA, Greenoug R et al. Current role of gallium scanning in the management of lymphoma. Eur J Nucl Med 1990; 16: 755-771.

7) Skillings JR, Bramwell V, Nicholson RL et al. A prospective study of magnetic resonance imaging in lymphoma staging. Cancer 1991; 67:1838-843.

8) Nyman R, Rehn S, Glimelius B et al. Magnetic resonance imaging for assessment of treatment effects in mediastinal Hodgkin's disease. Acta Radiol 1987;28:145-151.

9) Jochelson MS, Herman TS, Stomper PC, Mauch PM, Kaplan WD. Planning mantle radiation therapy in patients with Hodgkin's disease: role of gallium-67 scintigraphy. AJR 1988; 151:1229-1231.

10) Israel O, Front D, Lam M. Gallium-67 imaging in monitoring lymphoma response to treatment. Cancer 1988; 61:2439-2443.

11) Kostakoglu L, Yed SDJ, Portlok C et al. Validation of gallium-67 citrate single photon emission computed tomography and Computed Tomography in biopsy confirmed residual Hodgkin's disease in the mediastinum. J Nucl Med 1992; 33:345-350.

12) Hill M, Cunningham D, MacVicar V, et al. Role of Magnetic Resonance Imaging in predicting relapse in residual masses after treatment of lymphoma. J Clin Oncol 1993; 11:2273-2278.

13) Gasparini M, Balzarini L, Castellani MR et al. Current role of gallim scan and magnetic resonance imaging in the management of mediastinal Hodgkin lymphoma. Cancer 72; 2:577-582.

Radioactive Isotopes in
Clinical Medicine and Research XXII
ed. by H. Bergmann, A. Kroiss and H. Sinzinger
© 1997 Birkhäuser Verlag Basel/Switzerland

LYMPHOCYTIC IMMUNOPHENOTYPES IN GMCSF- ASSOCIATED JUXTAARTICULAR UPTAKE ON BONE SCINTIGRAPHY

R.M.Aigner and G.F.Fueger

Karl-Franzens-University of Graz, Department of Radiology, Divison of Nuclear Medicine,

Austria

Summary

This prospective study elucidated an uptake pattern seen on whole body bone scintigraphy (BS) in 45 oncologic patients. It consisted of a typically, symmetrically increased uptake pattern in the knees, the shoulders and sometimes the ankles in regions of former growth plates, just similar to activated growth plates. It was associated with peripheric bone marrow expansion seen on bone marrow scintigraphy, increased serum levels of GM-CSF, and increased CD4+T-helper cells and interleukin-2-receptor expressing cells. We believe that uptake pattern of BS to be most promising for early recognition of bone marrow activation or invasion. It should lead to oncologic examination with a view toward cytotoxic chemotherapy. The scintigraphic observation of activation of epiphyseal zones in adult life will require supplementary investigation to understand its nature. That uptake pattern may serve as a part in the evaluation of therapy, since it is reversible.

Introduction

This prospective study elucidated an uptake pattern seen on whole body bone scintigraphy (BS) which was observed in oncologic patients with associated scintigraphic peripheric diffuse bone marrow pathology and elevated serum GM-CSF levels. The aim of this study was to correlate these scintigraphic findings with immunophenotypic analysis of lymphocytes, i.e. the expression activation and differentiation state.

Materials and Methods

The patients comprised 45 cases, 32 female and 13 male, aged between 37 and 76 years. The bone marrow pathology was verified in 19/45 patients by biopsy. The bone marrow biopsies were carried out as a sternal puncture or as a punch biopsy of the iliac crest.

Radionuclide imaging consisted of whole body bone scintigraphy (BS) with the osteotropic tracer 99m-Technetium-methylen-di-phosphonate (MDP) in 45 patients, and of (additional) whole body bone marrow scintigraphy (MS) with 99m-Technetium-human-serum-albumine-nanocolloid (NNC) in 26/45 patients (57,7%). The time interval after tracer injection was 3 hrs for BS, and 30 - 60 min for MS. Wide-field-of-view scintillation cameras were used for scintigraphy, equipped with a general purpose collimator suitable for 99m-Tc. Twelve single images were obtained to cover the body from anterior and posterior.

Flow cytometry analysis was done on a FACScan (Becton- Dickinson, Mountain View, CA). Forward light scatter, orthogonal light scatter, and 2 fluorescence signals were determined for each lymphocyte. The cellcount/ mm3 bearing the following surface antigens were determined: CD3, CD4, CD8, CD16, CD19, CD25, CD56, CD57, HLA-DR, CD3/CD25, CD57/CD8, CD16/CD56, CD3/CD16+56+.

Results

The **clinical diagnoses** were: carcinoma of the breast (22/45 cases), carcinoma of the prostate (5/45 cases), non-Hodgkin lymphoma (7/45 cases), Hodgkin lymphoma (11/45 cases).

Bone marrow biopsy: The bone marrow pathology was classified on the basis of the bone marrow biopsy findings in one of the following categories: (a) diffuse malignant bone marrow infiltration by tumour cells (11/19 patients), (b) benign myeloproliferation (8/19 patients).

Bone scintigraphy: In all patients, regardless of the type of finding on marrow biopsy, we observed a characteristic pattern of osteotropic tracer distribution: it consisted of localized, increased uptake at certain sites: a transverse band of uptake in the distal femora symmetrically covering the region of the former distal epiphyseal growth plates: this occurred in all cases (100%); in more pronounced cases extension of the pathologically increased uptake to the entire distal articular extremity of the femora, and proximally in the diaphysis in 12/45 cases (26,6%). In the tibial plateau we saw enhanced tracer concentrations in 37/45 cases (82.2%), with some extension to the proximal tibial diaphysis in 8/45 cases (17.7%), in the ankles in 16/45 cases; involvement of the proximal humeri in 44/45 cases (97.7%), in the proximal diaphysis of the humeri in 9/45 cases (20%); in the convexity of the calvaria in 35/45 cases (77.7%); in the sternum in 24/45 cases (53.3%): this was tie-shaped in 19/45 cases (42.2%), diffuse in 5 cases

(11.1%), see fig. 1,2.

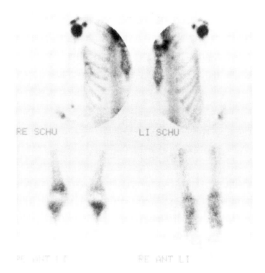

Figure 1. Bone scintigraphy: submetaphyseal activation of the shoulder-, and knee-joints and the ankles.

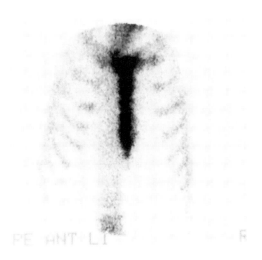

Figure 2. Distinct appearance of the sternum.

Bone marrow scintigraphy: MS revealed symmetrical bilateral peripheral bone marrow expansion in all cases confirming the diffuse involvement of the bone marrow suspected by BS. In the femura the MS revealed bilateral extension of the active marrow to the distal one half of the femoral diaphysis in 10/26 cases (38.5%), along the proximal one-third of the femur-shaft in 13/26 cases (50%); there was no NNC uptake in the femura in only 1 case. The tibiae revealed bilateral pathological NNC uptake in only 6/26 cases (23%), whereas it occurred in the proximal perimetaphysis and in the proximal half of the diaphysis in 3/26 (11.52%). The humeri showed bilateral pathological NNC uptake in all cases so studied: in the proximal diaphysis in 3/26 cases (11.5%), to the distal third of diaphysis in 13/26 cases (50%) and in the whole diaphysis in 10/26 cases (38.4%). The calvaria showed pathological NNC uptake in 5/26 cases (19.2%), and in 1 case it was significant. The sternum never revealed a pathological tracer uptake. The ankles did not show a pathological uptake pattern. The peripheral marrow expansion was regulary accompanied by reduced activity in the vertebral column and in the ribs (focal or diffuse). Well-circumscribed focal defects of activity in the humeral or femoral shaft created the need to differentiate between residual islets of yellow bone marrow from focal peripheral metastasis. This finding was recognized in 8/26 cases (30.7%), see fig. 3..

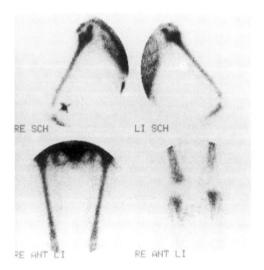

Figure 3. Bone marrow scintigraphy: Distinct peripheric expansion of the bone marrow in the femora and humeri, less in the proximal third of the radius and ulma and the tibiae.

Plain radiography: The radiography obtained in parallel to radionuclide imaging provided no signs of the pathological bone marrow conditions.

Flow cytometry analysis: The flow cytometry studies revealed elevated CD4+ T-helper cells and elevated interleukin-2- receptor expressing cells in all patients. The other lymphocyte distribution presented normal in all patients.

DISCUSSION

In patients with diffuse bone marrow pathology seen on MS, bone marrow biopsy and/or increased serum levels of GM-CSF we observed a localized increased uptake of MDP in areas of certain former growth plates in the distal femora, the proximal humeri, the proximal tibiae and the ankles, in the sternum and the calvaria. To our knowledge this uptake pattern has not been understood, so far.

The attempts at defence of the bone tissue against the invasion by malignant neoplastic cells results in the formation of immature osteoid causing locally enhanced osteotropic tracer uptake. Increased osteoid formation, callus or the intercellular matrix are well known substrates for osteotropic tracer uptake (1). During childhood and adolescence the osteotropic tracer uptake in epiphyseal zones is proportional to local blood flow to bone tissue, and to the affinity of the tracer to a tissue component or certain layers of the growth plates. It needs an explanation why former epiphyseal growth plates appear to become activated when they should remain non-reactive. Two phenomena need to be related: One is the fact that infiltrative or proliferative affections of the bone marrow triggered the peripheral expansion of the bone marrow. The other is the localized osteotropic tracer uptake in the mineralized bone tissue at certain sites, especially around former growth plates in adult life. It is reasonable to assume that the disease-provoked peripheral marrow expansion in adult life is facilitated by a process fundamentally similar to the seeding of the bone marrow in embryological or fetal life. Certain mechanisms seem to trigger the increased release of circulating (pluripotent) stem cells from the bone marrow and their increased nidation in certain skeletal parts in peripheral bone marrow expansion (2). Since we observed peripheral expansion of bone marrow and activation of former epiphyseal zones of bone tissue in patients with benign pathology of the bone marrow it is rather unlikely that oncogenes or growth hormones would directly cause the observed phenomena. One denominator is evidently the granulocyte- macrophage colony- stimulating factor (GM-CSF). McAfee et al. (3) described a juxtaarticular activity, as best observed in the knees and ankles, to be induced by GM-CSF in patients with locally advanced and metastatic breast cancer. GM-CSF is a multipotential hematopoietic growth factor, with relative lineage specific properties. It supports the differentiation and proliferation of progenitors already committed to the neutrophil or macrophage lineages. It appears to be required for optimal colony formation of human macrophages in vitro. On the other hand GM-CSF is said to be able to stimulate the growth and function of a variety of non- hematopoietic cells, normal bone marrow fibroblasts, and endothelial cells (4,5,6). The presence of CD4 functionally defines the helper/inducer T-cell subset for T-T, T-B, and T-macrophage interactions. In these interactions the CD4 molecule of the T-helper cell serves as the recognition structure for the HLA Class II molecules of the antigen presenting- cells or target cells and may also play a direct signaling role in T- cell activation (7,8). Functionally the T-helper cells are essential for the induction of B- lymphocyte differentiation, as well as for the development of T- suppressor cells which modulate the immune response. Lymphocyte subtyping with the anti- CD4 monoclonal antibodies has been employed in the phenotypic differentiation of hematopoietic neoplasms. The interleukin-2 (IL-2R) receptor is a well- established marker of lymphocyte activation. In vivo studies have demonstrated a potential role for IL-2 therapy in the treatment of adult metastatic tumors, and there is great interest in the utilization of other immunomodulatory agents. The action of IL-2 is the production of lymphokine- activated killer cells, which have the property of lysing autologous tumor cells without prior stimulation. Except for the erythropoietin mechanism the homeostatic mechanism guarding the integral functional capacity of the bone marrow is unknown. Local tumor growth factors or hormones may induce enhanced activity of the osteoblasts. Most, if not all oncogenes associated with malignant transformation, are components of the pathways normally stimulated by growth factors (9,10,11,12). It is known that the growth of malignancies is supported, at least in part, due to the aberrant activation of signalling pathways involved in the regulation of proliferation of normal cells (13,14). The pattern appeared as a persistent or a transient phenomenon. However, that scintigraphic uptake pattern appeared early and clearly.

CONCLUSION

Given the fact that radionuclide imaging plays an important role in oncology, it is important to remember that BS always detected in these patients bone marrow activation which was associated with increased serum levels of GM-CSF, CD4+ T-helper cells and IL-2-R expressing cells. We believe that uptake pattern most promising for early recognition of bone marrow activation or invasion. It should lead to oncologic examination with a view toward cytotoxic chemotherapy. The scintigraphic observation of activation of epiphyseal zones in adult life will require supplementary investigation to understand its nature.

References

1. McKillop JH, Fogelman I. In: Benign and Malignant Bone Disease, Clinician`s Guide to Nuclear Medicine, Series Editor: P.J. Ell. Churchill Livingstone, Edinburgh, London, Melbourne, New York: 1991: 30- 52.

2. Hart IR. The spread of tumours. In: Introduction to the Cellular and Molecular Biology of Cancer, Second Edition, edited by L.M.Franks and N.M.Teich, Oxford University Press, Oxford, New York, Tokyo: 1991: 31- 48.

3. McAfee JG, Carrasquillo JA, Camera L, O'Shaughnessy JA, Cowan KH, Neuman RD. Changes in skeletal images induced by granulocyte- macrophage colony- stimulating factor (GM-CSF) in patients with locally advanced and metastatic breast cancer. Abstract. J Nucl Med 1994; 35, 5: 89.

4. Ruff MR, Farrar WL, Pert CB. Interferon- Gamma and granulocyte/macrophage colony-stimulating factor inhibit growth and induce antigens characteristic of myeloid differentiation in small- cell lung cancer cell lines. Proc Natl Acad Sci USA 1986; 83:6613-6617.

5. Bussolino F, Wang JM, Defilippi P et al. Granulocyte- and granulocyte- macrophage colony-stimulating factors induce human endothelial cells to migrate and proliferate. Nature 1989; 337:471-473.

6. Dedhar S, Gaboury L, Galloway P, Eaves C. Human granulocyte- macrophage colony-stimulating factor is a growth factor active on a variety of cell types of non- hematopoietic origin. Proc Natl Acad Sci USA 1988; 85:9253-9257.

7. Biddison WE, Shaw S. CD expression and function in HLA class II-specific T- cells. Immunol Rev 1989; 109:5-15.

8. Janeway CA Jr. The role of CD4 in T-cell activation: Accessory molecule or co- receptor? Immunol Today 1989; 10:234-238.

9. Hunter R. Cooperation between oncogenes. Cell 1991; 64:249-270.

10. Simon MI, Strathmann M, Gautam N. Diversity of G proteins in signal transduction. Science 1991;252:802-808.

11. Cantely L, Auger K, Carpenter C, Duckworth B, Garziani A, Kapeller R, Soltoff S. Oncogenes and signal transduction. Cell 1991; 64:281-302.

12. Auerbach et al. Specificity of adhesion between murine tumor cells and capillary endothelium. Cancer Res 1987; 47:1492-1496.

13. Kaminsky R, et al.. Tumor cells are protected from natural killer cells mediated lysis by adhesion to endothelial cells. Int.J.Cancer 1988; 41: 847-849.

14. Roberts AB, Sporn MB. Principles of Molecular Cell Biology of Cancer: Growth Factors Related to Transformation; in Cancer. In: Principles and Practice of Oncology, DeVita V.T., S.Hellman, S.A.Rosenberg, J.B.Lippincott Company, Philadelphia, 1989: Vol.1, 68-78.

Neurology

Radioactive Isotopes in
Clinical Medicine and Research XXII
ed. by H. Bergmann, A. Kroiss and H. Sinzinger
© 1997 Birkhäuser Verlag Basel/Switzerland

NEUROACTIVATION AND VASOACTIVATION STUDIES IN PATIENTS WITH IMPAIRED COGNITIVE FUNCTION USING Tc-99m-HMPAO-SPECT

Dannenberg C., Marschall B., Zedlick D., Bettin S., Seese A., Knapp W.H.

Departments of Nuclear Medicine and Psychiatry, University of Leipzig, Germany

Summary: Early stages of dementia of Alzheimer type (DAT) often fail to show characteristic patterns of local cerebral blood flow (lCBF). The present study deals with the question whether characteristic lCBF deficits can be produced or enhanced by activation. 22 patients underwent vasomotor activation by 500 mg acetazolamide and 33 patients cognitive activation by labyrinth task prior to 500 MBq Tc-HMPAO administration. According to visual scoring vasomotor activation decreased the fraction of patients with abnormal patterns from 16/22 (73 %) to 7/22 (32 %.) In contrast, neuroactivation increased the number of definitely abnormal patient studies from 19 (58 %) to 27 (82 %) out of 33 studies.

INTRODUCTION

Since SPECT of local cerebral blood flow (lCBF) shows highly characteristic patterns in various types of dementia, it actually helps to identify those patients in whom disease may be treatable or reversible. In order to enhance the efficiency of treatment protocols it would be desirable to identify patients with neurodegenerative diseases in early stages.

We hypothesized that activating the vascular system or neuronal function could unmask local functional deficits.

MATERIALS AND METHODS

Subjects:

55 right-handed patients, 31 female and 24 male, mean age 66 ± 10.4 with probable DAT or mild cognitive impairment (MMS 24 ± 6) were enrolled.

Probable DAT was diagnosed according to NINCDS/ADRDA criteria [1]. Cerebrovascular disease was judged unlikely by Hachinsky Ischemic Scale scoring [2]. All patients had Computer Tomography and Transcranial Doppler Ultrasonography to exclude cerebral lesions or major vascular abnormalities. A Depression Screening scale [3] was used to exclude patients with depression.

Activation:

In addition to baseline studies 22 patients underwent vasoactivation and 33 patients cognitive activation studies. Age and sex distribution of both groups were similar. The two studies of one patient were performed on different days within one week. Vasoactivation: 500 mg acetazolmide were injected intravenously 25 min prior to injection of 500 MBq Tc-99m-HMPAO. Cognitive activation: The task consisted in drawing a continuous line from the center of a labyrinth [4] on a sheet of paper to the exit and to complete as many of the different labyrinths as possible without interruption within 7 min. 500 MBq Tc-99m-HMPAO were injected 2 min after onset of the task performance.

SPECT:

Photons were registered using a dual-detector scintillation camera (ADAC Laboratories, Vertex). Acquisition was started 15 min after injection of the radiopharmaceutical. Data were reconstructed by standard filtered backprojection using a Gaussian weighted ramp filter. For attenuation correction Chang's first order method was used.

For semiquantitative analysis of transversal and coronal slices 12 rectangular regions of interest were used. Cerebellar ROIs were selected in the center of each cerebellar hemisphere. Cortical count density was expressed as cortical-to-cerebellar activity ratio (c/c ratio). In addition tomgrams were visually classified by three experts using the following score system [5]: 0 homogenous distribution, 1 inhomogeneous in activity distribution, 2 activity deficits, 3 severe defects.

Statistical analyses:

Differences in c/c ratios between baseline and activation studies were examined utilizing the Wilcoxon-test. Since multiple tests were performed the results were subjected to a Bonferroni correction. Inter-rater reliability for visual scores was assessed by determining the degree of inter-rater concordance using Kendalls W-test.

RESULTS

There was a significant increase in right temporal activity and a slight increase in other cortical regions related to cerebellum by vasoactivation in 22 patients with mild cognitive impairment or DAT (Table 1) whereas neuroactivation produced the opposite effect. Temporal and parietal regions in 33 patients showed a significant reduction in c/c ratios (Table 2).

Table 1. Mean count density (%) in ROIs related to that of cerebellum (= 100 %) in patients at baseline (B) and vasoactivation (V) (n = 22). Significance testing: comparison between B and V (* p < 0.05, ** = p < 0.01, *** = p < 0.001, § = p < 0.05 using a Bonferroni correction for multiple comparisons (= 16)

	left B	left V	right B	right V
prefrontal	84.2 ± 9.8	89.1 ± 12.2 *	83.4 ± 8.5	88.4 ± 11.1 **
frontal	81.7 ± 7.7	87.3 ± 10.6 *	87.5 ± 9.0	93.4 ± 10.7 **
occipital	92.0 ± 7.6	93.0 ± 13.1	89.3 ± 12.6	93.0 ± 11.4 *
parietal	81.7 ± 7.0	84.3 ± 12.4	88.1 ± 9.6	94.0 ± 14.1 *
temporal inferior	72.3 ± 8.1	76.6 ± 9.7	77.1 ± 12.0	85.4 ± 11.9 **§
temporal lateral	79.6 ± 9.0	85.5 ± 12.3 **	83.2 ± 8.0	88.4 ± 13.3
temporal	79.4 ± 9.5	83.8 ± 8.2 **	78.2 ± 12.2	91.4 ± 11.0
temporo-parietal	81.6 ± 6.8	85.4 ± 11.0	84.9 ± 9.4	90.9 ± 10.8 *

Table 2. Mean count density (%) in ROI related to that of cerebellum (= 100 %) in patients at baseline (B) and neuroactivation(N) (n = 33). Significance testing: comparison between B and N (* = p < 0.05, ** = p < 0.01, *** = p < 0.001, § = p < 0.05 using a Bonferroni correction for multiple comparisons (= 16)

	left B	left N	right B	right N
prefrontal	80.9 ± 8.2	78.3 ± 8.8 **	81.0 ± 8.6	78.9 ± 8.3 *
frontal	79.2 ± 6.7	76.8 ± 7.8 **	84.2 ± 7.7	82.4 ± 8.9
occipital	88.5 ± 8.2	86.9 ± 7.6	86.9 ± 9.0	84.1 ± 11.4 *
parietal	78.3 ± 7.8	74.8 ± 8.8 ***§	85.3 ± 9.8	82.9 ± 9.2 *
temporal inferior	70.9 ± 7.9	68.3 ± 7.9 **§	75.6 ± 9.5	72.3 ± 8.2 **§
temporal lateral	78.6 ± 9.0	75.5 ± 8.2 ***§	83.7 ± 8.4	78.7 ± 7.7 ***§
temporal	76.4 ± 8.1	74.0 ± 6.8 *	84.6 ± 9.9	81.6 ± 9.1 *
temporo-parietal	79.5 ± 7.2	76.6 ± 7.3 **§	84.2 ± 7.6	81.9 ± 7.4 *

The mean values of visual scores differed by 0.09, 0.25, and 0.16 respectively. The degree of concordance (Kendalls Coefficient) was W = 0.79 (p < 0.0001).

According to visual scoring vasomotor activation decreased the fraction of patients with abnormal patterns (score ≥ 2) from 16/22 (73 %) to 7/22 (32 %.) In contrast, cognitive activation increased the number of definitely abnormal patient studies from 19 (58 %) to 27 (82 %) out of 33 studies.

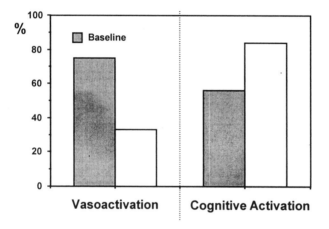

Percentage of patients with definite count deficiency (Score ≥ 2) in temporal or parietal cortex

DISCUSSION AND CONCLUSION

The aim of this study was to test the hypothesis that activating the vascular system or neuronal function could help to detect disease-releated lCBF deficits in patients with impaired cognitive function and probable DAT.

The effect of vasoactivation on regional blood flow was investigated, because special vascular involvement has been suggested in DAT [6]. Our results using acetazolamide stimulation clearly contradict the hypothesis that local perfusion deficits become more pronounced in patients without evidence of CVD. There was an increase in temporal and parietal activity uptake relative to cerebellum and a decrease in the number of activity deficits. This result indicates that there is increased local perfusion reserve in the temporal and parietal areas relative to other cortical territories and cerebellum. This appears to disagree with the study of Stoppe et al. [7] who found reduced cerebrovascular reactivity with increasing cognitive impairment using acetazolamide and HMPAO-SPET. When temporal and parietal areas show reduced baseline perfusion in DAT and an increased local perfusion reserve it appears unlikely that vascular disease was the primary cause for the typical DAT perfusion pattern. This view is supported by several vasoactivation studies in DAT patients. Bonte et al. [8] found no accentuation of flow inhomogeneity in 35 DAT patients in contrast to patients with cerebrovascular disorder using acetazolamide and the Xe-133 inhalation technique. Kuwabara et al. [9] did not find different responsiveness to CO_2 between 5 DAT and 5 control subjects using O-15-H_2O and PET.

For neuroactivation by cognitive task we chose the labyrinth test by which cerebral functions are activated in a complex manner [4]. This is in contrast to stimulation procedures that were employed using PET with the aim to identify reduced stimulation response by tasks specific for certain topograpic areas, e.g., memory or olfactory tasks [10-12]. Since SPET quantitation of absolute flow using HMPAO is not widely accepted, it appeared appropriate for this technique to activate a variety of different cerebral territories including those not being typically affected in DAT like motor, sensory and visual cortices, and cerebellum [13,14]. It was hypothesized that areas affected by DAT would be less activated than the others and accordingly show enhanced contrast in perfusion imaging.

This study provides evidence that neuroactivation by the labyrinth task does not only significantly reduce the corticocerebellar activity ratio in a number of territories, particularly in parietotemporal areas, but also increases the number of apparent defects when a complete set of tomograms is classified visually. Neuroactivation significantly increased the percentage of abnormal results and that of parietal/temporal regions classified abnormal.

Further studies have to define the diagnostic accuracy of neuroactivation SPET. This aim requires autopsy-confirmed diagnoses and a sufficient number of control subjects undergoing activation studies.

Acknowledgements

This work was supported by grants from the Bundesministerium für Bildung, Wissenschaft und Forschung to W.H.K. (FKZ 01 ZZ 9103/2.4) and to D.Z. (FKZ 01 ZZ 9103/2.24).

C. Dannenberg et al.

REFERENCES

1. McKhann G, Drachman D, Folstein M, Katzman R, Price D, Stadlan EM. Clinical diagnosis of Alzheimer's disease: report of the NINCDS-ADRDA Work Group under the auspices of Department of Health and Human Services Task Force on Alzheimer's disease. Neurology 1984; 34: 939-944.

2. Hachinski VC, Iliff LD, Zilkha E, DuBoulay GH, McAllister VL, Marshall J, Russel WR, Symon L. Cerebral blood flow in dementia. Arch Neurol 1975; 32: 632-637.

3. Yesavage JA, Brink TL, Rose TL, Lum O, Huang V, Adez M, Leirer V. Development and validation of a geriatric depression screening scale: A preliminary report. J Psychiat Res 1983; 17: 37-49.

4. Ostwald WD, Fleischmann VM. Der Labyrinthtest. In: Nürnberger Altersinventar Manual (NAI), Hogrefe Verlag, Göttingen-Bern-Toronto 1995; 64-82.

6. Scheibel AB, Duong T, Tomiyasu U. Denervation microangiopathy in senile dementia. Alzheimer type. Alzheimer Dis Assoc Disord 1987; 11: 19-37.

7. Stoppe G, Schütze R, Kögler A, Staedt J, Munz D, Emrich D, Rüther E. Cerebrovascular reactivity to acetazolamide in (senile) dementia of Alzheimers type: relationship to disease severity. Dementia 1995; 6: 73-82.

8. Bonte FJ, Devous MD, Reisch JS, Ajmani AK, Weiner MF, Hom J, Tintner R. The effect of acetazolamide on regional cerebral blood flow in patients with Alzheimer's disease or stroke as measured by single-photon emission computed tomography. Invest Radiol 1989; 24: 99-103.

9. Kuwabara Y, Ichiya Y, Otsuka M, Masuda K, Ichimiya H, Fujishima M. Cerebrovascular responsiveness to hypercapnia in Alzheimer's dementia and vascular dementia of the Binswanger type. Stroke 1992; 23: 594-598.

10. Miller JD, DeLeon MJ, Ferris SH, Kluger A, George AE, Reisberg B, Sachs HJ, Wolf HP. Abnormal temporal lobe response in Alzheimer's disease during cognitive processing as measured by C-11-2-deoxy-D-glucose and PET. J Cereb Blood Flow Metab 1987; 7: 248-251.

11. Buchsbaum MS, Kesslak JP, Lynch G, Chui H, Wu J, Sicotte N, Hazlette E, Teng E, Cotman CW. Temporal hippocampal metabolic rate during an olfactory memory task assessed by positron emission tomography in patients with dementia of the Alzheimer's type and controls. Preliminary studies. Arch Gen Psychiatry 1991; 48: 840-847.

12. Kessler J, Herholz K, Grond M, Heiss WD. Impaired metabolic activation in Alzheimer's disease. A PET study during continuous visual recognition. Neuropsychologia 1991; 29/3: 229-243.

13. Frackowiak RSJ, Pozzilli C. Legg NJ. Regional cerebral oxygen supply and utilization in dementia. A clinical and physiological study with oxygen-15 and positron tomography. Brain 1981; 104: 753-778.

14. Friedland RP, Budinger TF, Ganz E. Regional cerebral metabolic alterations in dementia of the Alzheimers type: Positron emission tomgography with F-18 fluorodeoxyglucose. J Comput Assist Tomogr 1986; 7: 590-598.

Radioactive Isotopes in
Clinical Medicine and Research XXII
ed. by H. Bergmann, A. Kroiss and H. Sinzinger
© 1997 Birkhäuser Verlag Basel/Switzerland

NEUROACTIVATION WITH SPECT AND SMOOTH PURSUIT EYE MOVEMENT IN SCHIZOPHRENICS

Pinkert J.[1], Gerdsen I.[2], Fötzsch R.[3], Franke W.-G.[1], Oehme L.[1], Felber W.[2]
University of Technology Dresden, Depts. of Nuclear Medicine[1] Psychiatry[2] and Neurology[3]
Fetscherstr. 74, Dresden, D-01307, Germany

SUMMARY: Schizophrenia and affective disorders are supposed to involve neural systems for information processing and biogenic amine transmission. In this context functional neuroimaging has been widely accepted for detecting possible cortical impairments. In our present study we performed functional neuroimaging using ^{99m}Tc-ECD SPECT for a paradigm on smooth pursuit eye movement and compared the results with resting patterns. Saccadic intrusions were monitored during an electronystagmographic examination. Reduced neuroactivaton during smooth pursuit eye movement in subjects with an elevated rate of catch up saccades was found in centers of the frontal lobe (FEF). This might indicate an impairment of higher cortical motor control.

INTRODUCTION

Abnormalities in biogenic amine transmission, cerebral perfusion and glucose metabolism may contribute to schizophrenic and affective disorders. Sensory information processing as well as motor control is affected. DIEFENDORF and DODGE (1908) firstly described in this context disorders of smooth pursuit eye movement in schizophrenic subjects during performance of a simple ocular motor task. Subsequent studies have reported abnormal smooth pursuit and saccadic eye movements in 50-85% of schizophrenic patients and 30% of non schizophrenic psychiatric patients. As a result eye movement function may be a promising vulnerability trait marker for schizophrenia and with minor significance also for affective disorders.

This phenomenon is considered to be independent of any drug treatment and clinical state and is also transmitted within families (HOLZMAN, 1974).

The ocular motor system, where higher cortical control could be impaired, involves a complex interacting neuronal network of cortical and subcortical structures. Cortical areas incorporating the frontal (FEF) and supplementary eye fields (SEF), the dorsolateral prefrontal cortex (DLPFC), posterior parietal cortex (PPC), medial superior and middle temporal area and striate cortex (SC) are part of this network. Neurons in the FEF, SEF, DLPFC and basal ganglia seem to discharge during saccadic eye movements. The cortical areas active during eye movements are shown in Fig. 1.

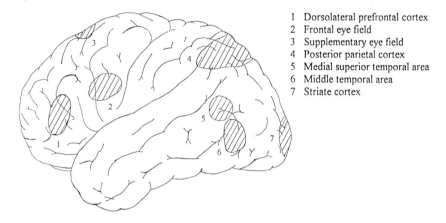

1 Dorsolateral prefrontal cortex
2 Frontal eye field
3 Supplementary eye field
4 Posterior parietal cortex
5 Medial superior temporal area
6 Middle temporal area
7 Striate cortex

Figure 1: Cortical areas active during ocular movements according to Goldberg, et al. (7)

Up to now the neurological and psychological substrates responsible for such impairments are entirely unknown.

Recent neuroactivation studies with SPECT (CRAWFORD, 1996) and with PET (NAKASHIMA, 1994) using saccadic paradigms have shown functional abnormalities in centers of the frontal lobe. To understand more about the functional anatomy underlying abnormalities in eye tracking pattern we performed functional neuroimaging using high resolution single photon emission computer tomography (SPECT) on a paradigm for smooth pursuit eye movement.

METHODS

Sixteen schizophrenic and 14 depressive patients aged from 20 - 60 years were recruited from our Psychiatric Department and diagnosed according to DSM-IV criteria. Patients with a history of any neurological disorder or substance abuse were not included. Psychopathological symptoms were assessed on the BPRS, SANS, SAPS and Hamilton Depression Rating Scale. Handedness was defined according to the Edinburgh Inventory. Neuroophthalmological and electronystagmographic examinations were carried out in all patients and the number of catch up saccades during smooth pursuit was counted. All patients were studied on a stable medication with neuroleptic and antidepressive drugs.

Following an activation for 3 minutes with a smooth pursuit tracking stimulus using a sinusoidally moving target on a lightbar (Nicolet Nystar Plus Task Design) in a dimed, quiet room 750 MBq ^{99m}Tc-ECD were administered intravenously via a long venous catheter so that the moment of injection was not noticed by the patient. Stimulation was continued for another two minutes after injection. The investigation under resting conditions was carried out two days later.

SPECT acquisitions were performed both at rest as well as following activation 1 h after injection using a dual head ADAC gamma camera equipped with low energy high resolution collimators with 40 seconds per projection, 64 projections in a 64x64 matrix. The system resolution was approximately 10 mm as FWHM (Full width at half maximum). After reconstruction (filtered back projection with a Butterworth filter) an attenuation correction using the CHANG-algorithm was carried out. A reorientation in the orbito-meatal-line and an image registration between the activation and rest study was performed. Neuroactivation images were calculated by subtracting images at rest from images after activation. All images were finally smoothed by a 5x5 spatial filter. The sites of hot spots due to activation were identified by overlaying neuroactivation and resting images. The activation pattern of all calculated neuroactivation images was visually analysed using a score comprising the categories „no activation", „questionable activation", „small activation" and „strong activation" taking into account SPECT slices from both studies.

RESULTS

SPECT slices of a 37 years old male schizophrenic patient are shown in fig. 2. Activation can be seen in the striate cortex, posterior parietal cortex, cerebellum, thalamus and clearly right fronto-parietal in the region of the frontal eye field. The number of catch-up saccades was within the normal range.

The SPECT images of a 21 years old male patient with first episode schizophrenia presenting increased rates of saccadic intrusions are shown in fig. 3. The enhancement of rCBF under stimulation in the frontal eye field was found to be reduced compared to other patients with low rate of catch-up saccades. In our study we found neuroactivation in the primary visual cortex, unilateral frontal in the region of the frontal eye field, the posterior parietal cortex and temporal. To a smaller extent activation was also observed in the basal ganglia, thalamus and cerebellum. This activation pattern is in coincidence with the known functional anatomy active during the generation of saccades, visual attention processing for saccades and visual motion processing.

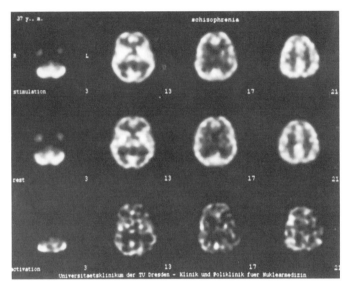

Figure 2: SPECT slices including substracted images of a 37 years old male schizophrenic patient

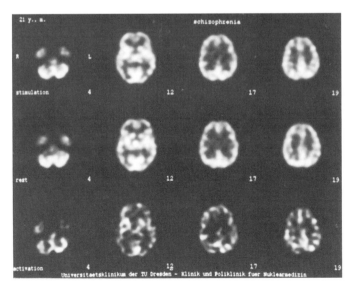

Figure 3: SPECT slices including substracted images of a 21 years old male schizophrenic patient

Reduced enhancement of rCBF in the FEF under stimulation was observed in several subjects presenting an increased number of saccadic intrusions. In addition the enhancement of rCBF as an index for neuroactivation was found to be significantly lower in the frontal eye field for the schizophrenic group compared with depressive patients (Chi-Square-Test, $p < 0,05$). A clear correlation of activation pattern with handedness was not found.

DISCUSSION

Our results support the hypothesis for an impairment of the frontal eye field to suppress inappropiate saccades towards a visual stimulus. This finding is consistent with theories that implicate frontal lobe pathology in schizophrenia and is supported by results published from NAKASHIMA et al. (10) obtained with ^{15}O water and PET. They reported a lack of activation in the frontal eye field (FEF) in schizophrenics during reflexive, volitional and memory-guided saccadic tasks. Other groups like BERMAN et al. and WEINBERGER et al. mention a so-called functional „hypofrontality" in schizophrenics with PET during prefrontal challenge tasks (1,5,6,9,11). Reduced activation of the frontal eye field (FEF) in our study has to be considered within the same functional context.

Our data also confirm the possibility to visualize functional well defined areas of the ocular motor system with high resolution SPECT by using a specific task design.

Further improvements for image calculation in our ongoing study will include registration of resting and activation images using a program for automatic registration.

In addition, image fusion for SPECT and MRI data will allow precise identification of anatomical structures. Image quality and resolution can be improved by using a triple head camera equipped with fan-beam collimators and by applying an iterative method for reconstruction of SPECT images. All data also will be evaluated by comparison of rCBF values by statistical parametric mapping (SPM 95).

We conclude that satisfying functional imaging can also be realized by using SPECT and does not exclusively require PET and fMRI equipment. SPECT studies are advantageously less costly and well tolerated by anxious or psychotic patients. Futurous functional studies with healthy volunteers or patients with other neuropsychiatric disorders using SPECT could be helpful to detect relevant pathomorphological substrates.

REFERENCES

1. Berman KF, Zec RF, Weinberger DR. Physiologic dysfunction of dorso-lateral prefrontal cortex in schizophrenia: II. role of neuroleptic treatment, attention, and mental effort. Arch Gen Psychiatry 1986; 43: 126-135.

2. Büttner-Ennever JA, editor. Reviews of Oculomotor Research, Volume 2: Neuro-anatomy of the Oculomotor System. Amsterdam-New York-Oxford: Elsevier, 1988.

3. Crawford TJ, Puri BK, Nijran KS, Jones B, Kennard C, Lewis SW. Ab-normal saccadic distractibility in patients with schizophrenia: a ^{99m}Tc-HMPAO SPECT study. Psychol Med 1996; in press.

4. Diefendorf AR, Dodge R. An experimental study of the ocular reaction of the insane from photographic records. Brain 1908; 31: 451-489.

5. Dolan RL, Bench CJ, Liddle FF, Friston KJ, Frith CD, Grasby PM, Frackowiak RSJ. Dorsolateral prefrontal cortex dysfunction in the major psychoses; symptom or disease specificity ? J Neurol Neurosurg Psychiatry 1993; 56: 1290-1294.

6. Franzén G, Ingvar DH. Absence of activation in frontal structures during psychological testing of chronic schizophrenics. J Neurol Neurosurg Psychiatry 1975; 38: 1027-1032.

7. Goldberg ME, Eggers HM, Gouras P. The ocular motor system. In: Principles of neural science. Third Edition, Kandel ER, Schwartz JH, Jessell TM, editors. New Jersey-London-Sydney-Toronto-Mexico City-New Delhi-Tokyo-Singapore-Rio de Janeiro: Prentice-Hall International Inc, 1991: 660-677.

8. Holzman PS, Proctor LR, Hughes DW. Eye tracking patterns in schizophrenia. Science 1973; 181: 179-181.

9. Ingvar, DH, Franzén G. Distribution of cerebral activity in chronic schizophrenia. Lancet 1974; 2: 1484-1486.

10. Nakashima Y, Momose T, Sano I, Katayama S, Nakajima T, Niwa SI, Matsushita M. Cortical control of saccade in normal and schizophrenic subjects: a PET study using a task-evoked rCBF paradigm. Schizophr Res 1994; 12: 259-264.

11. Weinberger DR, Bergman KF, Zec RF. Physiologic dysfunction of dorso-lateral prefrontal cortex in schizophrenia: I. Regional cerebral blood flow evidence. Arch Gen Psychiatry 1986; 43: 114-124.

Radioactive Isotopes in
Clinical Medicine and Research XXII
ed. by H. Bergmann, A. Kroiss and H. Sinzinger
© 1997 Birkhäuser Verlag Basel/Switzerland

USEFULNESS OF BRAIN PERFUSION SPET WITH Tc-99m ECD IN HIGH RISK NEONATES

A. Ahonen[1], M. Valkama[1], P. Torniainen[1], L. Vainionpää[2], M. Koivisto[2]

[1]Division of Nuclear Medicine, Oulu University Hospital, 90220 Oulu, Finland
[2]Department of Paediatrics, Oulu University Hospital, 90220 Oulu, Finland

Summary

Until now 21 neonates have been studied; 19 of them were preterm (born before 34 gestational weeks) and two asphyxiated new-borns. Imaging studies were carried out between 36 and 44 gestational weeks, at the same time when conventional imagings (ultrasound and magnetic resonance imaging) were performed. Imaging was carried out using a single head or a double head gamma camera with a slant or fan beam collimator. A new brain perfusion agent Tc-99m ethyl-cysteinate dimer (ECD) was used, a dose of 110 MBq was given. In all 6 neonates with proved cerebral palsy brain perfusion SPET results revealed some pathological changes. All these patients had perfusion abnormalities at least in one cranio-caudal ratio. Slight or substantial sensorimotoric cortical perfusion abnormalities were detected in five of six CP cases. In neonates with normal SPET results no brain damage related to CP could be found. US or MRI revealed pathological findings suggesting CP in four of six proved CP patients. These preliminary results encourage the selective clinical use of Tc-99m ECD brain perfusion SPET studies in high risk neonates.

Introduction

Functional development of the human brain: Typically, four brain regions visualised by PET are metabolically prominent in new-borns: the primary sensorimotor cortex, the thalamic nuclei, the brain stem and the cerebellar vermis (Chugani and Phelps 1986, Suhonen-Polvi et al. 1992). These structures are phylogenetically relatively old. It is generally accepted that the relatively limited behavioural repertoire of neonates is dominated by subcortical brain structure activity. Visuomotor function is only rudimentary form (Von Hofsten, 1982), and the cortical function is mostly limited to primary sensory and motor areas. The prominent metabolic activity of the sensorimotor cortex is also consistent with its relatively early morphological maturation compared to other cortical areas (Rabinowicz, 1979).

Hypoxic–ischemic encephalopathy: Hypoxic–ischemic brain injury is the single most important perinatal cause of neurological morbidity of both the premature and full term infant and in the premature infant it is usually complicated by intraventricular haemorrhage. Estimates suggest that between two and four out of every full–term new–born infants suffer asphyxiation at or before birth, and this incidence figure approaches 60% in small premature infants (Hill 1991; Mac Donald et al. 1980) The subsequent neurological deficits of concern are, principally, a variety of motor deficits, especially spasticity, but also choreoathetosis and ataxia, often grouped together as "cerebral palsy", with or without accompanying mental impairment, and seizures of both (Volpe 1987).

Cerebral palsy is defined as a group of non–progressive, often changing, motor impairment syndromes secondary to lesions or anomalies of brain arising in the early stages of its development. In high risk neonates it is often difficult to diagnose brain damage and to predict neurological sequelae on the basis of clinical examinations and conventional investigations. Asphyxiated and very low birth weight neonates are at enormous risk to develop cerebral palsy. Aim of this study was **to develop a semiquantitative SPET** method for brain perfusion studies in neonates and **to evaluate the prognostic value** of these perfusion studies in neonates.

Patients and methods

Until now 21 neonates have been studied; 19 of them were preterm (born before 34 gestational weeks) and two asphyxiated new–borns. Imaging studies were carried out between 36 and 44 gestational weeks, at the same time when conventional imagings (ultrasound and magnetic resonance imaging) were performed. To avoid movement artefacts neonates came to imaging room after feeding and during imaging they were wrapped in swaddling clothes on a stretcher in a quiet room. (Figure 1). Imaging was carried out using a single head rotating gamma camera with a slant collimator (Siemens/Orbiter) or a **double head** gamma camera equipped with a fan beam collimator (Adac/Vertex). In a single head 64 frames of 30 sec and in a double head 64 frames of 35 sec were acquired. Transaxial (parallel to the base of the brain), coronal and sagittal slices 2 pixels thick were reconstructed. No attenuation correction was applied.

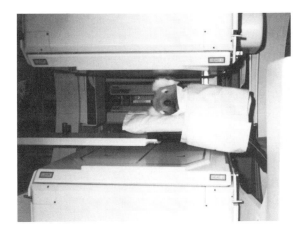

Figure 1. "Baby imaging system"

Visual interpretation: An interpretation was based on visual inspection of asymmetry between hemispheres as well as detection of abnormalities in cranio–caudal direction. Abnormalities were required at least in two consecutive slices. **Semiquantitation:** Right–left hemispheric asymmetries of more than 12% were defined as abnormals by analogy to adults values. (Podreka et al) (8) For assessment of the anterior–posterior abnormalities following cortico–cerebellar and cortico–thalamic rations on the middle sagittal slice were calculated. (Frontal (F), sensorimotor (SM), parietal (P), occipital (O), thalamostriatal (T–S), and brain stem (BS). Figure 2.) Findings were classified as abnormal when at least 2 of the rations were out of the reference values in neonates based on the previous works of Denay et al (10) and Chugan et al (9).

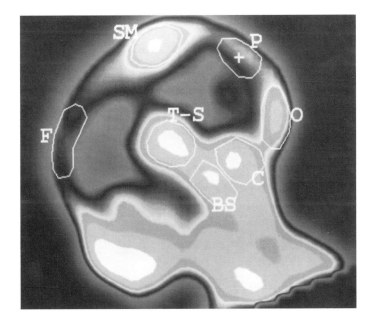

Figure 2. Brain perfusion ROI's on the middle sagittal slice.

Results

Results of visual interpretation and semiquantitative measurements were following: **Cranio–caudal abnormalities** were found in 9 (6 mild, 3 substantial) and hemispheric asymmetry in 12 (9 mild, 3 substantial) out of the **21** neonates. Details are shown in Table 1. In all 6 neonates with proved cerebral palsy brain perfusion SPET results revealed some pathological changes. All these patients had perfusion abnormalities at least in one cranio–caudal ratio. Slight or substantial sensorimotoric cortical perfusion abnormalities were detected in five of six new–borns. In neonates with normal SPET results no brain damage related to CP could be found. Example of normal and abnormal brain perfusion findings in neonates are shown in Figures 3 and 4.

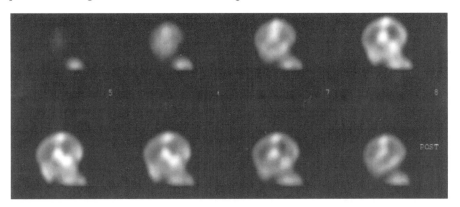

Figure 3. Case 1, a double head gamma camera. Normal brain perfusion in new–born; prominent cortical sensorimotor uptake. Sagittal slices.

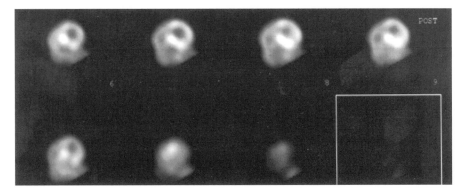

Figure 4. Case 16, a double head gamma camera. Thoroughly abnormal low brain perfusion in new–born. Sensomotor and occipital areas are not prominent. Proved CP. Sagittal slices.

US or MRI performed between 36 and 44 gestational weeks revealed pathological findings suggesting CP in four of six proved CP patients, whereas SPET was abnormal in all six CP cases.

Table 1. Brain perfusion SPET changes in details.

Case (gender)	GW (weeks)	BW (grams)	US (age)	MRI (age)	SPET normals s	SPET normals tr	SPET slight abnormals s	SPET slight abnormals tr	SPET substantial s	SPET substantial tr	Follow-up (motor development at the age when measured last time)
1 M	33	1210	normal (44)	normal (44)	1	1	s	tr	s	tr	normal (8 mos)
2 F	27	890	normal (40)	normal (40)	1	1					normal (1 yr)
3 M	31	1375	normal (42)	normal (42)	1	1	(p)		sm		suspected CP; mild left hemiparesis, physiotherapy (8 mos)
4 F	29	1145	normal (41)	normal (36)	1			(sin p)		dx, f sin sm	normal (1,5 yrs)
5 M	30	1380	normal (38)	suspect trigonal changes (42)	1	1					motor development delay, severe BPD, home oxygen therapy, physiother. (6 mos)
6 F	28	1085	left ICH and right PVL (36)	left parieto–occipital ICH 4,5 cm (37)					t–s, c, o, sm	t–s, p, o, c, t, sin all	CP; tetraplegia dystonica, hydrocephalus shunt, strabismus, physiotherapy (1 yr)
7 M	29	1430	normal (36)	normal (36)	1	1					normal (7 mos)
8 F	29	1150	mild ventricle dilatation (42)	mild ventricle dilatation (37)	1			dx t			normal (1 yr)
9 M	28	1365	mild left ventr. dilatation (39)	mild left ventricle dilatation (39)			o	sin f			CP; diplegia, dystonia musculorum, right predominance (1 yr)
10 M	42	3340	normal (42)	slight occipito–parietal defect (44)			t–s, c	sin t–s			mild hypotonia musculorum; physiotherapy, normal (1yr)
11 F	30	870	normal (44)	normal (44)	1	1					motor development delay, severe BPD, cor pulmonale, hearing defect, oxygen therapy, physiotherapy (10 mos)
12 F	31	1160	normal (38)	normal (38)	1		c, t–s	dx p			CP; right hemiparesis, physiotherapy (1,5 yrs)
13 M	36	3730	cystic lesions (42)	cystic PVL (41)				dx t–s sin p			CP; dystonia tetraplegica, retardation, epilepsia (1 yr)
14 F	26	790	left PIVH lost (40)	left PIVH (40)	1			t–s, p, t, o, p, dx all			mild hypertonia musculorum; physiotherapy, normal (1 yr)
15 M	26	960	PVL (39)	PVL (38)			sm				suspected CP; motor development delay, physiotherapy (10 mos)
16 F	28	1070	left ICH and cysts (38)	left ICH–defect and cysts (40)			sm	sin p			CP; right triplegia spastica strabismus, physiotherapy (1 yr)
17 M	30	1630	normal (38)	normal (37)			sm	sin o, f, dx t–s			mild hypertonia musculorum, physiotherapy (8mos)
18 M	30	1500	SEH l.a. (38)	SEH l.a. (37)			t–s o sm, c	dx t–s			mild hypertonia musculorum, physiotherapy (8mos)
19 M	27	1120	SEH (40)	SEH (40)	1						motor delay
20 M	27	650	mild ventric dilatation (40)	–	1						dystonia
21 M	21	760	normal (38)	SEH (38)		1	sm				CP, diplegia

Discussion and Conclusions

Denays et al (1993) have also studied cerebral palsy in high–risk neonates using Tc–99m HMPAO brain perfusion SPET. However, they could find anterior–posterior perfusion abnormalities only in four out of six neonates with proved CP contrary to our results with another one new perfusion agent Tc–99m ECD. All proved CP cases showed some abnormal brain perfusion changes whereas in five of six cases pathological changes in **sensorimotoric** cortical area could be found. In neonates with normal SPET results no brain damage related to CP (after one year follow–up time) could be found. However, these results should be considered very cautiously because of the small number of neonates. Our experiences are similar with Denays et al concerning the predictive value of normal anterior–posterior perfusion distribution; these neonates had good outcome. However follow–up time for some patients is too short for the reliable diagnosis of CP so that later on we will have more proved CP cases imaged with Tc–99m ECD. These brain perfusion findings in high risk neonates support the idea of the crucial role of the sensomotoric cortex abnormality in the development of CP. These preliminary results encourage the clinical use of Tc–99m ECD brain perfusion SPET studies in high risk neonates.

References
1. Chugani HT, Phelps ME. Maturational changes in cerebral function in infants determined by [18] FDG positron emission tomography. Science 1986;231:840–843.
2. Suhonen-Polvi H, Ruotsalainen U, Kero P, Korvenranta H, Bergman J, Haaparanta M, Simell O, Wegelius U. Functional development of the brain during the first months of life. A [^{18}F]FDG positron emission tomography study. Fetal Diagn Ther 1992;7:37–38.
3. Rabinowicz T: The differentiate maturation of the human cerebral cortex. In: Falkner R, Tanner JM (eds): Human growth, vol.3. Neurobiology and nutrition. New York, Plenum, 1979, pp 97–123.
4. Mac Donald HM, Mulligan JC, Allen AC et al. Neonatal asphyxia: I. Relationship to obstetric and neonatal complications to neonatal mortality in 30,405 consecutive deliveries. J Pediatr 1980;96:989–902.
5. Volpe J Neurology of the newborn. Philadelphia, WB Saunders, 1987.
6. Podreka I, Suess E, Goldenberg G, et al. Initial experience with technetium-99m HM-PAO brain SPECT. J Nucl Med 1987;28:1657–1666.
7. Chugani Harry T, Phelps Michael E, Mazziotta John C. Positron Emission Tomography Study of Human Brain Functional Development.. Ann Neurol 1987;22:487–497.
8. Denays R, Han H, Tondeur M, Piepsz A Noel P. Detection of bilateral and symmetrical anomalies in technetium-99m HMPAO brain SPECT studies. J Nucl Med 1992;33:485–490 (correction: J Nucl Med 1992;33;1282.
9. Denays R, Van Pachterbeke T, Toppet V, Tondeur M, Spehl M ,Piepsz A, Noêl P, Haumont D, Ham HR. Prediction of Cerebral Palsy in High-Risk Neonates: A Technetium-99m–HMPAO SPECT Study. J Nucl Med 1993;34:1223–1227.

Radioactive Isotopes in
Clinical Medicine and Research XXII
ed. by H. Bergmann, A. Kroiss and H. Sinzinger
© 1997 Birkhäuser Verlag Basel/Switzerland

Tc99m-ECD BRAIN SPET IN DIAGNOSIS OF CEREBRAL PERFUSION ABNORMALITIES IN
CHILDREN WITH THERAPY-RESISTANT EPILEPSY

A. Vattimo, L. Burroni, P. Bertelli, D. Volterrani, A. Vella

Department of Nuclear Medicine, University of Siena, Policlinico "Le
Scotte", Siena, Italy.

SUMMMARY: We performed Tc99m-ECD interictal SPET in 26 children with severe
therapy-resistant epilepsy. All children underwent detailed clinical
examination, EEG investigation and brain MRI. In 21/26 children, SPET
demonstrated brain blood flow abnormalities, 13 of them in the same
territories with EEG alterations. MRI showed structural lesions in 6/26
children. These data confirm that brain SPET is considerably sensitive in
detecting and localizing hypoperfused areas that could be associated with
epileptic foci in these patients, even when the MRI pattern is normal.

INTRODUCTION

Since 1965 in Italy epilepsy has been considered a social disease because
of its elevated prevalence and incidence (one per cent of total population
and 25000 new cases every year). Frequently the crisis occurs in childhood
due to perinatal causes such as asphyxia, intracranial hemorrhage , trauma or
genetic diseases and metabolic disorders. Rarely epilepsy is related to
encephalitis, endocranial neoplasm or drug intoxication. Cerebral
malformations are revealed only in 12% of clinical seizures. Unfortunately
the cause of epilepsy cannot be determined in almost the half of patients,
even if in many of them it is possible to classify exactly the kind of
seizure by means of an accurate clinical examination and an EEG performed
during the seizure and during the intervals between seizures. In fact
electrophysiological techniques, such as EEG, stereo-EEG,
electrocorticography and telemetry, are often able to identify the focus of
the seizure, but its accurate localization is required for the case of
surgical treatment. CT or MRI are effective in displaying structural brain
lesions associated with clinical manifestations, but these techniques often

fail to show any brain abnormalities. It has now become necessary to apply functional imaging techniques to the study of cerebral blood flow with SPET and glucose metabolism with PET. The usefulness of studying epilepsy with PET is now well established (1), but its use is limited to the interictal phase; moreover it is an expensive technique, not available in the majority of the medical centres. In previous studies Technetium99m-Hexamethyl-Propylene-Amine-Oxime (Tc99m-HMPAO) SPET imaging was used to evaluate the interictal and postictal periods in adults with intractable epilepsy (2-4). Post-operative evaluations have also been performed (5). Moreover, there exist only a few published studies concerning epilepsy in childhood (4,6). More recently Technetium99m-Ethyl Cysteinate Dimer (Tc99m-ECD) was introduced as a new agent for cerebral blood flow imaging with SPET. Nowadays it is demonstrated that Tc99m-ECD is a marker of regional cerebral perfusion (7) and probably an effective tracer for diagnostic assessment in epilepsy. Moreover, in comparison with Tc99m-HMPAO, Tc99m-ECD has the advantages of long radiochemical stability, rapid wash-out from extracerebral tissues and favourable radiation dosimetry (8,9). The aim of this study was to evaluate the accuracy of Tc99m-ECD SPET in studying the cerebral perfusion abnormalities in a group of children with therapy-resistant epilepsy and to compare the scintigraphic findings with data from neuroradiological techniques, clinical examination and EEG monitoring.

MATERIALS & METHODS

Twenty-six children (14 boys and 12 girls, aged 22 months to 16 years) with therapy-resistant epilepsy and referred for cerebral blood flow evaluation were examined: 8 of them presented Complex Partial Seizure (CPS), 5 Generalized Tonic Clonic Seizure (GTCS), 10 presented both of these conditions (CPS+GTCS), 2 displayed Infantile Spasm (IS), and one showed Simplex Partial Seizure (SPS). Twelve children presented a poor intellectual performance. All children underwent detailed clinical examination, EEG investigation and MRI. At one or two week intervals, brain SPET was performed in the interictal period using Technetium99-ECD (10 MBq/Kg) administered intravenously in a quiet environment. In twenty-one non-cooperative children the acquisition was performed under monitored sedation administered following injection of the tracer. Ninety-six frames (40 seconds/frame in a 64x64 pixel matrix; zoom=1.50) were acquired over 360 degrees with a dual-head rotating camera (Vertex, ADAC Laboratories, U.S.A.) fitted with Low Energy UHR (VXUR) collimators. Data was reconstructed 1 pixel thick using a Butterworth filter (order 10; cutoff 0.45) in the transaxial (O-M line), coronal and sagittal planes and were presented to two blinded observers: the findings were considered to be pathological if one or more areas of hypoperfusion in the regional brain flow were present in more than one view and slice and if the observers were concordant.

RESULTS

The results are summarized in the following table.

Table 1. Positive results in various type of seizures

	SPET	MRI	EEG
SPS	1/1	0/1	1/1
CPS	7/8	0/8	8/8
GTCS	3/5	1/5	5/5
CPS+GTCS	8/10	5/10	9/10
IS	2/2	0/2	2/2
Total	21/26	6/26	25/26
(%)	(80.76)	(23.07)	(96.15)

Out of a total of 26 cases, SPET demonstrated brain blood flow abnormalities in 21 cases (Fig.1), 13 of these displayed a correlation in the results obtained with EEG and SPET for the same areas. MRI illustrated 6 structural lesions while SPET confirmed only 5 of these, since one measured only three millimeters in diameter. In five symptomatic children with normal SPET, in one case EEG was normal; in the others, EEG showed diffuse and non-focal abnormalities. EEG abnormalities were found in all patients with pathological SPET: in 13/21 children the two methods show agreement in both lobe and side abnormalities, in 2/21 there was agreement in the lobe but not in the side, in 2/21 there was agreement in the side but not in the lobe and 4/21 show disagreement in both the lobe and the side. All the hypoperfused areas were evaluated and classified in table 2: the most frequently involved area was the temporal lobe.

Table 2. Anatomical localization of brain blood flow abnormalities revealed with brain SPET

	Right	Left	Total
Frontal lobe	4	2	6
Temporal lobe	8	11	19
Parietal lobe	4	5	9
Occipital lobe	1	1	2
Total	17	19	36

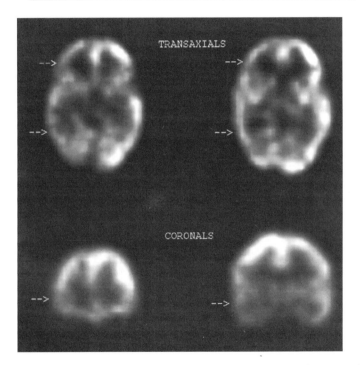

Figure 1. A representative patient with a diffuse right fronto-temporal hypoperfusion.

DISCUSSION

The management of patients with therapy-resistant epilepsy requires an objective and precise localization of the brain damage for an accurate diagnosis and for the appropriate treatment. Because SPET can utilize a conventional camera, this method is much less expensive and more widely available than PET. In accordance with literature (1,4,10), interictal SPET was superior to MRI in detecting brain abnormalities, even if MRI is able to reveal smaller lesions. Sometimes brain blood flow abnormalities were larger than MRI lesions. This phenomenon is probably related to the abnormal metabolism of the neurons around the focus which is decreased by perfusion (11). In accordance with other pubblications (2,4,10), our data confirm that the most frequently involved cerebral lobe is the temporal lobe. SPET and EEG agreed reasonably well. Eight children showed a discrepancy between the site of brain blood flow abnormalities and seizure foci revealed from EEG recordings. These non- concordant cases suggest the presence of multiple lesions or seizure propagation within the brain. The disagreement of the lateralization of SPET and EEG findings revealed in two children may be considered related to false lateralization of surface EEG, as other authors have suggested (10,12). In some cases it would be necessary to perform more sophisticated EEG studies (3). Tc99m-ECD is an effective marker of cerebral perfusion imaging, showing a rapid and high uptake by the brain. The results obtained with Tc99m-ECD may be correlated to those we obtained using Tc99m-HMPAO in our past study (4) to reveal brain blood flow abnormalities in therapy-resistant epilepsy, even if a different group of children was involved. Nevertheless Tc99m-ECD presents a high in vitro stability for up to 8 hours (8) and this is a great advantage in ictal studies. In non-cooperative or very young children it is highly convenient and allows us to work more comfortably, avoiding possible inconveniences such as losing the i.v. line. Moreover Tc99m-ECD is eliminated more rapidly than Tc99m-HMPAO from most tissues and more than 50% of Tc99m activity is excreted in the urine within two hours (8,9). For these reasons, radiation dosimetry is favourable to Tc99m-ECD and the use of this tracer in children is recommended. At last, in accordance with Léveillé et al. (9), Tc99m-ECD SPET images appear "better and easier to interpret" when compared to Tc99m- HMPAO images, probably because of reduced background facial uptake. Tc99m-ECD SPET procedure was considerably sensitive in detecting focal or diffuse brain blood flow abnormalities closely related to EEG alterations, even when the MRI pattern was normal. In non-cooperative children, head movement is the only drawback but in this situation mild sedation can be carried out. It may

be concluded that brain SPET with Tc99m-ECD is helpful in the clinical
assessment of therapy-resistant epilepsy, especially when neuroradiological
techniques are inconclusive.

REFERENCES

1. Ryvlin P, Philippon B, Cinotti L, Froment JC, Le Bars D, Mauguiere F:
    Functional neuroimaging strategy in temporal lobe epilepsy: a comparative
    study of 18FDG-PET and 99mTc-HMPAO-SPECT. Ann Neurol 1992; 31: 650-6.

2. Rowe CC, Berkovic SF, Austin MC, Saling M, Kalnins RM, McKay WJ, Bladin
    PF: Visual and quantitative analisys of interictal SPECT with Technetium-
    99m-HMPAO in temporal epilepsy. J Nucl Med 1991; 32: 1688-94.

3. Ho SS, Berkovic SF, Newton MR, Austin MC, McKay WJ, Bladin PF: Parietal
    lobe epilepsy: clinical features and seizure localization by ictal SPECT.
    Neurology 1994; 44: 2277-84.

4. Vattimo A, Burroni L, Bertelli P, Vella A, Volterrani D: Brain SPECT with
    99mTc-HMPAO in children with therapy-resistant epilepsy. J Nucl Biol Med
    1994; 38: 373-4.

5. Grunwald F, Durwen HF, Bockisch A, Hotze A, Kersjes W, Elger CE, Biersack
    HJ: Technetium-99m-HMPAO brain SPECT in medically intractable temporal
    lobe epilepsy: a post-operative evaluation. J Nucl Med 1991; 32: 388-94.

6. Abdel-Dayem HM, Nawaz MK, Hassoon MM, Abdel-Rahman M, Olofsson OE:
    Cerebral perfusion abnormalities in therapy- resistant epilepsy in
    mentally retarded pediatric patients: comparison between EEG, X-ray CT,
    and Tc-99m HMPAO. Clin Nucl Med 1991; 16: 557-61.
7. Knudsen GM, Andersen AR, Somnier FE, Videbaek C, Hasselbalch S, Paulson
    OB: Brain extraction and distribution of 99mTc- Bicisate in humans and in
    rats. J Cereb Blood Flow Metab 1994; 14 suppl.1: S12-8.

8. Vallbhajosula S, Zimmerman RE, Picard M, Stritze P, Mena I, Hellman RS,
    Tikofsky RS, Stabin MG, Morgan RA, Goldsmith: Technetium-99m ECD: a new
    brain imaging agent: in vivo kinetics and biodistribution studies in
    normal human subjects. J Nucl Med 1989; 30: 599-604.

9. Leveille J, Demonceau G, Walovitch RC: Intrasubject comparison between
    Technetium-99m-ECD and Technetium-99m-HMPAO in healthy human subjects. J
    Nucl Med 1992; 33: 480-4.

10. Heiskala H, Launes J, Pihko H, Nikkinen P, Santavuori P: Brain perfusion
    in children with frequent fits. Brain Dev 1993; 15: 214-8.

11. Mitsuyoshi I, Tamaki K, Okuno T, Mutoh K, Iwasaki Y, Konishi J, Mikawa H:
    Regional cerebral blood flow in diagnosis of childhood onset partial
    epilepsy. Brain Dev 1993; 15: 97-102.

12. Valmier J, Touchon J, Daures P, Zanca M, Baldy-Moulinier M: Correlation
    between cerebral blood flow variations and clinical parameters in
    temoporal lobe epilepsy: an interictal study. J Neurol Neurosurg Psych
    1987; 50: 1306-11.

Immunoscintigraphy; Inflammation

Radioactive Isotopes in
Clinical Medicine and Research XXII
ed. by H. Bergmann, A. Kroiss and H. Sinzinger
© 1997 Birkhäuser Verlag Basel/Switzerland

Striatal Dopamine Transporter in Parkinson's Disease Studied with [123I]β-CIT-FP SPET

J.T. Kuikka[1], J.O. Rinne[2], K.A. Bergström[1], H. Kilpeläinen[3], M. Lehtovirta[1], U.K. Rinne[2]

[1]Kuopio University Hospital, FIN-70210 Kuopio, [2]Turku University Hospital, FIN-20520 Turku, and [3]Savonlinna Central Hospital, FIN-57120 Savonlinna, Finland

SUMMARY: Six healthy controls and 13 patients with Parkinson's disease in different disability stages were studied with high resolution SPET using [123I]β-CIT-FP. The caudatus-to-cerebellum and putamen-to-cerebellum ratios were calculated at 3.5 hours after injection. Patients had the significantly lower ratio than that of the controls in the putamen (3.0 ± 1.0 vs. 4.7 ± 0.4) and in the caudatus (3.5 ± 1.1 vs. 4.9 ± 0.5), respectively. There was a significant negative correlation between the ratio and the Hoehn and Yahr stage in the putamen ($r = -0.74$) and in the caudatus ($r = -0.80$). Reduced striatal uptake demonstrates the loss of presynaptic nerve endings in the striatum of the patients with Parkinson's disease.

INTRODUCTION

Decreased dopamine transporter density in the basal ganglia has been observed in Parkinson's disease (1,2). There are several new cocaine analogs which have potential for imaging the striatal dopamine transporter density in vivo with PET and SPET (3-6). Here we report how the striatal dopamine deficiency in various disability stages of Parkinson's disease could be demonstrated by using SPET with [123I]-N-(3-fluoropropyl)-2β-carbomethoxy-3β-(4-iodophenyl)nortropane ([123I]β-CIT-FP) which is a fluoroalkyl derivative of β-CIT.

PATIENTS AND METHODS

Thirteen, right-handed patients with idiopathic Parkinson's disease were studied. Their mean age was 61 years (range: 43-82 years). The patients had various disability stages from recent-onset to advantage stage of Parkinson's disease. Five of the patients were de novo, and had received no antiparkinsonian medication whereas the rest of the patients were receiving levodopa (peripheral dopadecarboxylase inhibitor) with or without dopamine antagonist.

Six healthy volunteers with mean age of 52 years (range: 37-63 years) were also studied as controls. They were right-handed and they did not have any neurological diseases and were not on regular medication.

The precursor for labelling $[^{123}I]\beta$-CIT-FP was obtained from MAP Medical Technologies, Inc. (Tikkakoski, Finland). The labelling was performed as previously described (5). A dose of 150-210 MBq of $[^{123}I]\beta$-CIT-FP was diluted in a volume of 10 ml. The dose was slowly injected into the right antecubital vein in a dark and quiet room. High resolution SPET imaging was performed 3.5 hours after injection of tracer using a Siemens MultiSPECT 3 gamma camera with fan beam collimators (Siemens Medical Systems, Inc., Hoffman Estates, Illinois). The energy window was centered around the photopeak of ^{123}I (148-170 keV). A full 360° rotation was performed (40 views/camera head, each 40 s) and the total scanning time was 27 minutes. The imaging resolution was 7-8 mm.

Transaxial slices oriented in the orbitomeatal line, sagittal and coronal slices, all 3 mm thick, were reconstructed after Butterworth filtering (order of 8 and a cut-off frequency of 0.65 cm^{-1}). Figure 1 shows a typical set of slices. Two consecutive slices were summarized (total slice thickness of 6 mm), and three regions of interest for each hemisphere were semi-automatically selected from the putamen, from the head of the caudate nucleus and from the cerebellum using a brain quantification program of Siemens (ICON vol. 5.0, Siemens Medical Systems, Inc.). The average count densities were used in calculations. The putamen-to-cerebellum and the caudatus-to-cerebellum ratios were calculated for each hemisphere.

Six of the patients were previously scanned with $[^{123}I]\beta$-CIT using the same camera and computer settings as given above. These images were taken 4-8 hours after injection of tracer.

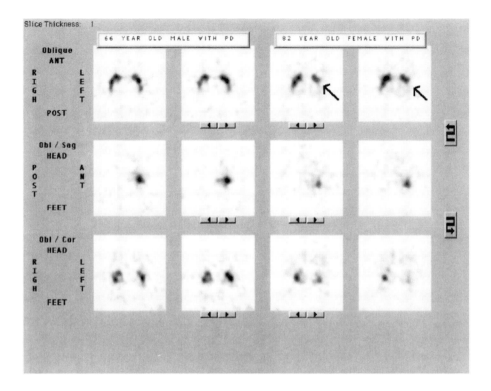

Figure 1. Transaxial (top), sagittal (middle) and coronal slices (bottom) of $[^{123}I]\beta$-CIT-FP scan in 2 patients with Parkinson's disease at very early stage. They both had symptoms on the right side. Note a completely normal finding of the patient on the left side whereas the patient on the right reveals a reduced uptake of $[^{123}I]\beta$-CIT-FP in her left putamen.

RESULTS

The mean region-to-cerebellum ratios of in the $[^{123}I]\beta$-CIT-FP are presented in Table 1. In patients with Parkinson's disease, the putaminal uptake was reduced to 60 % of the mean control value ($p < 0.001$). In the head of the caudate nucleus the decrease was on the average to 80 % of the control mean, but this difference was not statistically significant ($p > 0.05$).

Table 1.   Mean values and standard deviations of the striatal region-to-cerebellum ratios of
[^{123}I]β-CIT-FP in 6 controls and in 13 patients with Parkinson's disease.

Region of	Control	Patient	
Interest	(mean of left and right)	affected side	contralateral ' (Opposite to the symptoms)
Caudatus	4.9 ± 0.5	4.2 ± 1.2	3.9 ± 1.1
Putamen	4.7 ± 0.4	3.2 ± 1.0	2.7 ± 0.9

There was a significant negative correlation between the parkinsonian disability assessed
by Hoehn and Yahr scale (7) and the striatal uptake of [^{123}I]β-CIT-FP both in the putamen (r =
- 0.74) and in the head of the caudate nucleus (r = - 0.80).

Six of the patients had also previously scanned with [^{123}I]β-CIT (8). The striatal region-
to-cerebellum ratios were estimated at 7 hours after injection of tracer. In those cases the
average decline in the putamen was to 54 % of the control mean for [^{123}I]β-CIT, and to 45 %
for [^{123}I]β-CIT-FP. The corresponding figures for the head of the caudate nucleus were 61 %
and 66 %, respectively.

DISCUSSION

Our results demonstrate that [^{123}I]β-CIT-FP might be a useful ligand to visualize presynaptic
dopaminergic hypofunction in Parkinson's disease. The patients had more reduced uptake in
the putamen than in the caudate. These reductions were greater in advanced Parkinson's
disease than in early stage as shown by the negative correlation between the striatal region-to-
cerebellum ratio and the Hoehn and Yahr scale. Similar correlations have also been seen in
[^{18}F]fluorodopa PET (9) and in [^{123}I]β-CIT SPET (8,10). Reduced uptake of [^{123}I]β-CIT-FP

demonstrates the loss of presynaptic nerve endings in the striatum of the patients with Parkinson's disease.

One potential benefit of $[^{123}I]\beta$-CIT-FP is its much faster uptake (peak: 3-4 hours after injection) as compared with $[^{123}I]\beta$-CIT, which allows to use of a one-day imaging protocol. In addition, the radiation burden to the patient is lower and especially to the basal ganglia than that of $[^{123}I]\beta$-CIT. However, the findings of $[^{123}I]\beta$-CIT-FP are not as clear as using $[^{123}I]\beta$-CIT SPET. Sometimes, we had completely normal finding (see Fig. 1) although the patient had classified to suffer typical parkinsonian symptoms. Up to now we have had no atypical finding with $[^{123}I]\beta$-CIT. The best choice of these tracers for routine clinical SPET imaging is unquestionably $[^{123}I]\beta$-CIT as it has the highest target-to-background ratio.

$[^{123}I]\beta$-CIT-FP might be a useful ligand to demonstrate the presynaptic dopaminergic dysfunction in patients with Parkinson's disease. However, we need further studies with larger patient population in order to conclude its usefulness in clinical routine.

REFERENCES

1.   Kaufman MJ, Madras BK. Severe depletion of cocaine recognition sites associated with the dopamine transporter in Parkinson's diseased striatum. Synapse 1991; 9: 43-49.

2.   Brücke T, Kornhuber J, Angelberger P, et al. SPECT imaging of dopamine and serotonin transporters with $[^{123}I]\beta$-CIT. Binding kinetics in the human brain. J Neural Transm [Gen Sect] 1993; 94: 137-146.

3.   Rinne JO, Laihinen A, Någren K, et al. PET examination of the monoamine transporter with $[^{11}C]\beta$-CIT and $[^{11}C]\beta$-CFT in early Parkinson's disease. Synapse 1995; 21: 97-103.

4.   Kuikka JT, Tiihonen J, Bergström KA, et al. Imaging of serotonin and dopamine transporters in the living human brain. Eur J Nucl Med 1995; 22: 346-350.

5.   Kuikka JT, Bergström KA, Ahonen A, et al. Comparison of iodine-123 labelled 2β-carbomethoxy-3β-(4-iodophenyl)tropane   and   2β-carbomethoxy-3β-(4-iodophenyl)-N-(3-fluoropropyl)nortropane for imaging of the dopamine transporter in the living human brain. Eur J Nucl Med 1995; 22: 356-360.

6.   Kuikka JT, Åkerman K, Bergström KA, et al. Iodine-123 labelled N-(2-fluoroethyl)-2β-carbomethoxy-3β-(4-iodophenyl)nortropane for dopamine transporter imaging in the living human brain. Eur J Nucl Med 1995; 22: 682-686.

7.   Hoehn MD, Yahr MM. Parkinsonism: onset, progression and mortality. Neurology 1967; 17: 427-442.

8.   Rinne JO, Kuikka JT, Bergström KA, Rinne UK. Striatal dopamine transporter in different disability stages of Parkinson's disease studied with [^{123}I]β-CIT SPECT. Parkinsonism and Related Disorders 1995; 1: 47-52.

9.   Leenders KL, Palmer AJ, Quinn N, et al. Brain dopamine metabolism in patients with Parkinson's disease measured with positron emission tomography. J Neurol Neurosurg Psychiat 1986; 49: 853-860.

10.   Seibyl JP, Marek KL, Quinlan D, et al. Decreased single-photon emission computed tomographic [^{123}I]β-CIT striatal uptake correlates with symptom severity in Parkinson's disease. Ann Neurol 1995; 38: 589-598.

Radioactive Isotopes in
Clinical Medicine and Research XXII
ed. by H. Bergmann, A. Kroiss and H. Sinzinger
© 1997 Birkhäuser Verlag Basel/Switzerland

PATTERNS OF DIFFERENT BRAIN SPECT STUDIES IN PATIENTS WITH EXTRAPYRAMIDAL MOTOR SYMPTOMS (EPMS) AND THEIR POTENTIAL IMPACT ON CLINICAL MANAGEMENT

E. Donnemiller, J. Heilmann, G.N. Ransmayr°, R. Moncayo, G. Riccabona
Departments of Nuclear Medicine and Neurology°, University of Innsbruck, Austria

INDRODUCTION

Years ago already, when „Biochemistry of the brain" became visible by PET, the importance of receptors and transmitters for pathophysiology of EPMS became obvious (1). At the same time methods were developed to study regional cerebral blood flow (rCBF) by SPECT and PET (4,5), providing a possibility to correlate rCBF with data on basal ganglia (BG) dopamine metabolism. In recent years a variety of radiotracers has become available, which allow also transmitter and receptor studies with SPECT (10). The purpose of our study was to correlate BG perfusion based on SPECT obtained with 99mTc-HMPAO (perfusion marker) with those of 123 I-ß-CIT (presynaptic dopamine transporter marker) in patients belonging to different diseases with EPMS aiming also to clarify the pathophysiological mechanism of various brain disorders considering also possible consequenses for therapeutic decisions, e.g. L-dopa-therapy. This seemed important, as EPMS are frequent neurological problems which can only partially be attributed to classical Idiopathic Parkinson's Disease (IPD) (7). EPMS can also observed in many other brain disorders (6). Rigidity and/or dyskinesia, tremor, gait abnormalities are also observed in patients with Multiple System Atrophy (MSA), Alzheimer's Disease (DAT) and - of course - Huntington's Chorea (HC). Several reports also assume that a dysfunction of the dopaminergic system may be involved in the pathogenesis of the Periodic Movements of Sleep - Syndrome (PMS) and of the Sleep Apnea Syndrome (SAS) (8,9).

MATERIAL AND METHODS

We investigated 39 patients aged from 39-81 years (25 male,14 female), 6 patients with MSA (aged 63-73 years), 2 patients with HC (43 and 56 years), 7 patients with DAT (56-81 years), 10 patients with IPD (60-75 years), 4 patients with SAS (57-63 years) and 10 patients with PMS (39-74 years). Clinical classifications of the different diseases were based on neurological examination, CCT and/or MRI, EEG, EMG and polysomnography. In addition to the patients studies, 123I-ß-CIT SPECT reference studies were performed. A data set was obtained from 4 normal volunteers, 2 women and 2 men, aged 26-63; the younger ones were denominated group N1 (26 and 30 years) and the older patients, N2 (62 and 63 years) (Tab.1). All normal controls had an unevenful neurological examination.

We investigated rCBF with ^{99m}Tc-HMPAO SPECT and the dopamine reuptake with ^{123}I-ß-CIT SPECT in all patients. Thyroid uptake of iodine was blocked by administering 500 mg sodium perchlorate p.o. 30 minutes before tracer application. ^{99m}Tc-HMPAO was prepared from a non-radioactive kit according to the instructions of the manufacturers (Ceretec, Med-Pro, Amersham); 15 mCi (555 MBq) of 99mTc-HMPAO was injected i.v. into the patient within 15 min after preparation. The cocaine analog 2ß-carboxymethoxy-3ß-[4-iodophenyl]-tropane (ß-CIT) labeled with ^{123}I was obtained from the Österreichisches Forschungszentrum Seibersdorf (Austria). ^{123}I-ß-CIT, allows to investigate the presynaptic dopamine reuptake on dopamine transporters in the BG. A dose of 5 mCi (185 MBq) of ^{123}I-ß-CIT was injected i.v. ^{99m}Tc-HMPAO was administered i.v.. The patient had his eyes covered. Acoustic stimuli were avoided during application. Data aquisition was started 15 min after tracer application. Patients were placed in a supine position with covered eyes, their head fixed in a appropiate head holder. ^{123}I ß-CIT SPECT studies were performed 3 and 18 hrs after tracer application. The SPECT studies were done with a single head rotating Anger camera (Siemens Orbiter Digitrac ZLC 3700) equipped with a LEAP-collimator. The spatial resolution in z-direction (patient axis) was 18 mm FWH, given a rotation radius of the camera head of 20 cm. Raw data were aquired in 64 projections over an angle of 360°, equivalent to an angular sampling interval of less than 6°. An acquisition matrix of 64 x 64 was used, which results in a pixel size of 6,25 x 6,25 mm. For qualitative reporting the data were processed on a Siemens MicroDelta workstation connected to a MicroVax 3600 (MaxDelta configuration).

Transverse slices were reconstructed by backprojection using a Butterworth filter. Attenuation correction was done for ^{99m}Tc studies using the implemented Sörenson algorithm and the suggested linear attenuation coefficient for brain studies of $\mu = 0,11 cm^{-1}$. For semiquantitative analysis the projection data were transferred to a NUD Hermes workstation (processing software by Nuclear Diagnostics, U.K., running on a SUN Sparc 10/40). Data were reconstructed by back projection using a Wiener filter for ^{99m}Tc studies and a Metz filter for ^{123}I studies. Attenuation correction for ^{123}I was performed using the implemented method of Chang.

For semiquantitave analysis the program MultiModality from NUD was used. Irregular regions of interest (ROIs) were manually drawn arround the left and right BG and arround the cerebellum, which served as reference area for perfusion SPECT and the ^{123}I ß-CIT SPECT, as a nonspecific binding area for this tracer, in each of 4 reoriented transaxial slices. The ^{123}I ß-CIT stiatum/cerebellum (S/C) ratio was calculated from the mean count rates obtained in the BG and in the cerebellum. The calculation of the ^{123}J ß-CIT S/C count ratio was done on images obtained 3 hrs and 18 hrs after injection of the tracer. The difference between the 18 hrs-ratio and the 3 hrs-ratio represents the specific binding to the dopamine transporter in correlation to the transporter density in the BG (delta value).

RESULTS

Slice images were inspected visually for general pattern and for image quality. The results from semiquantitative analysis from patients and normal controls are shown in table 1. The mean delta value was lower in elderly than in young controls showing an age related decline in the striatal dopamine transporter binding (11) (Tab. 1).

123-I-ß-CIT SPECT	MSA n=6	HC n=2	DAT n=7	IPD n=10	SAS n=4	PMS n=10	N1 n=2	N2 n=2
S/C ratio 3hrs	1,33	1,44	1,39	1,74	1,88	2,02	2,99	2,43
S/C ratio 18hrs	1,65	2,21	2,49	3,43	3,75	5,25	7,88	6,86
delta S/C 18-3 hrs	0,32	0,81	1,09	1,67	1,87	3,22	4,89	4,43
99m-Tc-HMPAO SPECT	MSA n=6	HC n=2	DAT n=7	IPD n=10	SAS n=4	PMS n=10	normal	
S/C ratio	0,89	0,75	0,86	0,87	0,85	0,87	0,86-0,96	

Table 1: Results of the 123I-ß-CIT SPECT studies with S/C ratios after 3 hrs, 18 hrs and the difference between 18 hrs - 3 hrs ratios (delta) and the results of 99mTcHMPAO-SPECT studies.

Figure 1 shows representative cases of studies in patients with HC, IPD and MSA, including the semiquantitative values. The lowest delta values were found in MSA, whereas HC, DAT, IPD and SAS showed higher delta values. Slightly decreased delta values were observed in PMS. Striatal perfusion was reduced specially in HC. Normal striatal perfusion was found in PMS and MSA.

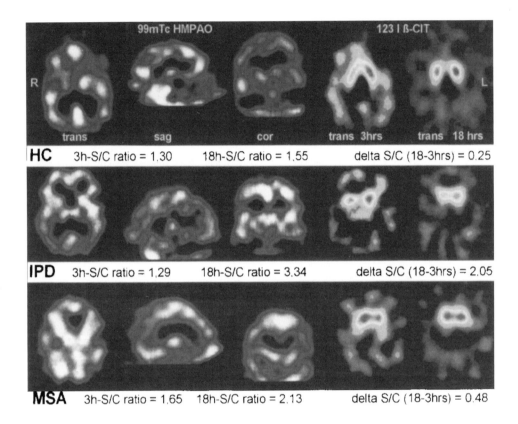

Figure 1: 99mTc-HMPAO SPECT and 123I ß-CIT SPECT in patients with HC, IPD and MSA.

DISCUSSION

Striatal uptake of ^{123}I-ß-CIT in healthy subjects peaks after about 8 hrs, whereas in patients with dopamine transporter abnormalities uptake peaks earlier. Uptake appears to be limited by its delivery to target sites in the striatum and shows slow accumulation for up to 8-15hrs in healthy subjects. After reaching the peak values, striatal activity is stable in both patients and healthy subjects (12). This study demonstrated a disturbance of the dopamine transporter system. in patients with EPMS, sometimes combined with striatal and other cortical perfusion defects belonging to different diseases in comparison to normal control subjects. In patients with PMS homogeneous symmetrical striatal uptake of 123 I ß-CIT and normal striatal perfusion was observed by visually inspection, but there was a lesser increase of striatal activity of 123 I ß-CIT from 3 to 18 hrs compared with the increase of uptake obtained in healthy controls. The normal findings by visual inspection of striatal perfusion could be confirmed by semiquantitave analysis. In patients with IPD there was marked reduction of bilateral 123 I ß-CIT uptake already at the initial investigation. Inhomogeneity in distribution of the tracer, persisting until 18 hrs, was associated only to a small increase of striatal accumulation of 123 I-ß-CIT. The striatum seems to be much more severely affected in longstanding IDP, than in PMS (2). In patients with IPD we also found a reduced perfusion in the BG and in other cortical areas, probably also related to disease duration (3). In patients with SAS there was initially low striatal uptake of 123 I ß-CIT with inhomogeneous distribution of the tracer. On images 18 hrs after tracerapplication only a moderate increase of striatal uptake became visible, and a reduction for delta value could be measured (average value for delta in this group was 1,87). Striatal perfusion seemed to be normal (9).

In HC most severe hypoperfusion in the BG bilaterally was found (with a characteristic "pear-shaped" pattern of the ventricles in the axial view) (3), combined with other cortical perfusion deficits and with coexisting striatal dopamine transporter defects with very low delta values. In MSA we found normal striatal perfusion, perfusion defects in the left temporoparietal and occipitoparietal regions, but with a severely reduced striatal uptake of 123 I ß-CIT bilaterally or unilateral. In the patients with DAT there was slight reduced striatal perfusion (disease duration related) and markely decreased perfusion frontobasal, temporoparietal and occipitoparietal perfusion bilaterally (3). The striatal uptake of 123I ß-CIT was inhomogeneous and reduced already initially with only a small increase of striatal activity at 18 hrs.

In conclusion an impaired dopamine re-uptake seems therefore be combined with inadequate striatal perfusion in HC. This appears also to occur in DAT, SAS, and IPD, whereby disease duration of IPD seems to be a determining factor. Perfusion is normal in MSA and PMS, while dopamine transporter kinetics are altered.

REFERENCES

1. Laihinen A.O. et al, PET-Studies on the presynaptik Dopamine reuptake mechanism using (11C)ß-CIT in human brain, VIII. Böttstein Colloquium, Workshop of COST-B3-Action on „New Radiotracers and Methods of Quality Assurance for Nuclear Medicine Application", Abstracts, Oktober 6/7, Paul Scherrer Institute,1994

2. Vermeulen et al, Evaluation of 123-J-ß-CIT binding with SPECT in controls, early and late Parkinson's disease, VIII. Böttstein Colloquium, Workshop of COST-B3-Action on „New Radiotracers and Methods of Quality Assurance for Nuclear Medicine Application", Abstracts, Oktober 6/7, Paul Scherrer Institute,1994

3. Costa D.C., Ell P.J., Brain Blood Flow in Neurology and Psychiatry, Clinician's Guide to Nuclear Medicine, Churchill Livingstone, London 1991

4. Nakamura K. et al. The behavior of ^{99m}Tc hexamethylpropyleneamineoxime (99-Tc-HMPAO) in blood and brain., Eur J Nucl Med,1989,15,100-7

5. Costa D.C.,Ell P.J., Cullum I.D., Jarritt P.H., The in vivo distribution of 99-m-Tc HMPAO in normal man, Nucl Med Comm, 1986, 7, 647-58

6. Seeman P. et al, Human D1 and D2 Dopamine receptors in Schizophrenia, Alzheimer's, Parkinson's and Huntington's diseases, Neuro Psycho Pharmacol, 1987,1, 5-15

7. Poewe W. et al, Klinische Subtypen der Parkinson-Krankheit, Wiener Medizinische Wochenschrift, 1986,15, 384-87

8. Akpinar S., Restless legs syndrome treatment with dopaminergic drugs, Clin Neuro-pharmacol, 1987, 10, 69-79

9. Feistl H. et al, Schlafapnoe und Tc-99m-HMPAO SPECT, Nucl Med, 1994,33,49-56

10. Kuikka JT et al, Initial experience with SPET examinations using [^{123}I]-2ß-carbomethoxy-3ß(4-iodophenyl) tropane in human brain. Eur J Nucl Med 1993;20:783-786

11. Christopher H. van Dyck et al.: Age-related decline in striatal Dopamine transporter binding with Iodine-123-ß-CIT SPECT. J Nucl Med 1995;36:1175-1181

12. Innis et al, SPECT imaging demonstrates loss of striatal dopamine transporters in Parkinson's disease. Proc Natl Acad Sci USA 1993;90:11965-11969

Radioactive Isotopes in
Clinical Medicine and Research XXII
ed. by H. Bergmann, A. Kroiss and H. Sinzinger
© 1997 Birkhäuser Verlag Basel/Switzerland

IMPACT OF SOMATOSTATIN RECEPTOR SCINTIGRAPHY IN PATIENTS WITH SUSPECTED MENINGEOMA

K.H. Bohuslavizki, W. Brenner, A. Behnke, N. Jahn, H.-H. Hugo, C. Sippel, H. Wolf,
S. Tinnemeyer, M. Clausen, H.M. Mehdorn and E. Henze

Clinics of Nuclear Medicine and Neurosurgery, Christian-Albrechts-Universitiy,
Arnold-Heller-Str. 9, 24105 Kiel, Germany

SUMMARY: To evaluate the usefulness of somatostatin receptor scintigraphy (SRS) in patients with suspected meningeoma, 58 patients were investigated prior to surgery receiving standard MRI and SRS following i.v. injection of 200 MBq In-111-octreotide. SRS was true positive in 44/58, true negative in 5 neurinoma, and false negative in 9 patients. In the latter tumor volume was < 10 ml. MRI was decisive for meningeoma in 39/58 patients. In 14/58 patients MRI could not differentiate between meningeoma and neurinoma. Of these, positive SRS confirmed meningeoma in 9 patients, and negative SRS excluded meningeoma in the remaining 5. In conclusion, SRS has significant clinical impact in patients with suspected meningeoma following MRI.

INTRODUCTION

Somatostatin receptors have been described in meningeoma both *in vivo* by scintigraphy (1-3) and *in vitro* in cell culture studies (4-6). This does not hold true for neurinoma (1, 7). Therefore, somatostatin receptor scintigraphy (SRS) was suggested by various authors for differential diagnosis neurinoma versus meningeoma (1). However, we observed negative scintigrams in some patients with histologically proven meningeoma. In consequence, the exclusion of meningeoma by a lack of tracer uptake seems questionable. Therefore, the aim of this study was to reassess the clinical impact of SRS in patients with suspected meningeoma.

MATERIALS AND METHODS

In this study 58 patients were included in whom meningeoma was either proven or suspected by MRI. 17 were male, 41 were female. Their median age was 57 yrs, ranging from 28 to 81 yrs. All patients underwent surgery and subsequent histological evaluation. Results of both MRI and SRS were compared to histology.

Surgical specimen were fixed in 4 % formaldehyde and embedded in paraffin for histopatho-logical examination. Sections of 4 μm thickness were stained both with Hematoxylin-Eosin and Elastica van Gieson.

MRI was performed on a 1.5 T machine acquiring both T1- (TR=500 ms, TE=12 ms) and T2-weighted (TR=3600 ms, TE=98 ms) spin-echo sequences with a slice thickness of 6-8 mm. Gadolinium was administered for contrast enhancement in a quantity of 0.2 mg/kg body weight. Tumor volumes were calculated from MRI images under assumption of a rotational ellipsoid, and ranged from 0.3 to 112.8 ml.

After an intravenous injection of 200 MBq In-111-octreotide digital whole-body acquisitions in anterior and posterior projection were obtained at 10 min, 1, 4, and 24 hrs. Single photon emis-sion computed tomography was performed at 4 and 24 hrs. Regional uptake was quantified by ROI-technique. Relative percental tumor uptake was calculated after correction for background ac-tivity as geometric mean of anterior and posterior projections. Results are given as mean ± one standard deviation.

With respect to histological diagnosis patients were divided in true positive (SRS positive when histology revealed menigeoma), true negative (SRS negative when histology revealed ab-sence of menigeoma), and false negative (SRS negative when histology revealed meningeoma).

RESULTS

Evaluation of SRS with respect to histology, tumor volume and location did not yield any cor-relation between detailed histological analysis, scintigraphic results and anatomical location. Therefore, pooled data are given only.

In 16 patients with a tumor volume of < 10 ml and in 28 patients with a tumor volume of >10 ml true positive somatostatin receptor scintigrams could be shown in planar images resulting in an increasing T/B-ratio over time. This is illustrated in Figure 1 (filled squares) and table 1. In 9 out of 44 patients significant information could be added by positive somatostatin receptor imaging when compared to MRI.

A lack of somatostatin receptors could be demonstrated correctly negative in 5 patients. The corresponding lack of an increase of T/B ratio and uptake is shown in Figure 1 (filled circles) and table 1, respectively. Tumor volume was > 10 ml in all patients. Significant clinical information could be added by SRS in all 5 of them when compared to MRI. In all of them MRI showed tu-mors with criteria of both neurinoma and meningeoma, thus, MRI was not decisive. However, SRS clearly demonstrated a lack of somatostatin receptors. Histological examination confirmed presence of 5 neurinoma.

In 9 patients with histological proven meningeoma SRS yielded false negative results. Consequently, T/B ratio and uptake values did not increase with time as shown in Figure 1 (open circles) and table 1, respectively. While there was neither correlation with location nor with histological type of the meningeoma tumor volume was < 10 ml in all patients as shown in Figure 2.

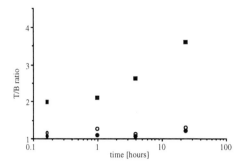
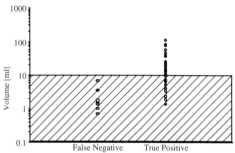

Fig 1: Tumor-to-background ratio of SRS in 58 patients with suspected meningeoma versus logarithm of time post injection in hrs. Filled squares: 44 true positive; open circles: 9 false negative; filled circles: 5 true negative. For standard deviation see table 1.

Fig 2: Tumor volume of patients with false negative and true positive somatostatin receptor scintigraphy. Observe, all patients with false negative somatostatin receptor scintigraphy have tumor volumes of < 10 ml (shaded area).

Table 1. Tumor-to-background ratio of somatostatin receptor scintigraphy with respect to histology at different time post injection of In-111-octreotide. Data represent mean ± standard deviation.

	T/B ratio ( )		
time p.i.	True positive n=44	False negative n=9	True negative n=5
10 min	1.96 ± 0.81	1.13 ± 0.44	1.05 ± 0.10
1 hr	2.14 ± 0.62	1.23 ± 0.41	1.09 ± 0.11
4 hrs	2.61 ± 0.83	1.17 ± 0.52	1.07 ± 0.05
24 hrs	3.68 ± 1.99	1.25 ± 0.33	1.18 ± 0.17

DISCUSSION

While meningeoma and neurinoma are tumors which have similar predelection sites surgical treatment may require different strategies due to their differing biological behaviour. Therefore, preoperative discrimination is mandatory for the neurosurgeon. Usually, meningeoma and neurinoma can be discriminated sucessfully by MRI (8), but not in all patients. MRI could prove meningeoma in 39 of our 58 patients. However, in 14 patients MRI alone could only limit differential diagnosis to meningeoma versus neurinoma.

Somatostatin receptors are expressed in nearly 100 % both in cell cultures of meningeoma independent of tumor size (5, 6). Consequently, uptake of In-111-octreotide could be shown by scintigraphy in all meningeoma reported (1-3, 8). On the other hand, it is known from autoradiographic studies (4, 7) that neurinoma do not express somatostatin receptors on their surface. Consequently, our five neurinoma exhibited true negative somatostatin receptor scintigrams in consistance with the literature (1, 8). Functional imaging using In-111-octreotide was suggested to clearly discriminate meningeoma and neurinoma (1). This was shown successfully in 4 patients suffering from both multiple meningeoma and neurinoma on the basis of neurofibromatosis (1).

In conflict with the literature (1, 3-5) we found false negative SRS in 9 patients with histologically proven meningeoma. Neither histological type nor localization of the meningeoma correlated with their negative tracer uptake. Therefore, exclusion of meningeoma by a negative somatostatin receptor scintigram is not longer permitted. However, in a larger series of patients varying expression of somatostatin receptors should be tested for any differences in biological behaviour.

In contrast to histology and localization, tumor volume was associated with tracer uptake. While all large meningeoma could be imaged positively, SRS was positive in small meningeoma in 65 % only (Figure 2). The critical tumor size is given with either 10 ml volume or 2.7 cm diameter. Thus, the known sensitivity of near 100 % (1-3, 8) needs to be qualified with respect to tumor size. Our data are consistant with the literature (1, 3-5) for large meningeoma only.

As this paper reports on somatostatin receptor free meningeoma in vivo technical reasons for negative SRS had to be excluded. First, whole body images performed in our SRS negative patients showed typical normal distribution of In-111-octreotide. Second, our study group included a patient with both simultaneous exhibition of SRS positive and negative meningeoma. Thus, the SRS positive meningeoma proves normal and exspected tracer behaiviour and thereby validated the SRS negative meningeoma within the same patient. Third, a relationship between the detection of uptake and size might be expected from physical principles but probably not with such a large threshold. Even a relatively poor SPECT system should be able to detect tumors much smaller than 2.7 cm in diameter. However, our smallest SRS positive meningeoma was 0.5 cm in diameter corresponding to a volume of about 1 ml. Thus, reasons of radiopharmacy or image acquisition can be excluded for our SRS negative meningeoma.

In the light of these findings the clinical benefit of SRS in preoperative work-up of patients with suspected meningeoma has to be re-defined carefully. MRI is mandatory during clinical work-up. In most tumors final diagnosis can be established by MRI alone. However, in some cases MRI is not decisive and yields two possible differential diagnoses. When these two tumors under consideration have different expression of somatostatin receptors they can be discriminated by functional imaging using SRS. In our study this holds for 9/47 patients. In five out of these nine patients SRS could correctly diagnose meningeoma. In 4 patients with large tumors a lack of somatostatin receptors enabled to exclude meningeoma. Histologically neurinoma were found which fail to express somatostatin receptors on their surface (4-8).

In our study all patients who benefitted from SRS had large tumors. With the preselection by MRI as mentioned above positive SRS will confirm meningeoma independent of tumor size. With small tumors negative SRS will carry no clinically usefull information. Thus, patients with small meningeoma benefitted from positive SRS only.

In this study the usefullness of SRS in the differential diagnosis of meningeoma versus neurinoma is documented. It remains to be established whether SRS helps in the differentiation of meningeoma versus other disease entities located in the skull base, e.g. chordoma, ependymoma, ganglion Gasseri tumors, and scar tissue. This may be examplified in a single patient observation in which MRI could not discriminate between recurrent meningeoma and scar tissue. However, positive SRS correctly identified tumor recurrency and, thus, assisted in clinical decision-making.

CONCLUSIONS

Functional imaging by somatostation receptor scintigraphy has significant impact in differential diagnosis of patients with suspected meningeoma. Large meningeoma can be excluded by scintigraphy alone, while meningeoma of any size may be confirmed in combination with specific MRI results only.

ACKNOWLEDGMENT

We thank C. Bahr, A. Bauer, R. Bradtke, C. Fock, I. Hamann, D. Hundt, W. Latendorf, G. Mester, K. Nielsen, S. Ossowski, M. Reymann and E. Schmidt for perfect technical assistance.

REFERENCES

1.   Maini CL, Cioffi RP, Tofani A, Sciuto R, Fontana M, Carapella CM, Crecco M. In-111-octreotide scintigraphy in neurofibromatosis. Eur J Nucl Med 1995; **22**: 201–206.

2. Hildebrandt G, Scheidhauer K, Luyken C, Schicha H, Klug N, Dahms P, Krisch B. High sensitivity of the in vivo detection of somatostatin receptors by ^{111}Indium-(DTPA-octreotide)-scintigraphy in meningeoma patients. Acta Neurochir Wien 1994; **126**: 63–71.

3. Maini CL, Tofani A, Sciuto R, Carapella C, Cioffi R, Crecco M. Scintigraphy visualization of somatostatin receptors in human meningiomas using 111-indium-DTPA-D-Phe-1-octreotide. Nucl Med Commun 1993; **14**: 505–508.

4. Reubi JC, Maurer R, Klijn JGM, Stefanko SZ, Foekens JA, Blaauw G, Blankenstein MA, Lamberts SWJ. High incidence of somatostatin receptors in human meningiomas: biochemical characterization. J Clin Endocrinol Metab 1986; **63**: 433–438.

5. Reubi JC, Kvols L, Krenning EP, Lamberts SWJ. In vitro and in vivo detection of somatostatin receptors in human malignant tissue. Acta Ocol 1991; **30**: 463–468.

6. Reubi JC, Laissue J, Krenning EP, Lamberts SWJ. Somatostatin receptors in human cancer: incidence, characteristics, functional correlates and clinical implications. J Steroid Biochim Molec Biol 1992; **43**: 27–35.

7. Reubi JC, Lang W, Maurer R, Koper JW, Lamberts SWJ. Distribution and biochemical characterization of somatostatin receptors in tumors of the human central nervous system. Cancer Res 1987; **47**: 5758–5764.

8. McConachie NS, Worthington BS, Cornford EJ, Balsitis M, Kerslake RW, Jaspan T. Review article: Computed tomography and magnetic resonance in the diagnosis of intraventricular cerebral masses. Br J Rad 1994; **67**: 223–243.

9. Haldemann AR, Rösler H, Barth A, Waser B, Geiger L, Godoy N, Markwalder RV, Seiler RW, Sulzer M, Reubi JC. Somatostatin receptor scintigraphy in central nervous system tumors: role of blood-brain barrier permeability. J Nucl Med 1995; **36**: 403–410.

Radioactive Isotopes in
Clinical Medicine and Research XXII
ed. by H. Bergmann, A. Kroiss and H. Sinzinger
© 1997 Birkhäuser Verlag Basel/Switzerland

BACTERIAL SPECIFIC INFECTION IMAGING

Britton, K.E., Vinjamuri, S., Hall, A., Kashyap, R., Das,
S.S., Solanki, K.K.,
St. Bartholomew's Hospital

Departments of Nuclear Medicine and Microbiology

London

INTRODUCTION

The question at issue is whether one wishes to diagnose the
site of an inflammation or the site of an infection. In
different clinical circumstances, one may be preferred to the
other. For example, a pyrexia of unknown origin may be due to
a bacterial infection or some other cause of acute
inflammation. For this a catch all technique using a
sensitive but not necessarily a specific agent for
inflammation will be preferred to one with a more restricted
specificity. However, if a clinical problem is that of
searching for a source of bacterial infection when for example
a blood culture is positive, then an agent specific to
bacterial infection may be the more appropriate.

Many causes of inflammation may have an associated infection.
Thus trauma to bone clearly causes a local inflammatory
response but whether it is infected or not with bacteria will
determine its subsequent management. Diagnosis of specific
bacterial infection is particularly important when the therapy
may be long lasting as in endocarditis or in acute or chronic
osteomyelitis. To this end, the search for an appropriate
method of imaging bacteria infection specifically has been
pursued and has resulted in the development and evaluation of

Tc-99m Infecton. This new radiopharmaceutical is based on a
synthetic broad-spectrum antiobiotic Ciprofloxacillin, which
is a 4-fluoroquinolone. Solanki et al (1) noted that the
efficacy of this antibiotic is impaired by the presence of
iron due to its chelating properties, and therefore postulated
that such a compound would bind Tc-99m. He also noted the
wide distribution of this antibiotic and its ability to bind
to living bacteria and remain bound through the inhibition of
the DNA gyrase enzyme which is present in most bacteria. Tc-
99m Infecton has been patented.

MATERIAL AND METHODS

Am ampoule containing 2mg of the antibiotic Ciprofloxacillin
in sterile solution is opened and the contents are mixed with
400ug of Formamidine sulphonic acid with 1,000MBq of
Technetium - 99m solution in a sterile nitrogen filled vial.
The mixture is then boiled for 10 minutes at 100 C. It is
allowed to cool and then passed through a Sephadex column
attached to a 0.5micron filter. The resulting pharmaceutical
preparation has a radiochemical purity of over 95% with about
3% free Tc-99m. The method can be used for other
fluroquinolone antibiotics. Patients attending for routine
white cell imaging were asked if they would participate in a
comparative study. This study had been passed by the East
London & City Health Authority Ethics Committee and by the
Administration of Radioactive Substances Advisory Committee.
The patients gave informed signed consent. The presenting
problems included skeletal complaints, suspected endocarditis,

pyrexia of unknown origin, abdominal and gastrointestinal problems and chest diseases.

IMAGING PROTOCOL

About 400 MBq of Tc-99m Infecton is injected intravenously over 30 seconds. Anterior and posterior whole body static images are acquired at approximately 1 and 4 hours and occasionally 22 hours post injection using a large field of view gamma camera with a low energy general purpose, parallel hole collimator. The camera is peaked to 140 KeV with a 15% window. Image data is transferred on line to a Nuclear Diagnostics Hermes Sun Workstation. For comparison many patients were either injected with 20 MBq of Indium-111 white cells, WBC, with images at 4 hours and 24 hours, the labelling being performed conventionally; or else with Tc-99m-HMPAO labelled WBC, labelled according to the method of Solanki et al (2) with images acquired at 1 and 4 hours and occasionally 22 hours after injection. The normal distribution of Tc-99m Infecton is to show high uptake in the kidneys with excretion to the urinary bladder, a moderate uptake in the liver and spleen with no bone marrow uptake.

At the site of bacterial infection there is diffuse uptake. It is interesting to compare an abscess imaged with the white cells where there is focal uptake at the site of the abscess whereas with the Tc-99m Infecton there is no uptake in the pus, which of course contains dead bacteria, but uptake around the site of pus where the living bacteria are proliferating,

and indeed in a limb there is uptake seen in the direction of
the draining lymphatics. The clinical evaluation was
undertaken in the following way: Concordant positive or
concordant negative white cell/Infecton images were considered
correct. For discordant findings between the white cell image
and the Infecton image, microbiological data indicating active
bacterial infection was taken as correct. In the cases where
there was absence of adequate microbiological data, the
clinical management and outcome analysis was taken as
demonstrating bacterial infection to be present or not.

RESULTS

No adverse effects were observed in response to intravenous
injection of Tc-99m Infecton in over 120 patients studied.
Comparisons were undertaken both with radiolabelled white
cells and with microbiological data. Information about the
persistence of antibiotic therapy at the time of imaging with
Tc-99m Infecton was obtained and whether the antibiotic
therapy was successful or not. 20% of patients could not be
evaluated because of lack of adequately recorded comparative
data. The following conclusions can be drawn. In obvious
infections there was concordance between positive white cells
and positive Infecton imaging and in patients shown not to
have infection there was concordant negative white cell and
Tc-99m Infecton imaging. The discordant results were of
interest. Diseases where it was reasonable to assume that the
inflammation was not due to infection such as Crohn's disease,
showed positive white cell uptake and negative Infecton

uptake. However, there were a number of patients with clear
microbiological evidence of infection but who had been on
antibiotic therapy and in whom the Infecton scan was negative,
particularly if the antibiotic therapy had been prolonged for
more than 5 days. Other patients in whom antibiotic therapy
of a similar length of time has been unsuccessful still showed
persistent positive Infecton imaging. The overall accuracy in
89 out 102 evaluated patients was 87% when allowing for
successful antiobiotic therapy.

DISCUSSION

An agent that is capable of imaging infection has many
advantages over radiolabelled white cells. In contrast to the
formal labelling of white cells, no blood has to be withdrawn
from the patient but this is also true of the injection of
anti white cell antibodies, white cell binding peptides and
radiolabelled human immune globulin. The definition of Tc-99m
infecton sites of bacterial infection are usually clear cut.
The lack of bone marrow uptake makes the evaluation of bone
infection in the spine and proximal limbs more effective than
white cells. The lack of reaction in non infected
inflammatory bowel disease and the positive uptake in infected
inflammatory bowel disease and abdominal and pelvic abscess
are advantages. Although there is a little bilary excretion
and intestinal activity seen after 4 hours, it is not as much
as is seen with Tc-99m HMPAO labelled white cells. The agent
can be used when there is leucopenia. In some patients Tc-99m
Infecton imaging was positive when white cell imaging was

negative, yet microbiological confirmation of infection was obtained.

The most interesting area is whether a negative Infecton scan can be taken to represent successful antibiotic therapy in a known infection or whether a positive Infecton scan on antibiotic therapy can be used as evidence that there is antibiotic resistance.   This has still to be evaluated.

The move from non specific but sensitive agents to specific and sensitive agents in nuclear medicine is a trend not only in cancer but in the evaluation of the complex elements of the inflammatory response.   Autoimmune diseases can be identified due to the uptake by activated T-lymphocytes of radio-labelled Interleukin-2 with I-123 or Tc-99m (3).   Alternatively anti-CD4 radio-labelled monoclonal antibody may be used (4). Activated monocytes may be imaged with Tc-99m J001X (5). Endothelial activation may be imaged with radio-labelled E-selectin (6) and amyloid with I-123-serum amyloid protein (7).   Various infections may also be imaged specifically, such as pneumocystis carinii (8) or potentially tuberculosis (9).

In conclusion, Tc-99m Infecton imaging contributes to the evaluation of infection in the differential diagnosis of inflammation.   Imaging should be performed before appropriate antibody therapy is initiated, however, it still has to be tested as to whether it has a role in evaluating the effectiveness of antibiotic therapy.

Bacteria specific imaging with Tc-99m Infecton has now been
reasonably well validated clinically and should encourage the
development of yet more specific and sensitive agents for the
in-vivo characterisation of the many causes of inflammation.

REFERENCES

1.   Solanki KK, Bomanji J, Siraj Q, et al.
      Tc-99m-Infecton: a new class of radiopharmaceutical for
      imaging infection.
      J Nucl Med 1993; 34: 119P.

2.   Solanki KK, Mather SJ, Al-Janabi M, Britton KE.
      A rapid method for the preparation of Tc-99m-HMPAO
      labelled leucocytes.
      Nucl Med Commun 1988; 10: 753-761.

3.   Chianelli M, Signore A, Ronga C et al.
      Labelling, purification and biodistribution of ^{99m}Tc
      Interleukin-2 a new radiopharmaceutical for in vivo
      detection of activate lymphocytes.
      Eur J Nucl Med 1994; 21: 807.

4.   Kinne RW, Bicker W, Schwab J et al.
      Imaging Rheumatoid Arthritis joints with technetium-99m
      labelled specific anti-CD4- and non specific monoclonal
      antibodies.
      Eur J Nucl Med 1994; 21: 176-180.

5.   Perin F, Pittet J-C, Hoffschir D et al.
      ^{201}Tl and ^{99}Tc^m-J001X macrophage scintigraphy: Two
      radionuclides imaging techniques for the surveillance of
      acute localised radiation over exposures.
      Nuc Med Commun 1995; 16: 608-614.

6.   Jamar F, Chapman BT, Haskard DO, Peters AM.
      Imaging using anti E selectin antibody as a marker of
      endothelial activation in inflammatory arthritis.
      J Nucl Med 1994; 35: 45P.

7.   Hawkins PN, Myers MJ, Lavender JP.
      Diagnostic radionuclide imaging of amyloid: biological
      targeting of circulating human serum amyloid P component.
      Lancet 1988; 6: 1413-1418.

8.   Goldenberg DM, Sharkey RM, Udun S et al.
      Immunoscintigraphy of Pneumocystis Carinii pneumonia in
      AIDS patients.
      J Nucl Med 1994; 35: 1028-1034.

9.   Hazra DK, Lahiri VL, Saran S et al.
      In vivo tuberculoma creation and its radioimmunoimaging.
      Nucl Med Commun 1987; 8: 139-142.

Radioactive Isotopes in
Clinical Medicine and Research XXII
ed. by H. Bergmann, A. Kroiss and H. Sinzinger
© 1997 Birkhäuser Verlag Basel/Switzerland

IN VIVO DETECTION OF ACTIVATED LYMPHOCYTES IN IMMUNE-MEDIATED DISEASES BY ^{123}I-INTERLEUKIN-2 SCINTIGRAPHY

A. Signore, M. Chianelli, A. Picarelli, E. Procaccini, R. Barone,
M. Greco, A. Annovazzi, M. De Vincenzi*, P. Pozzilli and G. Ronga

Institute of Clinica Medica II, University "La Sapienza" and
*Istituto Superiore di Sanità, Rome, Italy

Summary: In this study we describe the use of ^{123}I-interleukin-2 scintigraphy in patients affected by chronic inflammatory diseases as a non invasive technique for in vivo detection and quantitation of the severity and extent of the inflammatory process. We conclude that ^{123}I-IL2 scintigraphy is a specific and sensitive non-invasive technique to quantify in vivo the severity of the mononuclear cell infiltrate in tissues. It provides information of the whole affected organ and may have relevant clinical implications for early diagnosis of several autoimmune diseases as well as to evaluate the severity and extent of inflammation during the follow-up.

Introduction

Several human chronic inflammatory diseases, such as organ specific autoimmune diseases, are characterized by a chronic, slowly progressing, mononuclear cell infiltration of the target organ, with little increase of vascular permeability. This infiltrate can anticipate of several months or years the onset of clinical symptoms. Tissue biopsies may not be easily applicable to every organ and may poorly represent the condition of the whole organ particularly in inflammatory bowel diseases and in Type 1 diabetes (IDDM). Thus, the possibility to detect in vivo the presence and the extent of a mononuclear cell infiltration by a simple scintigraphy may be of considerable clinical utility for diagnosis and follow-up of several chronic inflammatory diseases. Immunohistochemical studies of tissue biopsies in several chronic inflammatory diseases have revealed that the target tissue is infiltrated by mononuclear cells (mainly T-lymphocytes) and that 10 to 50% of these cells express interleukin-2 receptors (IL2R) as sign of cell activation[1-3].

We previously described the labelling of IL2 with ^{123}I and we validate its use in two animal models of Type 1 diabetes, the BB/W rat[4] and the NOD mouse[5].

Aims of this study were: 1) to correlate results of IL2 scintigraphy with histological findings in Coeliac Disease (CD) patients; 2) to apply this technique to detect tissue infiltrating lymphocytes in several immune-mediated diseases.

Patients and methods

a) <u>10 patients with Coeliac disease</u> diagnosed by jejunal biopsy and by the presence of anti-gliadin (AGA, IgG and IgA) and/or anti-endomysium (EMA) antibodies, were studied at time of diagnosis. Samples for jejunal biopsy were taken with a Quinton multipurpose hydraulics biopsy tube and presence of IL2R+ cells in the intestinal mucosa was investigated by immunohistochemical staining on cryostat sections of biopsy specimens using an anti-CD25 monoclonal antibody (2A3, Becton Dickinson). Positive cells per mm of mucosa were counted using a microscope grid. Patients were studied again by biopsy with immunohistochemical staining of sections and by scintigraphy after 12-18 months of a gluten free diet.

b) <u>13 patients with ileal Crohn's disease</u> (8 active and 5 in remission) diagnosed by conventional radiology, endoscopy and histology. In all patients the disease activity was assessed according to the Crohn's Disease Activity Index (CDAI) and to the Bristol Simple Index (SI) supplemented by laboratory measurements. Active patients were defined by a CDAI > 210 (range 210-310) and a SI > 5 (range 5-9).

c) <u>8 patients affected by IDDM</u> of recent diagnosis within 90 days from the first insulin injection. ICA and AGA were measured in all patients.

d) <u>5 first degree relatives of IDDM patients</u> selected by the presence of ICA and/or IAA autoantibodies and a reduced first phase insulin secretion after IVGTT.

e) <u>8 patients with Hashimoto's thyroiditis</u> diagnosed by ultrasound scan, ^{131}I scintigraphy and all had high titre of anti-TPO and thyroglobulin antibodies. All patients were under L-thyroxin (2.0 µg/kg/day) therapy at time of study with suppressed TSH values and suppressed ^{131}I uptake.

f) <u>4 patients with Graves' disease</u> of recent diagnosis diagnosed by ^{131}I scintigraphy and all had high titre of anti-TSHr, TPO and thyroglobulin antibodies. All patients were under methimazole (15 to 20 mg/day) and L-thyroxin (2.0 µg/kg/day) therapy at time of study and with normal TSH and thyroid hormones.

f) <u>10 normal subjects</u> with no history for autoimmune diseases.

Labelling of IL2, gamma camera imaging and data analysis: Human recombinant IL2 (EuroCetus, The Netherlands) was labelled using an enzymatic method as described elsewhere[6].

Subjects were fasting for at least 8 hours and received 400 mg of $KClO_4$ orally 20 min before the study to prevent stomach and thyroid uptake of free [123]I. Approximately 2 mCi of ^{123}I-IL2 (<5 µg IL2) were administered i.v. and images were acquired with a single head Elscint SP4 gamma camera fitted with a low energy and medium resolution collimator. Planar antero-posterior images (collected in a 256x256 pixel matrix) and tomographic (SPET) images (collected in a 64x64 pixel matrix acquiring 60 frames of 20 seconds each during a 360° rotation) were acquired 1 hour after injection. Transaxial sections of 10 pixel thickness were reconstructed for studying the bowel and sections of 3 pixel for studying the pancreas, along the abdomen. Images were then filtered using a Hanning filter (0.5 cycles) and a pre-attenuation correction (0.125 cm^{-1} attenuation coefficient). For quantitative analysis of bowel radioactivity, 6 regions of interest (ROI) were considered in the abdomen and drawn as follows: three squared, 10 by 10 pixel ROI were drawn on the right, central and left part of each of two consecutive abdominal transaxial sections cut between the lower kidney poles and the bladder. A circular region of interest was also drawn over the spinal marrow as background. Bowel/marrow radioactivity ratios (B/M) were calculated for each of the 6 ROI after normalisation of counts per ROI area.

For analysis of pancreatic radioactivity, a ROI was drawn in SPET section over the pancreas, guided by the corresponding CT image, and a circular ROI over the spinal marrow as background. Pancreas/marrow radioactivity ratio (P/M) was calculated after normalisation of counts per ROI area.

For analysis of ^{123}I-IL2 thyroid uptake a ROI was drawn over the thyroid and a rectangular ROI was drawn above the thyroid for background. After normalization of counts per area, the thyroid/background (T/B) radioactivity ratio was calculated.

The ^{123}I-IL2 uptake in each ROI (B/M, P/M or T/B) was considered statistically significant when higher than the mean of values of the corresponding region in normal subjects + 2 SD.

Results

No significant gastrointestinal or pancreatic uptake was detectable in normal subjects. We found a variable degree of liver and spleen uptake which can be explained by the physiological presence of IL2R bearing mononuclear cells in these tissues. There was some thyroid radioactivity in normal subjects (T/B = 3.43±0.7) probably due to the presence of some free ^{123}I despite the administration of $KClO_4$. A variable degree and extent of intestinal uptake of radiolabelled IL2 was found in patients with newly diagnosed Coeliac disease which was statistically reduced in 5 out of 6 regions after 1 year diet (table 1). Immunohistochemical analysis of intestinal biopsies showed that all patients at diagnosis had partial atrophy of intestinal villi and extensive mononuclear cell infiltration and a positive correlation was found between the number of IL2R+ve cells per mm of jejunal mucosa and the B/M ratio calculated in the jejunal region (left ROI of the upper section) by ^{123}I-IL2 scintigraphy (r^2=0.727; p<0.0001).

Intestinal uptake of ^{123}I-IL2 in active Crohn's disease patients showed focal and patchy distribution within each ROI. Overall, intestinal uptake was significantly higher than in normal subjects and patients in remission phase in all ROI, with exception of the left ROI of the upper transaxial section (table 1). All patients had at least one intestinal ROI (range 1-4) with a significantly high B/M ratio.

Table 1. Bowel/Marrow (B/M) radioactivity ratios in the 6 intestinal ROI in Coeliac and Crohn's disease patients and in normals 1 hour after i.v. injection of ^{123}I-IL2

	Coeliac after diet (n=7)	Coeliac at diagnosis (n=10)	Normal subjects (n=10)	Active Crohn's disease (n=8)
Upper right ROI	1.25±0.24	2.13±0.65	1.18±0.29	1.50±0.35
	p = 0.03*	p = 0.001	p = 0.04	
Upper central ROI	1.74±0.13	2.58±0.74	1.54±0.21	1.76±0.22
	p = 0.02*	p = 0.0001	p = 0.04.	
Upper left ROI	1.36±0.18	2.68±0.71	1.46±0.29	1.62±0.22
	p = 0.02*	p = 0.0001	p = n.s.	
Lower right ROI	1.14±0.30	1.69±0.59	1.10±0.18	1.21±0.25
	n.s.	p = 0.003	p = 0.04	
Lower central ROI	1.60±0.28	2.51±0.89	1.44±0.25	1.74±0.26
	p = 0.03*	p = 0.002	p = 0.02	
Lower left ROI	1.15±0.02	2.25±0.84	1.09±0.14	1.39±0.19
	p = 0.01*	p = 0.0001	p = 0.001	

Data are mean ± SD. Statistical analysis was performed by Student's t test for paired* or unpaired data. n.s. = not significant.

In IDDM patients a wide range of pancreatic uptake was observed (P/M range: 2.36-10.77) and overall we found an average P/M ratio significantly higher than in normal subjects in both diabetics and pre-diabetic subjects (3.05±0.4 and 3.87+0.8 vs 2.12±0.5; p=0.02 and p=0.01, respectively vs NS), (table 2). However, only 4 out of 8 IDDM patients, had a significantly high pancreatic uptake of ^{123}I-IL2 and 4 out of 5 pre-diabetic subjects.

Furthermore, all pre-diabetics with positive scintigraphy developed clinical diabetes, between 1 to 12 months after scintigraphy. No correlation was found between P/M ratios and ICA or IAA levels.

Finally, thyroid uptake of ^{123}I-IL2 was variable and disomogeneous in both patients with Graves' and Hashimoto's thyroiditis (table 2). In all patients we found a significantly higher uptake than in normal subjects which can not be attributed (or only to a minor extent) to free ^{123}I uptake since all patients had blocked thyroid function.

Table 2. Target/Background (T/B) radioactivity ratios in thyroid and pancreas of normals and patients with IDDM, pre-IDDM and thyroiditis 1 hour after ^{123}I-IL2

	Hashimoto's thyroiditis (n=8)	Normal subjects (n=10)	Graves' disease (n=4)
Thyroid/Background *n° of positive patients*	10.7±3.1 (8/8)	3.4±0.7 (0/10)	15.0±2.5 (4/4)
	I_____II_____I		
	p = 0.0001	p = 0.0001	

	IDDM at diagnosis (n=8)	Normal subjects (n=10)	Pre-IDDM subjects (n=5)
Pancreas/Background *n° of positive patients*	3.05±0.4 (4/8)	2.12±0.5 (0/10)	3.87±0.8 (4/5)
	I_____II_____I		
	p = 0.02	p = 0.01	

Data are mean±SD. Statistical analysis was performed by Student's t test for unpaired data. Positivity was defined for T/B ratios heigher that normal mean+2SD.

Discussion

In summary, here we validated the use of ^{123}I-IL2 scintigraphy for in vivo detection of tissue infiltrating mononuclear cells in Coeliac disease patients by comparing the scintigraphic results with histopathological findings. Moreover, we applied this technique to several other chronic inflammatory diseases including: i) Crohn's disease, characterized by a marked infiltration of activated mononuclear cells within the gut wall[2]; ii) IDDM, a localised T-cell mediated autoimmune disease characterized by a mononuclear cell infiltration of a deep parenchymal organ as the pancreas (*insulitis*[7]) and iii) as positive controls, Graves' and Hashimoto's thyroiditis in which IL2R+ve massively infiltrate the thyroid which is an easily accessible organ to be studied by scintigraphy[3].

Our results showed that ^{123}I-IL2 significantly accumulates in the bowel of all Coeliac disease patients at diagnosis and the degree of uptake significantly correlates with the number of IL2R+ve lymphocytes present per mm of jejunal mucosa. Moreover, after 1 year diet the reduction of autoantibody titre and of gut wall infiltration is reflected by the negative IL2 scintigraphy in all patients. Thus, our results support the use of ^{123}I-IL2 scintigraphy for correct assessment of disease activity, instead of the invasive jejunal biopsy, as ^{123}I-IL2 scintigraphy provides information on the entire intestinal tract.

In Crohn's disease, it is likely that this technique will be of clinical value for assessing disease activity (even sub-clinical), for monitoring the response to treatment and for early detection of post-operative recurrence.

In IDDM patients the wide range of pancreatic uptake observed may reflect a different degree of mononuclear cell infiltration at the time of diagnosis, as described by histological investigation of human insulitis. In this respect, it is remarkable that IDDM patients with negative scintigraphy had the longest duration of the disease (data not shown), suggesting a reduction of the inflammatory process after diagnosis and implementation of insulin therapy.

In thyroid autoimmunity we demonstrated the possibility to detect in vivo the presence of IL2R+ve cells in the thyroid of patients with Graves' and Hashimoto's thyroiditis. This may have important implications to follow-up the efficacy of different therapies and for the differential diagnosis of thyroid disorders.

In conclusion, we have shown that by ^{123}I-IL2 scintigraphy is possible to detect in vivo IL2R+ve mononuclear cells infiltrating tissues affected by chronic inflammatory diseases, thus allowing a non-invasive "histological examination" of the whole target organ. This may have important clinical implications for diagnosis, prevention and follow-up therapy in these diseases.

References

1.   Pallone F, Fais S, Squarcia O, Biancone L, Pozzilli P, Boirivant M. Activation of peripheral and intestinal lamina propria lymphocytes in Crohn's Disease. in vivo state of activation and in vitro response to stimulation as defined by the expression of early activation antigens. *Gut* 1987; 28: 745-49.

2.   Choy MY, Walker-Smith JA, Williams CB, Mc Donald TT. Differential expression of CD25 (interleukin-2 receptor) on lamina propria T cells and macrophages in the intestinal lesions in Crohn's Disease and Ulcerative Colitis. *Gut* 1990; 31: 1365-70.

3. Wall JR, Baur R, Schleusener H, Bandy-Dafoe P. Peripheral blood and intrathyroidal mononuclear cell populations in patients with autoimmune thyroid disorders enumerated using monoclonal antibodies. *J Clin Endocrinol Metab* 1983; 56: 164-68.

4. Signore A, Parman A, Pozzilli P, Andreani D, Beverley PCL. Detection of activated lymphocytes in endocrine pancreas of BB/W rats by injection of 123-interleukin-2: an early sign of type 1 diabetes. *Lancet* 1987; 2: 537-40.

5. Signore A, Chianelli M, Ferretti E, Negri M, Andreani D, Pozzilli P. A new approach for in vivo detection of insulitis: activated lymphocyte targeting with 123I labelled interleukin-2. *Eur J Endocrinol* 1994; 131: 431-37.

6. Signore A, Chianelli M, Toscano A, Ronga G, Monetini L, Nimmon CC, Britton KE, Pozzilli P, Negri M. A radiopharmaceutical for imaging areas of lymphocytic infiltration: 123I-interleukin-2. Labelling procedure and animal studies. *Nucl Med Commun* 1992; 13: 713-22.

7. Foulis AK, Liddle CN, Farquharson MA, Richmond JA, Weir RS. The histopathology of the pancreas in type 1 (insulin-dependent) diabetes mellitus: a 25-year review of deaths in patients under 20 years of age in the United Kingdom. *Diabetologia* 1986; 29: 267-74.

Cardiology

Radioactive Isotopes in
Clinical Medicine and Research XXII
ed. by H. Bergmann, A. Kroiss and H. Sinzinger
© 1997 Birkhäuser Verlag Basel/Switzerland

QUANTITATIVE EVALUATION OF MYOCARDIAL BLOOD FLOW AND CORONARY RESERVE IN PATIENTS WITH CORONARY ARTERY DISEASE: A DOBUTAMINE STRESS - [O-15] H_2O PET STUDY

D. Moka, E. Voth, C.A. Schneider, F.M. Baer, J. A. Melin, A. Bol,
R. Wagner, U. Sechtem, H. Schicha

Departments of Nuclear Medicine and Internal Medicine III (Cardiology),
University of Cologne, Germany
Max-Planck-Institut für Neurologische Forschung, Cologne, Germany
University of Louvain Medical School, Brussels, Belgium

SUMMARY

In order to assess changes in myocardial blood flow and coronary reserve during dobutamine stress, 14 patients with coronary single vessel stenosis (> 70 % by angiography) were examined by O-15 water positron emission tomography (PET) at rest and during maximal dobutamine stress (maximal dosis 40 µg/kg/min). Control regions (myocardium supplied by a normal artery) showed a 2.5 fold increase in myocardial blood flow during dobutamine stress due to a reduction of coronary resistance. In contrast, myocardial blood flow in regions supplied by a stenosed coronary artery did not increase significantly.

INTRODUCTION

In patients with coronary artery disease a hemodynamic difference between percent area stenosis detected by angiography, fractional flow derived by intracoronary pressure measurements and coronary perfusion derived by positron emissions tomography (PET) is often found. Myocardial blood flow estimated with O-15 water PET was not significantly different from that measured with radio labeled microspheres (3). De Bruyne et al. showed that there is a better correlation between fractional flow reserve and relative flow reserve derived from PET-data than between fractional flow reserve and angiographic percent area stenosis (2). Most measurements of cardiovascular function during resting state are poor predictors of circulatory performance during vigorous exercise.

However up to now, there are only rare data concerning exact quantitative changes of myocardial blood flow in patients with coronary artery disease, especially under stress conditions.

The objective of this study was the non-invasive quantitative evaluation of myocardial blood flow and flow reserve in these patients at rest and under pharmacological stress.

PATIENTS AND METHODS

We examined 14 patients (9 male, 5 female), mean age of 54 ± 7 years, with angiographically documented, coronary single vessel disease. Luminal diameter reduction was greater than 70 %. Eight of the patients had a stenosis of left anterior descending artery, 6 patients a stenosis of circumflex artery. All patients had angiographically normal left ventricular function.

Measurements were performed after withdrawal of antiischemic medication for at least 48 hours. Dobutamine as a sympathomimetic agent was used for stress testing (6). The maximum dosage for dobutamine stress was determined by a stress ECG with dobutamine in increasing dose (10, 20, 30, 40 µg/kg/min).

For acquisition of the PET-data we used a whole body positron emission tomograph (CTI ECAT Exact 921) with an axial field of view of 16 cm and 47 slices of 3.5 mm.

First, a dynamic PET scan at rest after i.v. injection (slow bolus) of 30 mCi O-15 water (1.1 GBq) was performed over 180 sec (5). Then, patients underwent dobutamine stress as determined by dobutamine ECG. After i.v. injection of another 30 mCi O-15 water a second dynamic scan was carried out during maximal dobutamine stress. Each examination was terminated by a transmission scan (30 min) and an emission scan (30-60 min) after injection of 10 mCi (370 MBq) F-18 FDG.

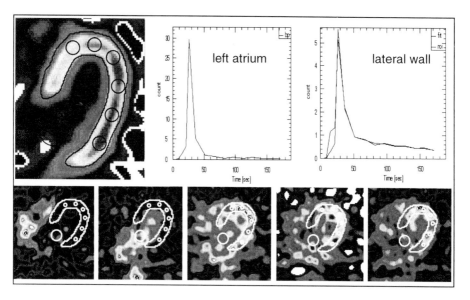

Fig. 1   ROIs positionated in the apical and lateral myocardial wall (left). Time activity curves of left atrium and lateral wall (right). O-15 water scans (representative study - bottom).

6 ROIs (regions of interest) were placed in the apical and lateral wall of the heart defined on the FDG tomogram (Fig. 1) for data analysis . Then, the ROIs were transfered to the dynamic water scans. Myocardial blood flow was calculated using a **single compartment model for tracer kinetics,** published by Bol et. al. (1). Input function was determined from the dynamic scans by placing a ROI over the left atrium. Ischemic regions were defined as territories of stenosed artery, control regions were defined as territories of non-stenosed coronary artery.

RESULTS

During dobutamine infusion none of the patients showed severe clinical side effects. Four patients had signs of angina pectoris and 6 patients showed ECG-changes (ST-segment depression, new arrhythmias). Heart rate increased from 67 ± 11 beats/s to 114 ± 18 beats/s. Systolic blood pressure rose from 130 ± 14 mm Hg at rest to 151 ± 21 mm Hg at maximum stress. The double product (rate-pressure-product) as a reliable index of heart workload and oxygen consumption increased from 8800 ± 2200 to 17100 ± 3400 mm Hg/min. All changes were statistically significant (p<0.001).

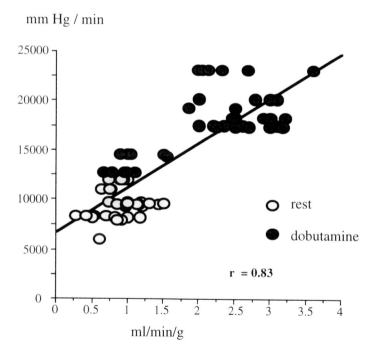

Fig. 2   Myocardial blood flow versus rate pressure product (control regions, supplied by a non-stenotic coronary artery)

Comparing PET-data with hemodynamic parameters there was a good positive correlation between calculated myocardial blood flow and rate pressure product in control regions (Fig. 2). Myocardial blood flow increased significantly from 0.9 ± 0.2 ml/min/g at rest to 2.6 ± 1.0 ml/min/g at maximum dobutamine stress (p<0.001) (Fig. 3). In contrast, ischemic regions showed an insufficient increase of myocardial blood flow (from 1.0 ± 0.3 ml/min/g to 1.3 ± 0.7 ml/min/g; p = n.s.).

The coronary flow reserve, defined as myocardial blood flow under dobutamine stress devided by myocardial blood flow at rest, was 2.6 ± 0.7 in control regions. In contrast, the coronary flow reserve was only 1.3 ± 0.5 in ischemic regions. The total coronary resistance, defined as (1/3 systolic blood pressure + 2/3 diastolic blood pressure)/myocardial blood flow, declined significantly under stress conditions in control regions. However, ischemic regions showed only a slight non significant decrease from 93 to 77 mm Hg min g/ml (Fig. 3 - right graph).

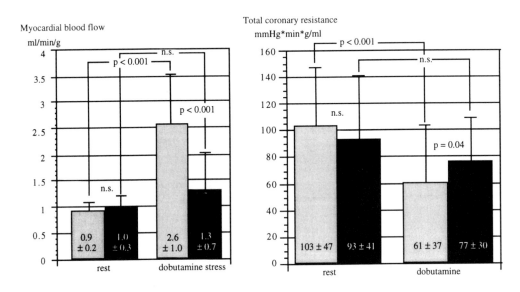

Fig. 3   Left graph: Myocardial blood flow: resting state versus maximal pharmacological stress (high dose dobutamine infusion).
Right graph: Total coronary resistance (TCR): resting state vs. high dose dobutamine infusion (TCR = (1/3 systolic blood pressure (BP) + 2/3 diastolic BP)/myocardial blood flow)

☐ control regions   ■ ischemic regions

DISCUSSION

O-15-water as perfusion marker has the advantage of a short halflife time (122 sec), so repeated measurements, especially under stress and resting conditions are possible without movement of the patient. The additional use of a single compartment model for data evaluation makes an arterial cannulation for clinical studies unnecessary (4, 5). Thus, the impairment of patients was moderate.

The non invasive measurements of myocardial blood flow by use of 15-O labeled water in patients with coronary artery disease validated the hemodynamic importance of angiographically documented coronary artery stenosis with luminal diameter reduction > 70 %. At rest there was a normal myocardial perfusion in regions supplied by stenotic vessels as well as in control regions (6). Under stress conditions, however, myocardial blood flow increased by a factor of 2.9 in control regions and did not change in ischemic regions. This is in agreement with data from Krivokapich et. al., who determined a flow reserve of 2.9 during dobutamine stress in controls (6).

The main reason for these alterations was likely the inadequate decline of total coronary resistance in ischemic territory during exercise because of lacking vasodilatating capacity and disturbed coronary autoregulation (7).

Our findings have practical implications for the treatment of a coronary artery vessel disease with a luminal diameter reduction higher than 70 %. There is a hemodynamical importance at least during maximal or near-maximal exercise. So, a angioplastic intervention or revascularisation can be useful for the maintenance of viable myocardium and can provide ischemic injury. Non invasive measurements of myocardial blood flow have an important predictive value for appreciating the severity of coronary artery disease.

Finally, dobutamine is capable to raise myocardial workload and oxygen consumption suffiently as to be shown in the increase of the hemodynamic stress predictor: the rate-pressure-product (6). So, dobutamine stress is a good alternative for e.g. myocardial scintigraphy if standard stress procedures like ergometric exercise or dipyridamole application are contraindicated.

CONCLUSION

Dynamic O-15 water PET is capable to quantify regional myocardial blood flow and flow reserve. The technique can therefore be used for non-invasive studies of coronary pathophysiology.

High-dose dobutamine infusion increases myocardial oxygen demand. This is followed by a proportional increase in myocardial blood flow in control regions. In contrast, the increase in myocardial blood flow is inadequate in ischemic regions supplied by a coronary artery with hemodynamic important stenosis.

REFERENCES

1. Bol A., Melin J. A., Vannoverschelde J.-L., Baudhuin T., Vogelaers D., De Pauw M., Michel C., Luxen A., Labar D., Cogneau M., Robert A., Heyndrickx G. R. and Wijns W. Direct comparison of [13N]ammonia and [15O]water estimates of perfusion with quantification of regional myocardial blood flow by microspheres. Circulation 1993; 87:512-525.

2. De Bruyne B., Baudhuin T., Melin J. A., Pijls N. H., Sys S. U., Bol A., Paulus W. J., Heyndrickx G. R. and Wijns W. Coronary flow reserve calculated from pressure measurements in humans. Validation with positron emission tomography. Circulation 1994; 89:1013-22.

3. Herrero P., Staudenherz A., Walsh J. F., Gropler R. J. and Bergmann S. R. Heterogeneity of myocardial perfusion provides the physiological basis of perfusable tissue index. J Nucl Med 1995; 36:320-7.

4. Iida H., Rhodes C. G., de Silva R., Araujo L. I., Bloomfield P. M., Lammertsma A. A. and Jones T. Use of the left ventricular time-activity curve as a noninvasive input function in dynamic oxygen-15-water positron emission tomography. J Nucl Med 1992; 33:1669-77.

5. Iida H., Takahashi A., Tamura Y., Ono Y. and Lammertsma A. A. Myocardial blood flow: Comparison of oxygen-15-water bolus injection, slow infusion and oxygen-15-carbon dioxide slow inhalation. J Nucl Med 1995; 36:78-85.

6. Krivokapich J., Huang S.-C. and Schelbert H. R. Assessment of the effects of dobutamine on myocardial blood flow and oxidative metabolism in normal human subjects using nitrogen-13 ammonia and carbon-11 acetate. Am J Cardiol 1993; 71:1351-1356.

7. Nitenberg A. and Antony I. Coronary vascular reserve in humans: a critical review of methods of evaluation and of interpretation of the results. Europ Heart J 1995; 16:7-21.

Radioactive Isotopes in
Clinical Medicine and Research XXII
ed. by H. Bergmann, A. Kroiss and H. Sinzinger
© 1997 Birkhäuser Verlag Basel/Switzerland

PREDICTION OF IMPROVEMENT IN GLOBAL AND REGIONAL VENTRICU-LAR FUNCTION AFTER REVASCULARIZATION WITH FDG SPECT.

J.J. Bax, J.H. Cornel*, F.C. Visser, P.M. Fioretti*,
R. Lengauer, A. van Lingen, C.A. Visser.

Free University Hospital Amsterdam, *Academic Hospital Rotterdam, The Netherlands.

SUMMARY: This study evaluated the role of ^{18}F-fluorodeoxyglucose (FDG) imaging with SPECT to assess functional recovery after revascularization. Twenty-one with a poor left ventricular function (LVEF 31±8%) patients were studied. Functional improvement was assessed by 2D echo 3 months after revascularization. FDG SPECT had a sensitivity of 89% and a specificity of 71% to assess improvement of regional function. Global function improved after revascularization in 12 patients with 3 or more viable segments on FDG SPECT.

INTRODUCTION

In patients with extensive coronary artery disease, impaired ventricular function is not necessarily an irreversible process; Nesto et al demonstrated improvement in contractile function after revascularization when viable myocardium was present (1). Thus, identification of viable may be of importance in patients considered for revascularization.

Detection of viable myocardium is possible with ^{18}F-fluorodeoxyglucose (FDG) and positron emission tomography (PET) (2) or single photon emission computed tomography (SPECT) and 511 keV collimators (3). To validate the FDG SPECT approach, the diagnostic value for functional outcome after revascularization needs to be studied. Hence, aim of the present study was to investigate whether FDG SPECT can predict reversibility of wall motion abnormalities after revascularization.

METHODS

Study population. We prospectively studied 21 patients (19 men, mean age 64±8 yrs) with a left ventricular ejection fraction (LVEF) <40% (mean 31±8%) and regional wall motion abnormalities on resting echocardiography. All patients had a previous infarction but not within 1 month of the SPECT study. Subsequent to SPECT imaging, the patients underwent surgical revascularization. The decision to revascularize was not influenced by the SPECT results.

Study protocol. The patients underwent an early resting [201]thallium (Tl) SPECT, followed by FDG SPECT during a hyperinsulinemic euglycemic clamp as described previously (3). A resting echocardiogram was performed to assess regional wall motion abnormalities before and 3.2±1.2 months after the operation. None of the patients experienced a myocardial infarction or required hospitalization for unstable angina during the entire study period. Each patient gave informed consent to the study protocol that was approved by the Ethical Committees.

SPECT image analysis. Circumferential count profiles (60 radii, highest pixel activity/radius) from FDG and Tl short-axis slices were generated and displayed in a polar map format (divided into 13 segments). One region was positioned at the center (apex), 6 segments (anterior, anteroseptal, inferoseptal, inferior, inferolateral and anterolateral) at the midportion and 6 at the periphery of the polar map (4).

A region of normal perfusion was manually drawn on the Tl polar map (defined as the area with the highest Tl uptake associated with normal wall motion on echo). The activity of this area was normalized to the mean activity of the same area of a normal data base (5) and the correction factor was applied to all other segments. The region of normal perfusion was projected on the FDG polar map and the same normalization procedure was followed, except that a normal FDG database was used (5). The Tl and FDG activities were expressed as percentage of the corresponding normal reference values. A myocardial region was considered a perfusion defect when the Tl activity was <2SD below the normal reference value. A segment was considered viable if the perfusion on Tl SPECT was normal, or if the FDG uptake was ≥7% increased in a perfusion defect (6). The 7% cutoff level of increased FDG uptake was defined by receiver operating characteristic analysis in a previous study in patients undergoing revascularization (6).

Two-dimensional echocardiography. For comparison with the SPECT data the left ventricle was divided into 13 comparable segments (4). Each segment was assigned a wall motion score (WMS) of 0 to 3: normal=0, hypokinetic=1, akinetic=2 or dyskinetic=3. Post-interventional improvement of regional wall motion was considered if systolic thickening was detected in a segment that was a-/dyskinetic or if normal wall motion was detected in segments that were hypokinetic at baseline. A wall motion score index (WMSI) was utilized to evaluate the effect of revascularization on global LV function. The WMSI was calculated by dividing the sum of the segmental scores by the total number of segments analyzed per patient. A good relation existed between the LVEF (assessed angiographically) and the WMSI before revascularization: WMSI = -0.024*LVEF + 1.67 ($r=0.-82$, $P<0.005$), suggesting that the WMSI can be used as an indirect measure of global LV function.

Statistical analysis. All results were expressed as mean±1 SD. Patient data were compared using the Student's t-test for paired and unpaired data when appropriate. A P-value <0.05 was considered significant.

RESULTS

The total number of segments analyzed in the 21 patients was 273; 123 (45%) had normal wall motion and 150 (55%) abnormal wall motion before the operation. The mean number of dyssynergic segments per patient was 6.9±3.2. Ten segments were excluded from the analysis because of inadequate revascularization. Hence 140 dyssynergic segments remained for the final analysis, including 70 hypokinetic, 67 akinetic and 3 dyskinetic segments. Improvement in wall motion post-operatively was observed in 47 (34%) segments. Seven segments improved 2 grades in wall motion and 40 improved 1 grade. No change in wall motion was detected in 89 (64%) segments and 4 (2%) segments showed deterioration in wall motion post-operatively. SPECT imaging demonstrated viability in 42 of 47 improved segments (sensitivity 89%). Conversely, SPECT classified 66 of 93 non-improved segments as scar tissue (specificity 71%).

Subsequently, the patients were divided into 2 groups (see Figure 1). The WMSI decreased significantly from 1.02±0.36 before to 0.75±0.39 (P<0.01) after revascularization in 12 patients with 3 or more viable segments on SPECT (group A). In contrast, the WMSI did not change significantly (0.52±0.23 before versus 0.46±0.27 after revascularization, NS) in 9 patients with 2 or less viable segments on FDG SPECT (group B).

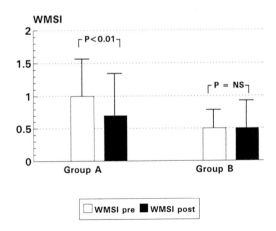

Figure 1. Changes in wall motion score index (WMSI) after operation in patients with ≥3 (group A) or ≤2 (group B) viable segments on FDG SPECT.

DISCUSSION

This study demonstrates that quantitative FDG SPECT can predict reversibility of regional contractile function after revascularization.

Findings in the present study. In the present study, 34% of the segments with abnormal wall motion improved after revascularization. The segments that improved in function, demonstrated either normal perfusion or increased FDG uptake. The results obtained with FDG SPECT are in line with previous results obtained with FDG PET. In 8 FDG PET studies the mean sensitivity and specificity to assess functional recovery after revascularization were 88% and 74% respectively (7).

FDG SPECT had a high sensitivity (89%), but a somewhat lower specificity (71%), indicating "overestimation" of functional recovery. Several factors may have resulted in failure of recovery of segments that were viable on FDG SPECT. It has been demonstrated that morphological degeneration occurs in viable myocytes before actual cell death occurs (8). Marwick et al (9) suggested that despite the increased FDG uptake, some segments may contain myocytes that are too severely injured to recover. Graft patency was not certain in our study and reocclusion may have lead to incomplete recovery in contractile function in segments that were viable on FDG SPECT.

Another interesting observation in this study was that the presence of 3 or more viable segments on FDG SPECT resulted in improvement of global function, although this parameter was only indirectly determined from the change in WMSI.

Methodologic considerations. In this study early resting Tl SPECT was used to measure regional perfusion, since regional FDG uptake needs to be compared with regional perfusion. In the present study no redistribution Tl image was acquired, although redistribution of Tl provides an important contribution to the identification of viable myocardium (10). However, preliminary results from our group have demonstrated superiority of FDG SPECT over Tl rest-redistribution for the prediction of functional recovery (11).

Viability was assessed by comparing regional perfusion with FDG uptake. However, Tl and FDG have different photon energies that may lead to differences in attenuation especially in the inferoseptal region of the myocardium. In a study performed in normal individuals however, it was shown that no differences between tracer activities occurred in the different regions of the myocardium (5). A future study using attenuation correction is needed to elucidate this problem.

Conclusions. The finding that FDG SPECT can predict reversibility of wall motion abnormalities after a revascularization procedure has important clinical implications, especially in patients with severe left ventricular dysfunction. These patients have a poor long-term survival on medical therapy, which may improve after surgical revascularization, but also have high surgical risks. Therefore, the detection of dyssynergic but viable myocardium (which is likely to recover after revascularization) with FDG SPECT may help in the identification of patients who will benefit most from a revascularization procedure.

REFERENCES

1. Nesto RW, Cohn LH, Collins JH et al. Inotropic contractile reserve: A useful predictor of increased 5 year survival and improved postoperative left ventricular function in patients with coronary artery disease and reduced ejection fraction. Am J Cardiol 1982;50: 39-44.

2. Schwaiger M, Hicks R. The clinical role of metabolic imaging of the heart by PET. J Nucl Med 1991;32:565-578.

3. Bax JJ, Visser FC, van Lingen A et al. Feasibility of assessing regional myocardial uptake of 18F-fluorodeoxyglucose using SPECT. Eur Heart J 1993;14:1675-1682.

4. Jaarsma W, Visser CA, Eenige van MJ et al. Prognostic implications of regional

hyperkinesia and remote asynergy of noninfarcted myocardium. Am J Cardiol 1986;58:3-94-398.

5. Bax JJ, Visser FC, van Lingen A et al. Relation between myocardial uptake of thallium-201 chloride and FDG imaged with SPECT in normal individuals. Eur J Nucl Med 1995; 22:56-60.

6. Bax JJ, Cornel JH, Visser FC et al. Quantitative analysis of FDG and Tl-201 SPECT for the prediction of functional outcome after revascularization. J Nucl Med 1995;36:36P.

7. Schelbert HR. Metabolic imaging to assess myocardial viability. J Nucl Med 1994;35 (Suppl):8S-14S.

8. Flameng W, Suy R, Schwartz F, Borgers M. Ultrastructural correlates of left ventricular contraction abnormalities in patients with chronic ischemic heart disease: Determinants of reversible segmental asynergy post revascularization surgery. Am Heart J 1981;102: 846-857.

9. Marwick TH, MacIntyre WJ, Lafont A, Nemec JJ, Salcedo EE. Metabolic responses of hibernating and infarcted myocardium to revascularization. Circulation 1992;85:1347-1353.

10. Dilsizian V, Perrone-Filardi P, Arrighi JA et al. Concordance and discordance between stress-redistribution-reinjection and rest-redistribution thallium imaging for assessing viable myocardium. Comparison with metabolic activity by positron emission tomography. Circulation 1993;88:941-952.

11. Bax JJ, Cornel JH, Visser FC et al. Comparison of Tl rest-redistribution and FDG SPECT in predicting functional recovery after revascularization. J Am Coll Cardiol 1996; in press.

Radioactive Isotopes in
Clinical Medicine and Research XXII
ed. by H. Bergmann, A. Kroiss and H. Sinzinger
© 1997 Birkhäuser Verlag Basel/Switzerland

MYOCARDIAL METABOLISM IN THYROID DYSFUNCTIONS OBSERVED BY PHOSPHOROUS-31 SPECTROSCOPY

P. Theissen, D. Moka, E. Voth, H. Schicha

Clinic for Nuclear Medicine
University of Cologne
D-50924 Cologne, Germany

SUMMARY

In the recent study it was proved whether metabolic changes of the myocardium in hypo- and hyperthyroid patients can be verified by in-vivo phosphorous-31 nuclear magnetic spectroscopy. Furthermore, it was evaluated whether there was a diminished left ventricular function at rest at the same time. The spectroscopic results showed a diminished intermediate phosphorous energy metabolism mainly determined by creatine phosphate decrease in hypo- and hyperthyroid patients. These deviations, however, were quantitatively more marked in the hyperthyroid patients and were fully reversible under hormone substitution in hypothyroid patients. Despite the changes of energy metabolism no decrease of left ventricular function occurred at rest.

INTRODUCTION

The skeletal muscle and the myocardium are preferred target organs of thyroid hormones. It is known that under both hyperthyroid and hypothyroid conditions functional changes of the myocardium can be observed by EKG, echocardiography, and radionuclide ventriculography. Phosphorous-31 magnetic resonance spectroscopy offers the unique opportunity to measure the phosphorous energy metabolism of cells non-invasively and in-vivo (1). Earlier spectroscopic studies could demonstrate quantitative changes of the phosphate energy metabolism of the skeletal muscle with hypothyroidism as well with overt and latent hyperthyroidism (2,3). Therefore, the present study should clarify whether changes of the phosphate energy metabolism can also be measured in myocardium as potential origin of the functional changes in hypo- and hyperthyroid patients which were observed by other authors In case of measurable changes of the phosphorous metabolism, it had to be proved whether they are reversible and accompanied by changes of the left ventricular function at rest conditions.

PATIENTS AND METHODS

Up to now, the recent study consisted of 13 hyperthyroid patients (4 male, 9 female) with a mean age of 40.4 ± 13.5 years. Eight patients were suffered from Graves disease and 5 from an autonomous goitre. The spectroscopic examination was done before start of treatment. The mean values of the thyroid hormone parameters are shown in table 1..

Table 1. Values of thyroid hormones for patients and healthy volunteers

	Euthyroid volunteers and patients	Hyperthyroid patients	Hypothyroid patients
TSHbasal (0.5 - 3.5 μIE/ml)	1.3 ± 0.5	≤ 0.1	57.7 ± 26.1
fT4 (0.8 - 2.3 ng/100ml)	1.4 ± 0.4	3.5± 1.9	0.6 ± 0.5
fT3 (2.0 - 5.0 pg/ml)	2.9 ± 0.5	7.4 ± 2.8	1.2 ± 0.8

The twenty-nine hypothyroid patients with thyroid carcinoma all had had thyroidectomy and were under hypothyroid conditions before a repeated radio iodine therapy. Of these patients 9 were male and 20 female. Their mean age was 46 ± 12 years. To prove the reversibility of changes in the hypothyroid patients a second spectroscopy was performed after 1 - 3 weeks of thyroid hormone substitution. For comparison 15 healthy volunteers were also examined by spectroscopy of the heart (mean age 34 ± 7 years; 9 women and 6 men). The hormone parameters are summarized in table 1..

The acquisition of the spectra and of the cardiac imaging was performed within a 1.5-Tesla whole body magnet (Gyroscan S15, Philips). The spectra were acquired by an image guided volume selection method using sagittal and transverse spin-echo slices of entire heart. The volume of interest comprized the myocardium of the anterior left ventricular wall, the anterior parts of the septum, of the diaphragmatic and lateral wall. The repetition time was 3000 ms. The data acquisition was triggered by EKG within systole to minimalize the contamination of the spectra by ATP from blood. The analysis of the spectra was done by an iterative deconvolution program. Corrections of the spectra were induced for partial saturation and for contamination with blood ATP by the known blood-specific 2,3-diphosphoglycerate (DPG)/ATP ratio (see figure 1.)(4). Because an external standard as in spectroscpoy of the skeletal muscle cannot be applied for technical reasons (2,3), the creatine phosphate (Pcr)/β-ATP and phosphodiester (PDE)/β-ATP ratios were used as parameter of the phosphate energy metabolism of the myocardium. This procedure assumes that ATP stays constant and is accepted in common practice (1,5).

Dynamic magnetic resonance imaging was used for the assessment of left ventricular function with sagittal and transverse midventricular gradient-echo slices at rest with a temporal resolution of 54 ms. The left ventricular ejection fraction was calculated by the area length method (normal range EF $\geq$ 55 compared to the values of the 15 healthy volunteers). For the assessment of left ventricular dilatation and myocardial thickness, measurements of the left ventricular diameter (normal: $\leq$ 60 mm) and of the thickness of the interventricular septum (IVS; normal range: 7 - 12 mm) at enddiastole were performed.

RESULTS

Significant changes of myocardial phosphorous metabolism with a decrease of the PCr/ATP ratio occurred in patients with hyper- and hypothyroidism. These changes are qualitatively simi-

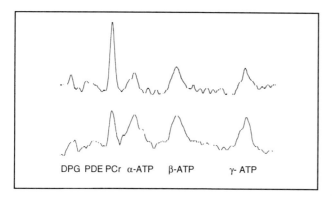

DPG PDE PCr α-ATP   β-ATP   γ- ATP

Figure 1.
Phosphorous-31spectra of a euthyroid volunteer (upper row) and of a hypothyroid patient (bottom row)

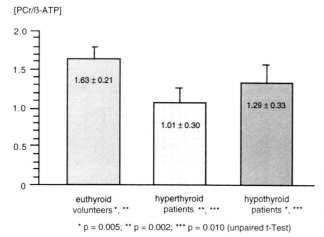

[PCr/ß-ATP]

euthyroid volunteers *, ** 1.63 ± 0.21

hyperthyroid patients **, *** 1.01 ± 0.30

hypothyroid patients *, *** 1.29 ± 0.33

* p = 0.005; ** p = 0.002; *** p = 0.010 (unpaired t-Test)

Figure 2.
PCr/ATP-ratio in hyper-thyroid patients compared to the euthyroid volunteers and the hypothyroid patients

lar in hyper- and hypothyroidism, but are quantitatively more marked in hyperthyroid patients (figure 1. and 2.). Comparing the peaks of PCr, figure 1. shows that in hyperthyroid patients

especially the intermediate metabolism of PCr seems to be affected. Hyperthyroid patients with
Graves disease showed a more intense PCr/ATP diminishing compared to the patients with
autonomous goitre (figure 3.). In patients with hypothyroidism an additional PDE/ATP increase
was observed in contrast to hyperthyroid patients (figure 5.).

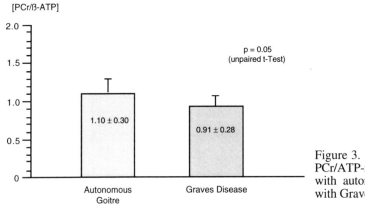

Figure 3.
PCr/ATP-ratio in patients
with autonomous goitre and
with Graves disease

Despite the metabolic changes no decrease of the left ventricular function could be found at rest
conditions. Hypo- and hyperthyroid patients showed normal LV ejection fraction (EF; 69 ± 9
%; MRI normal range ≥ 55 %) at rest as well as normal LV diameters and IVS thickness.
Neither a correlation between LVEF and PCr/ATP ratio (r = 0.31 resp. 0.23) nor between
PCr/ATP ratio and fT4 resp. fT3 (r = 0.29; 0.12 resp. 0.43; 0.25) could be found.

The PCr decrease and the PDE increase observed in hypothyroid patients were fully reversible
during hormone substitution (figure 4. and 5.).

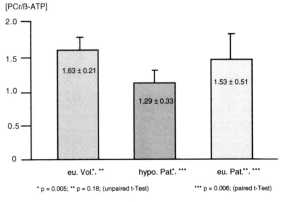

Figure 4.
PCr/ATP-ratio in hypothyroid
(hypo) patients compared to
euthyroid (eu) volunteers and
patients under hormone
substitution

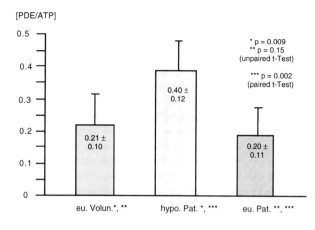

Figure 5.
PDE/ATP-ratio in hypothyroid patients compared to euthyroid (eu) volunteers and patients under hormone substitution

DISCUSSION

Since nuclear magnetic resonance spectroscopy can be applied also in-vivo it allowed important insights into pathophysiological aspects of different diseases as coronary artery disease, cardiomyopathy, and heart failure without invasive methods (6,7,8). Especially the significant decrease of the intermediate metabolite creatine phosphate in hypo- and hyperthyroidism which plays a direct role in the energy provision of myocardial contraction explains some aspects of the symptoms and clinical findings in these patients. Because both, skeletal muscle and myocardium are two of the preferred target organs of the thyroid hormones, it is understandable that these changes are similar in both organs in hyper- and in hypothyroidism. However, the increase of fT3 and fT4 seems to have a more intense influence on the phosphate energy metabolism in hyperthyroid patients (figure 2.). Up to now, it could not be clarified whether the decrease of PCr is due to changed mitochondrial function, a change of membrane transport capacity for phosphate ions in combination with diminished cellular phosphate concentrations, or changes of membrane receptor status. The recent findings may reflect (reversible) changes of enzymatic processes (e.g. of the creatine kinase), which are combined with cellular resp. mitochondrial remodelling processes in thyroid dysfunction. These processes are of special interest because also patients with ischaemic heart disease show a PCr decrease. Therefore, these change seem not to be specific for patients suffering from thyroid dysfunctions (7,8).

In contrast, until now only in hypothyroidism an increase of the phosphodiesters could be observed. This effect was comparable to that in the spectroscopic study on the skeletal muscle in hypothyroid patients (2).

In accordance with other studies concerning thyroid dysfunctions also the recent examination found no decrease of the LVEF or changes of the LV dimensions at rest conditions despite the described metabolic changes.

The observed changes in hypothyroid patients seemed to be fully revesible under hormone substitution. The reversibility also of the PDE increase in the hypothyroid patients may reflect passager catabolic changes of membrane metabolism without evidence of permanent cell damage.

REFERENCES

1. Bottomley PA, Hardy CJ, Roemer PB. Phosphate metabolite imaging and concentration measurements in human heart by nuclear magnetic resonance. Magn Reson Med 1990; 14:425-34
2. Moka D, Theissen P, Linden A, Waters W, Schicha H. Einfluß von Hyper- und Hypothyreose auf den Energiestoffwechsel der Skelettmuskulatur - Eine Untersuchung mit 31P-Kernspinspektroskopie. Nucl.-Med. 1991; 30:77-83
3. Theissen P, Kaldewey S, Moka D, Bunke J, Voth E, Schicha H. 31Phosphor-Kernspinspektroskopie: Gestörter Energiestoffwechsel bei latenter Hyperthyreose. Nucl.-Med. 1993; 32:134-9
4. Moka DC, Koppelmann S, Hahn J, Theissen P, Schicha H. Quantification of phosphate metabolites in human whole blood by 31-P-MRS. Eur. J. Nucl. Med. 1994; 21/10 (Suppl.): 164
5. Robitaille PM, Merkle H, Sako E, Lang G, Clack RM, Bianco R, From AH, Foker J, Ugurbil K. Measurement of ATP synthesis rates by 31P-NMR spectroscopy in the intact myocardium in vivo. Magn Reson Med 1990; 15:8-24
6. de Roos A, Doornbos J, Luyten PR, Osterwaal LJMP, van der Wall EE, den Hollander JA. Cardiac Metabolism in Patients with Dilated and Hypertrophic Cardiomyopathy: Assessment with Proton-decoupled P-31 MR Spectroscopy. J Magn Reson Imaging 1992; 2:711-9
7. Dilsizian V, Bonow RO. Current diagnostic techniques of assessing myocardial viability in patients with hibernating and stunned myocardium. Circulation 1993; 87:1-20
8. Neubauer S, Krahe T, Schindler R, Horn M, Hillenbrand J, Entzeroth C, Mader H, Kromer EP, Riegger GA, Lackner K. 31P magnetic resonance spectroscopy in dilated cardiomyopathy and coronary artery disease. Altered cardiac high-energy phosphate metabolism in heart failure. Circulation 1992; 86:1810-8

Radioactive Isotopes in
Clinical Medicine and Research XXII
ed. by H. Bergmann, A. Kroiss and H. Sinzinger
© 1997 Birkhäuser Verlag Basel/Switzerland

STRUCTURAL ALTERATIONS AND THE EFFECT OF CORONARY
REVASCULARIZATION ON MYOCARDIAL FUNCTION IN REGIONS WITH
MODERATE OR SEVERE PERSISTENT THALLIUM-201 DEFECTS

R. Zimmermann[1], J. Zehelein[1], B. Bubeck[2], G. Mall[3] and H. Tillmanns[4]

Departments of Cardiology[1], Nuclear Medicine[2], and Pathology[3], University of Heidelberg,
and Department of Cardiology[4], University of Gießen, Germany

SUMMARY: The extent of interstitial fibrosis and the effect of successful coronary artery bypass grafting on left ventricular function in myocardial regions with preoperatively reversible or persistent thallium-201 defects was investigated in 35 patients with coronary artery disease. The results provide additional evidence that the majority of regions with only mild-to-moderate persistent thallium-201 defects represents reversibly ischemic myocardium rather than myocardial scar tissue.

INTRODUCTION

Previous studies suggest that a part of myocardial regions with only moderate persistent thallium defects represents reversibly ischemic myocardium rather than myocardial scar tissue (1,2). Purpose of the present study was, therefore, to compare the structural alterations and the effect of coronary artery bypass surgery on left ventricular performance in myocardial segments with reversible and mild-to-moderate or severe persistent thallium-201 defects.

PATIENTS AND METHODS

The investigations were performed in 35 patients (5 female) with chronic coronary artery disease. The majority of the patients was suffering from multiple-vessel disease: 20 patients had triple-vessel disease, 18 patients two-vessel disease, and 7 patients had single-vessel disease.

Patients with a global left ventricular ejection fraction $< 35\%$ were not included because of a potentially higher risk for biopsy related complications. All patients had stable angina pectoris, mean age was 57 ± 7 years.

Patients underwent cardiac catheterization and stress thallium-201 scintigraphy with tracer reinjection within 2 months prior to coronary artery bypass grafting. During cardiopulmonary bypass, two transmural biopsy specimens were taken from the anterior left ventricular wall (before cardioplegia was begun) for the determination of the volume fraction of myocardial interstitial fibrosis. Cardiac catheterization was repeated 6 to 10 weeks after surgery.

The left ventricular performance before and after surgery was determined from the left ventricular angiograms obtained in the right anterior oblique view. The quantification of the anterolateral and inferior wall motion was performed using the centerline method as previously described (3).

Thallium scintigraphy was performed after symptom limited stress. Planar images were acquired in the anterior, LAO 30 degrees and LAO 60 degrees views immediately after stress and again after 4 hours of redistribution. Tracer reinjection was performed immediately after redistribution imaging and a third set of images was acquired 30 minutes later.

For quantitative assessment of the regional tracer uptake, for each projection, 9 regions of interest were automatically drawn by a computer program; the mean tracer activity in each of the vascular beds was related to the peak activity within the respective scintigram (4).

During aortocoronary bypass, but before instillation of cardioplegia, two transmural biopsy specimens were obtained from the anterior left ventricular wall using a biopsy needle with 1.5 mm diameter. As previously described (3), biopsies were fixed, dehydrated and embedded in epoxy resin. Semithin sections ($0.5~\mu m$) were then doublestained and the volume fraction of interstitial fibrosis - indicating the individual extent of irreversible myocardial damage - was determined using standard light microscopy (3).

RESULTS

Figure 1 demonstrates the results of the morphometric analyses in the different subgroups of patients according to their scintigraphic results. Defects were classified as mild-to-moderate if the residual tracer activity in the redistribution images remained between 65 and 80% of peak activity. Defects were classified as severe if the tracer activity remained below 65% of the peak activity. Patients with persistent defects were further subdivided into those who showed an improved tracer activity after reinjection (left bars) and into those who showed an unchanged tracer activity after reinjection (right bars).

Patients with reversible defects and patients with mild-to-moderate defects had a similar degree of interstitial fibrosis in the poststenotic myocardium (approx. 30 Vol%). Interstitial fibrosis was also similar in patients with severe defects at redistribution imaging, who showed an improvement in tracer activity after thallium reinjection. Interstitial fibrosis was significantly increased ($p < 0.05$) only in patients with severe persistent defects at redistribution imaging that remained unchanged after thallium reinjection (right bar).

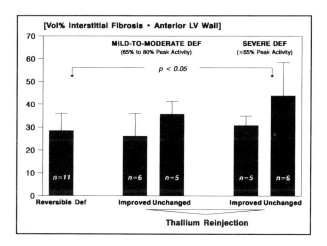

Figure 1. Mean interstitial fibrosis (± 1 SD) in the different subgroups of patients according to their scintigraphic results. Patients with reversible defects at the time of redistribution imaging are shown on the left, patients with mild-to-moderate defects in redistribution images are shown in the middle, and patients with severe persistent defects at the time of redistribution imaging are shown on the right.

Figure 2 demonstrates the changes in regional wall motion after coronary artery bypass grafting in the anterolateral and inferior left ventricular segments. Postoperative improvement in regional wall motion - indicated by the dark portion of the bars - was similar in patients with reversible defects, mild-to-moderate defects and severe defects that improved after reinjection. Improvement in regional wall motion was considerably less frequent only in patients with severe defects that persisted after thallium reinjection.

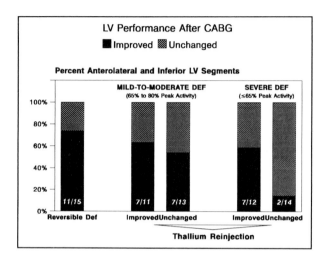

Figure 2. Changes in regional left ventricular (LV) performance after coronary artery bypass grafting (CABG) in the anterolateral and inferior LV segments.

CONCLUSION

In summary, the data provide additional evidence that the majority of myocardial regions with only mild-to-moderate persistent thallium-201 defects at the time of redistribution imaging represents reversibly ischemic myocardium rather than myocardial scar tissue. Only severe persistent defects after reinjection are associated with an higher degree of interstitial fibrosis. In these segments, regional myocardial function also improves less frequently after coronary revascularization.

REFERENCES

1. Bonow RO, Dilsizian V, Cuocolo A, Bacharach SL. Identification of viable myocardium in patients with chronic coronary artery disease and left ventricular dysfunction. Comparison of thallium scintigraphy with reinjection and PET imaging with 18F-Fluorodeoxyglucose. Circulation 1991; 83: 26-37

2. Dilsizian V, Freedman NMT, Bacharach SL, Perrone-Filardi P, Bonow RO. Regional thallium uptake in irreversible defects. Magnitude of change in thallium activity after re-injection distinguishes viable from nonviable myocardium. Circulation 1992; 85:627-634

3. Zimmer G, Zimmermann R, Hess OM, Schneider J, Kübler W, Krayenbuehl HP, Hagl S, Mall G. Decreased concentration of myofibrils and myofiber hypertrophy are structural determinants of impaired left ventricular function in patients with chronic heart diseases: a multiple logistic regression analysis. J Am Coll Cardiol 1992; 20: 1135-1142

4. Zimmermann R, Mall G, Rauch B, Zimmer G, Gabel M, Bubeck B, Tillmanns H, Hagl S, Kübler W. Residual thallium-201 activity in irreversible defects as marker of myocardial viability. Clinicopathological study. Circulation 1995; 91: 1016-1021

Radioactive Isotopes in
Clinical Medicine and Research XXII
ed. by H. Bergmann, A. Kroiss and H. Sinzinger
© 1997 Birkhäuser Verlag Basel/Switzerland

IMAGING OF MYOCARDIAL AMYLOID INVOLVEMENT
WITH 99m - Tc APROTININ

C. Aprile, M.G.Marinone, R. Saponaro, G. Cannizzaro,
G. Calsamiglia, E. Anesi, G. Merlini

Fondazione S.Maugeri,IRCCS- Nuclear Med. Serv; Policlinico
S.Matteo,IRCCS-Inst. of Clinical Med. II and Research Lab.
Biotechnology. Pavia-Italy

SUMMARY: We report on the use of 99m Tc-Aprotinin in the
detection of myocardial amyloid involvement in a population of
45 pts with amyloidosis and 22 control subjects with renal and
cardiac disease. Positive scans were obtained in 19 pts, no
cardiac uptake was observed in the remaining 25 and in the
controls. These results ,confirmed by histology in 4 pts and by
clinical-instrumental follow-up in 38, indicate TcA as a low-
cost readily available tracer for cardiac amyloidosis detection.

INTRODUCTION

Clinically overt heart involvement is oberved in about 55% of

pts with AL-amyloidosis and represents the most powerful

prognostic factor(1,2). We recently reported (3) on the

possibility to image extrasplanchnic amyloid deposits with the

antiserine protease inhibitor Aprotinin labelled with Tc-99m

(TcA). The aim of this study was to evaluate the possible role

of this tracer in the detection of myocardial involvement, in

view also of new therapeutical possibilities (4,5).

MATERIALS AND METHODS

Fiftysix scintigraphic studies were performed in 45 pts(median

age 57 years, range 32-80), 43 of them presenting with the light

chain form (AL) and the remaining two with the hereditary type

(AF). Twenty-two pts (median age 57, range 28-74) with renal and

cardiac disease served as control group. The following echo and

electrocardiographic parameters were considered: voltage (V, sum

in mm of S in V1 plus R in V5); CSA (cross sectional area, sq
cm/sq m BSA); interventricular septum thickness (IVS) in cm;
percent ejection fraction (EF); presence of granular sparkling
(GS);Voltage to Mass ratio (V/M); V-M relation according to
Carrol (6),where CSA >10 and V <15 indicates the pathological
area. On the basis of clinical and conventional diagnostic
modalities, myocardial involvement was judged to be unlikely
(score 0), suspected (sc.1), probable without (sc.2) or with
(sc.3) heart failure.The results of endomyocardial biopsy were
available for 3 pts and of a post-mortem examination for 1 pt.
In 34 pts the follow-up time was longer than 6 months.

Anterior and LAO views (preset time:5 and 10 min respectively)
of the thoracic area were taken 90 min after i.v. administration
of 350-400 MBq of TcA ,corresponding to 500-1200 KIU of
aprotinin). In addition, six pts were studied with 131 I
labelled SAP (serum amyloid P component) within one week (7).

Non parametric statistics tests (Kruskall-Wallis and Mann-
Whitney) were employed.

RESULTS

Significant cardiac uptake was detected in 19 pts with
amyloidosis (18 AL and 1 AF)(H+); LAO views confirmed that the
observed uptake was related to the myocardial wall and was not
due to the blood pool (Fig.1). The ratio between posterolateral
wall and apparently non involved lung ranged between 1.6 and
2.3. Usually, the activity was uniform throughout the ventricle,
and the apparently higher uptake in the inferior wall was due to
the scattering photons from the relatively higher liver
activity.In the remaining amyloid pts (H-), as well as in the
control group (C),no myocardial uptake was detectable. One of
the 6 pts studied with iodine labelled SAP,had a positive TcA
heart scan while all the SAP studies were negative. Positive
heart scans were confirmed by histology in 3 pts; in the fourth
pt, who had a negative myocardial histology, TcA scan was

negative but a pathological uptake could be recognized in the pericardium and pleuro-pulmonary structures; this finding also was confirmed by biopsy.

The relationship between scan results and echo and ECG parameters is shown in Table I: IVS thickness,V/M and EF were found significantly different in the three groups compared. These differences were significant even if pts with amyloidosis were taken into account, but not when H+ and C were compared.

Table I. Median values and range observed in amyloidosis pts with positive (H+),negative (H-) TcA heart scan and controls (C). The percentage of pathological findings is shown.

	H+ median (range)	%	H- median (range)	%	C median (range)	%	significance H+,H,C	H+,H-	H+ C
V	16 (8-22)	73	17 (9-25)	33	20 (5.5-41)	36	ns	ns	ns
IVS	1.5 (1.1-1.8)	84	1.7 (.8-1.7)	28	1.2 (.7-1.6)	35	.028	.003	ns
CSA	11.6 (8.2-18)	83	11.2 (6.2-16)	62	12 (8-14.8)	70	ns	ns	ns
EF	47 (25-60)	55	58 (46-69)	5	55 (14-68)	29	.0003	.0001	ns
GS	-	31	-	5	-	0	-	-	-
V/M	.96 (.6-1.8)	87	1.21 (.8-2.1)	50	1.9 (.8-31)	43	.03	.01	ns
V-M	-	73	-	22	-	36	-	-	-

Table II compares the cardiac involvement assesed by clinical and conventional instrumental findings with the results of TcA scintigraphy and the actual assesement of the presence of disease.The question point in the table indicates pts in whom a final diagnosis could not be reached because of short follow-up time or because the pts were lost for further follow-up.Two pts with score 0 had a positive scan and both showed later signs of cardiac involvement,with sudden death of 1 pt attributable to cardiac causality. In the score 1 group, a pt with positive scan did not show significant changes 8 mo after the scan, while in the other the elapsed time was too short to draw any conclusion; in another scan results were confirmed by biopsy. Four H- pts did not show clinical/instrumental changes in the observation

time ranging from 6 to 18 mo, one too had a negative SAP scan
and the last had only 1 mo follow-up time. Among the pts with
score 2, H+ evolved toward heart failure in 5 cases, in one
cardiac involvement was confirmed by nechroscopy and one died of
accidental death about 3 mo after scan when a deterioration of
the cardiac function was appearing. One H- pt did not show
myocardial uptake with SAP scintigraphy; the other did not
change his clinical status 6 mo after the scan, thereafter he
was lost for further follow-up. All scans in group 3 gave
positive findings, confirmed by clinical evolution.

Table II. Comparison among the pre-test clinical and
conventional diagnostic modalities (CDM), TcA myocardial scan
results and the actual assessement of infiltrative disease

CDM	TcA Scan		Actual Disease Status		
	−	+	−	?	+
score 0	18	2	18	0	2
score 1	6	3	6	2	1
score 2	2	10	1	1	10
score 3	0	4	0	0	4

Figure 1: Positive TcA scan in amyloidosis pts with cardiac
involvement. H- indicates a pt with negative scan.

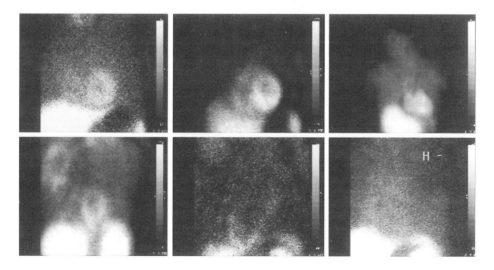

DISCUSSION

The rapid blood clearance of TcA (8) allows a sufficient contrast between target myocardium and background and,consequently, a significant imaging may be attained. The liver uptake is proportionally higher and is inversely related to renal function. Diffuse lung amyloid involvement may constitute a problem because of lowering heart to lung ratio; this problem however was observed only in one pt.

Conventional echo and ECG paremeters show an acceptable sensitivity. However statistical differences in IVS,CSA and EF are significant among the groups under study and betwen H+ and H-, but not between H- and C, there is a wide overlapping of values thus lowering the specificity of these parameters. Only granular sparkling appearance seems quite a specific parameter; however, it shows a low sensitivity, being appreciable only in 31% of H+. In addition, a low EF means only that contractile impairement is more probable in pts with infiltrative disease. In a similar way the voltage-mass relation in our series provides an index of disease severity in symptomatic pts,but does not offer sufficient specificity (6,9,10).

When TcA scan results are compared with the conventional clinical and instrumental assessement of infiltrative disease, it is interesting to note how positive scan were obtained and further confirmed by the clinical course in 2 pts without any sign of cardiac involvement at the time of the study. Conversely, in two cases TcA failed to confirm the clinical impression, both pts had a negative iodine labelled SAP study, but in both cases the follow-up time was too short to classify them as false or true negative results. On the other side SAP failed to image cardiac involvement in one pt with positive TcA scan.

It is not yet possible to draw final conclusions from the data obtained, because a longer follow-up period is mandatory to assess the accuracy of the test. However, some aspects must be regarded with interest,that is the ability of the tracer to depict early organ involvement before clinical or instrumental findings of disease are present, aiding in the differentiation of pts with suspected disese. In addition technetium single-step labelling and the short time interval between injection and scan, indicates TcA as a potential tracer of amyloidotic myocardial involvement.

REFERENCES

1.Kyle RA,Gertz MA. Cardiac amyloidosis. Int J Cardiol 1990;28:139-141.

2.Merlini G, Marinone MG,Anesi EF,Ascari E. Report of an italian study protocol of AL amyloidosis. Blood 1994;84(suppl):179a.

3. Aprile C, Marinone MG, Saponaro R,Bonino C,Merlini G. Cardiac and pleuropulmonary AL amyloid imaging with technetium-99 labelled Aprotinin. Eur J Nucl Med 1995;22:139-1401

4.Merlini G. Treatment of primary amyloidosis. Semin Haematol 1995;32:60-79.

5.Gianni L,Bellotti V,Gianni AM,Merlini G. New drug therapy of amyloidoses: Resorption of AL-type deposits with 4'-iodo-4'-deoxydoxorubicin. Blood 1995;86:855-861

6.Carrol JD,Gaasch WH,Mc Adam KPWJ. Amyloid cardiomyopathy: carachterization by distinct voltage/mass relation. Am J Cardiol 1983;52:137-146.

7.Hawkins PN,Lavender JP,Pepys MB. Evaluation of systemic amyloidosis by scintigraphy with 123-I-labeled serum amyloid P component. N Engl J Med 1990;325:508-513.

8.Aprile C,Saponaro R,Villa G, Lunghi F. 99mTc-Aprotinin: comparison with 99mTc-DMSA in normal and diseased kidneys. Nucl Med 1984;23:22-26.

9.Simons M, Isner JM. Assesment of relative sensitivities of non invasive tests for cardiac amyloidosis in documented cardiac amyloidosis. Am J Cardiol 1992;69:425-427.

10.Falk RH, Plehn JF,Deering T et al. Sensitivity and specificity of the echocardiographic features of cardiac amyloidosis. Am J Cardiol 1987;59:418-422.

Radioactive Isotopes in
Clinical Medicine and Research XXII
ed. by H. Bergmann, A. Kroiss and H. Sinzinger
© 1997 Birkhäuser Verlag Basel/Switzerland

THROMBORESISTANCE IS A VASCULAR PROPERTY

Sinzinger H., Karanikas G., Kritz H., Granegger Susanne, Mosing Bettina

Department of Nuclear Medicine, University of Vienna, Austria

SUMMARY: Platelet - vessel wall interaction is of key importance in regulating hemostatic balance. In order to examine, whether platelets or the vessel wall are the key determinant we performed in-vitro and in-vivo (perfusion and cross-perfusion) studies in rabbits, where either the vessel wall or the platelets have been pretreated with prostaglandins or prostaglandin-synthesis stimulating agents. The resulting platelet deposition was determined among others (e.g. morphometry) by counting the radioactivity of deposited ^{111}In-oxine labeled platelets. In-vitro perfusion studies reflect platelet function as important regulator of hemostasis, while - in contrast - in-vivo perfusion and cross-perfusion clearly demonstrate that the vessel wall rather than the platelets is responsible for preventing vascular deposition. It thus can be concluded, that the prostaglandin (I_2)-synthetizing capacity of the arterial wall is the main thromborepellant regulator of hemostasis in-vivo.

INTRODUCTION

Vascular endothelial cells are regulating hemostasis and are therefore of key importance for atherogenesis. Earlier studies examining platelet - vessel wall interaction perfusing citrated blood through a perfusion chamber (1) discovered relevant factors leading to platelet adhesion and platelet aggregation. They found biological factors, the chemical and in particular the physical properties of the exposed surface and platelet function as most relevant parameters. Prostaglandins (PG) as well as the inhibition of their synthesis (acetylsalicylic acid; ASA) have been shown to be of critical relevance for hemostatic balancing (2). While a great many studies are available on regulating factors, the extent to which platelets and / or the vessel wall are contributing to thromboresistance in-vivo, however, still needs to be examined.

It was thus the aim of this study to assess

    * whether intact endothelial vascular mediator production regulates thromboresistance

    * the effect of platelet pretreatment and / or

    * vascular pretreatment on thromboresistance and

    * the effect on PGI_2-synthesis stimulation on thromboresistance.

MATERIAL AND METHODS

Human and rabbit arterial and venous segments mounted on a rod (Fig. 1) were perfused in a Baumgartner chamber (3) under standardized conditions (RR 120/60 mmHg, 60 Hz, pulsatile flow, 37° C) using citrated (3.8 %) human blood.. Flow conditions were similar to the ones in human femoral artery (Fig. 2). Platelets were derived from human blood and radiolabelled using 111In-oxine as described earlier (4). In-vivo (cross-) perfusion (Fig. 3, 4) was performed in 6 months aged male rabbits under the same perfusion conditions as outlined in figures 1 and 2. Deposition of radiolabeled platelets was counted (cts/mm^2/min).

Statistical methods: Values are given as mean ± SD; calculation for significance was performed using Student´s t-test. A $p < 0.01$ was considered as being significant.

Figure 1: Baumgartner in-vitro perfusion

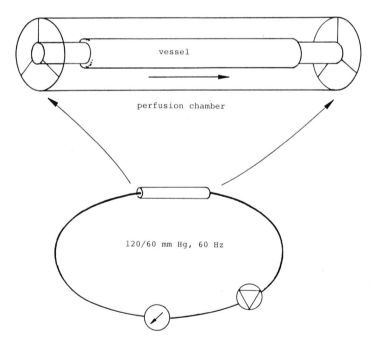

In-vitro perfusion of an everted vessel mounted on a rod under standardized flow conditions. The vessel is no longer able to produce prostaglandins, nitric oxide and other thromborepellant mediators. This system, thus nicely reflects platelet function, but not hemostatic balancing.

Figure 2: Volume rate flow

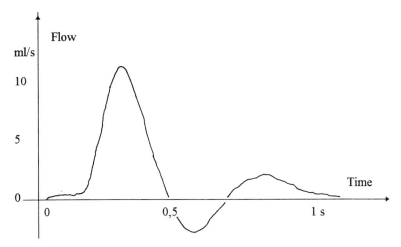

The volume rate flow achieved in the perfusion system is comparable to the one in human femoral arteries.

Figure 3: In-vivo perfusion

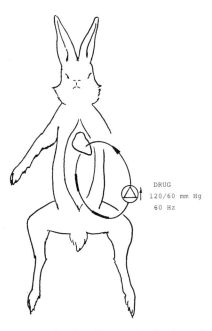

Rabbit aorta and iliac artery were perfused under standardized conditions in-vivo allowing to assess interaction of intact local mediators producing vessel wall with platelets.

Figure 4: In-vivo cross-perfusion

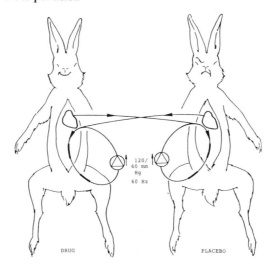

The cross perfusion system allows to monitor thrombogenicity in-vivo and to assess the interaction of drug treated vessel wall with placebo treated platelets and vice versa and thereby to identify the key hemostatic regulator under in-vivo conditions.

RESULTS

Platelet deposition during vascular in-vitro perfusion in absence of endothelial (vascular) mediator production is almost exclusively dependent on platelet function and not on the vessel wall. Within 10 minutes (table 1) platelet adhesion to any kind of vascular (arterial vs. venous) surface (intact vs. deendothelialized) of any species (rat, rabbit, human at least) reaches a maximum.

Table 1. Time course of aortic ^{111}In-oxine platelet deposition

minutes	intact	deendothelialized	n
1	9 ± 4 *	107 ± 31 *	6
2	14 ± 3 *	153 ± 26 *	8
3	17 ± 4	169 ± 28	6
5	23 ± 5	201 ± 28	6
10	25 ± 6	254 ± 23	8
15	24 ± 4	251 ± 26	5
20	25 ± 5	260 ± 22	6

$x \pm SD$; * $p < 0.01$ (vs. 10 min.); values in cts/mm^2/min
After an about 10-minutes perfusion a steady platelet deposition is achieved.

No difference in actual deposition of platelets is observed between arterial and venous tissue (table 2). In-vivo perfusion, however, clearly shows that - in contrast to the in-vitro findings - the intact vascular mediator production (table 3) is the key regulator of thromboresistance. In-vivo cross-perfusion shows that stimulating vascular PGI_2-production improves, while its blockade deteriorates hemostatic balance. Testing the same compounds (PGI_2, PGE_1, isradipine (stimulation of PGI_2-production), acetylsalicylic acid (blockade of cyclooxygenase) as well as placebo) on their role on platelets indicates, that they are only of minor relevance as compared to the vessel wall. Substances stimulating vascular PGI_2-formation (calcium antagonists, ACE-inhibitors and others) and physiological regulators (plasma factor) are improving hemostatic balance.

Table 2. In-vitro platelet interaction with subendothelium

vessel	species	n	adhesion[1]	^{111}In-oxine platelets[2]
a	H	8	81.0 ± 3.7	255.0 ± 34.1
v	H	7	83.4 ± 5.2	268.9 ± 41.2
a	R	16	89.7 ± 3.6	327.5 ± 30.7
v	R	9	88.6 ± 4.2	316.7 ± 29.8

$x \pm SD$; a......arteries, v......veins, H......human, R......rabbit; [1] % surface covered with contact and spread platelets, [2] $cts/mm^2/min$
In absence of endothelial mediators in-vitro no differences between arterial and venous tissue and only small ones between human and rabbit source can be found.

Table 3. Effect of endothelial lining on ^{111}In-oxine platelet deposition

	I	D
aorta	24 ± 5	256 ± 22
iliac artery	24 ± 4	318 ± 13

$x \pm SD$; n = 6 each; I......intact, D......deendothelialized
Platelet deposition on deendothelialized segments is about one order of magnitude higher as compared to intact areas.

Pretreatment of vascular tissue with acetylsalicylic acid (inhibition of PGI_2-synthesis) does not only abolish the beneficial effect of PGI_2 (table 4) on thromboresistance, but to a certain extent even also induce hemostatic imbalance.

Although the absolute values are somewhat differing (table 3), the findings for the abdominal aorta and the iliac arteries in all the in-vivo experiments are quite comparable. Morphometric data counting adhering and aggregating platelets as well as platelet thrombus formation revealed comparable results to radioactive counting of 111In-oxine labeled platelets (tables 2, 5).

Table 4. Deposition of ^{111}In-oxine labeled platelets and denuded aortic PGI$_2$-formation

	deposition[1]	PGI$_2$-synthesis[2]
isradipine	163 ± 25*	32.6 ± 4.6*
+ ASA	286 ± 41	1.3 ± 0.4*
control	271 ± 38	21.7 ± 3.6
ASA	326 ± 39	1.1 ± 0.3*

x ± SD; n = 8 each; [1] in cts/mm^2/min; [2] in pg/mg/min; * p < 0.01 (vs. control)
ASA abolishes PGI$_2$-synthesis and enhances platelet deposition.

Table 5. Quantification of platelet deposition on deendothelialized aorta. Comparison between morphometric results and radioactive counting.

	C	C + S	cts/mm^2/min
isradipine	9.3 ± 2.1*	71.4 ± 4.4*	176 ± 41*
+ ASA	19.9 ± 3.3*	94.6 ± 6.1*	297 ± 57
control	14.7 ± 2.0	84.9 ± 5.6	265 ± 41
ASA	20.6 ± 3.2*	99.8 ± 5.3*	324 ± 57*

x ± SD; n = 6 each group; * p < 0.01 vs. control
C......contact platelets, C + S......C + spread platelets (% surface involved)
There is a strong correlation between morphometric and radioisotopic findings.

These beneficial effects found on thromboresistance after PGE$_1$, for example, are surprisingly long-lasting and can still be monitored if the treatment has been done 6 hours before or even longer.

Table 6. Relevance of pretreatment (PGE$_1$) using in-vivo cross-perfusion of deendothelialized aorta

vessel/platelets	cts/mm^2/min
PGE$_1$/PGE$_1$	138 ± 21*
PGE$_1$/vehicle	189 ± 34*
vehicle/PGE$_1$	221 ± 45
vehicle/vehicle	261 ± 36

x ± SD; n = 6 each group; * p < 0.01 vs. respective control
Platelet deposition is significantly lower with pretreated vessels as compared to pretreated platelets.

DISCUSSION

These perfusion experimental findings clearly reveal (table 6) that the preserved mediator production (and in particular of PGI_2) by the vessel wall, even if deendothelialized, is of central importance (5, 6, 7, 8) for regulation of hemostasis. Perfusion of 10 minutes duration is sufficient in order to elucidate the respective behaviour and avoids relevant biochemical changes (pO2, PCO2; pH) seen after longer duration of the experiments (9).

Figure 5: Gammacamera image of ^{111}In-oxine labeled platelets

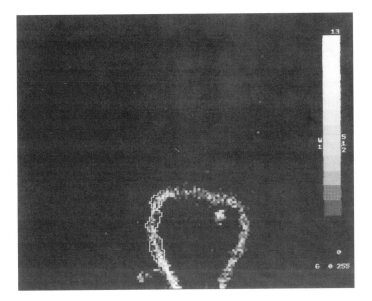

Outlook

The model established also allows in-vitro as well as in-vivo perfusion under controlled conditions of stenosis, surface conditions etc. Monitoring platelet deposition engymetrically as well as by gamma-camera images (fig. 5) using this model especially might contribute to a better understanding of how positively imaged areas are morphologically in-vivo looking alike.

REFERENCES

1. Baumgartner HR, Muggli R, Tschopp TB, Turitto VT. Platelet adhesion, release and and aggregation in flowing blood: effects of surface properties and platelet function. Haemost. 1976; 35: 124-138.

2. Moncada S, Gryglewski R, Bunting S, Vane JR. An enzyme isolated from arteries transforms prostaglandin endoperoxides to an unstable substance that inhibits platelet aggregation. Nature 1976; 263: 663-665.

3. Tschopp TB, Baumgartner HR, Silberbauer K, Sinzinger H. Platelet adhesion and platelet thrombus formation on subendothelium of human arteries and veins exposed to flowing blood in vitro. A comparison with rabbit aorta. Haemost. 1979; 8: 19-29.

4. Sinzinger H., Kolbe H., Strobl-Jäger E, Höfer R. A simple and safe technique for sterile autologous platelet labeling using monovette vials. Eur. J. Nucl. Med. 1984; 9: 320-322.

5. Sinzinger H, Keiler A, O´Grady J. The arterial wall rather than the platelets is responsible for the diminished thrombogenicity during isradipine therapy. J. Cardiovasc. Pharmacol. 1995; 25: 453-458

6. Buchanan MR, Dejana E, Gent M, Mustard JF. Enhanced platelet accumulation onto injured carotid arteries in rabbits after aspirin treatment. J. Clin. Invest. 1981; 67: 503-509.

7. Adelman B, Stemerman MB, Mennell D, Handin RI. The interaction of platelets with aortic subendothelium: inhibition of adhesion and secretion by prostaglandin I_2. Blood 1981; 58: 198-205.

8. Tschopp TB, Baumgartner HR. Platelet adhesion and mural platelet thrombus formation on aortic subendothelium of rats, rabbits and guinea pigs correlate negatively with the vascular PGI_2 production. J. Lab. Clin. Med. 1981: 98: 402-411.

9. Huber L., Karanikas G., Sinzinger H., Schima H. Simulation des Blutflusses in peripheren Arterien mit einem Kreislaufmodell mit minimalem Füllungsvolumen. Abstract, BMT-Kongress 1996, Universität und ETH Zürich.

Physics

Radioactive Isotopes in
Clinical Medicine and Research XXII
ed. by H. Bergmann, A. Kroiss and H. Sinzinger
© 1997 Birkhäuser Verlag Basel/Switzerland

ATTENUATION CORRECTION IN CARDIAC SPET
USING TWO GD-153 LINE SOURCES - FIRST CLINICAL RESULTS

R. Kluge, A. Seese and W.H. Knapp

Department of Nuclear Medicine, University of Leipzig, Germany

SUMMARY: The aim of the study was to assess the benefit of simultaneous transmission
and emission imaging using two Gd-153 line sources (ADAC Vertex, Vantage system). 35
patients without evidence of cardiac disease and 10 patients with posterolateral wall
infarctions under-went SPET with and without attenuation correction after administration of
400 MBq Tc-99m-Tetrofosmin. The non-uniformity of the mean count profile in polar maps
decreased in normal subjects significantly (range in non-corrected studies: 35.8 ± 10.8 %,
in attenuation corrected studies: $20.9 \pm 3,3$ %). In patients with CAD, extent and severity
of defects were more clearly represented.

INTRODUCTION

Photon attenuation by different layers of tissue between heart and body surface is a
well known problem in myocardial perfusion scintigraphy (3). In particular, the complex
and irregular geometry of tissues with different densities (lungs, bone, soft tissue) and the
variable location of the heart in the chest are responsible for interindividually varying non-
uniform attenuation artifacts (2).

Generally, attenuation produces a non-uniform representation of the activity distribution
within the myocardium, especially in SPET studies (6). Attempts to correct for non-uniform
attenuation have been made in order to improve sensitivity and specificity of myocardial
scintigraphy (1, 7).

This present study deals with the effects of the attenuation correction using a dual-head
camera and two movable Gd-153 line sources on myocardial scintigrams. In particular,
following questions are to be answered:

(a)   Does attenuation correction decrease segmental differences in count density in
        patients without heart disease?

(b)   Is the degree by which images are corrected, related to body mass or gender?

(c)   Does attenuation correction result in a reduced variability of normal
            circumferential profiles, thus facilitating the quantitative discrimination between
            normal and abnormal scintigrams?
(d)   Does attenuation correction result in an enhanced pathological activity
            distribution in CAD?

PATIENTS AND METHODS

        A group of 35 patients (20 female and 15 male) with low likelihood for CAD
underwent myocardial SPET with and without attenuation correction. A second patient
group was formed by 10 male patients after posterolateral or inferior wall infarction.
The patients underwent Tc99m-Tetrofosmin stress imaging using 360° data acquisition.
During the acquisition two Gd-153 line sources (200 mCi, 100 keV, $t_{1/2} = 242$ d) are
opposite to the two 90 ° detector heads and are moved along two planes parallel to those of
either detector surface. The transmission data are acquired in an electronically controlled
window (5 cm wide) moving synchronously with the line source over the detector. This
allows simultaneous acquisition of emission data outside the window using different energy
channels.
For reconstruction of the attenuation tomograms filtered back projection (Butterworth
filter, cut off 0.5, order 5) was used. Transversal slices were calculated from emission data
using an iterative reconstruction algorithm. During the iteration the algorithm made use of
the attenuation images pixelwise. Using 12 iterations about 1 min was required for
reconstruction.

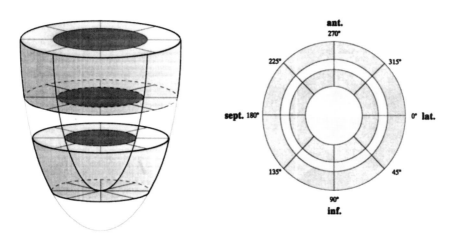

Figure 1.   Schematic representation of wall segments quantitated. Left: Myocardial
                short axis slices near apex and basis. Right: Wall segments are represented by
                8 equidistant wall segments

For quantification of the effects, profiles of circumferential counts in short axis slices were calculated in a basis-near and an apex-near slice. These two slices were further analysed by counting the events within 8 wall segments (Fig. 1).

RESULTS AND DISCUSSION

By visual evaluation, non-corrected studies frequently revealed reduced count density of the inferior wall, while attenuation corrected count densities of the inferior wall equaled those of the other wall segments in the same individuals. The activity distribution thus appeared more homogeneous. In female patients there was an additional visual effect: apart from increased activity representation of the inferior wall by attenuation correction, the relative count density of the anterior wall was also increased.
In men, non-corrected studies showed the lowest count rates in the inferior wall segments, followed by the inferoseptal wall segments whereas the highest count rates were observed in the anterior, and anterolateral segments. Minima in females were located in the inferior, inferoseptal and septal segments. The maxima were located in the lateral wall. The maximal differences in segmental count rates of each individual averaged 38.6 % in men and 33.4 % in women. In attenuation corrected studies the respective segmental differences averaged only 20,9 % (Fig. 2). In both male and female patients relative count density increased significantly in the inferolateral, inferior, inferoseptal and septal wall segments. The reduction of segmental count differences by attenuation correction produces a considerable reduction of the interindividual variability in normals. Thereby an improved definition of the

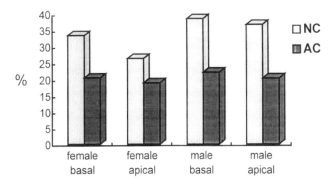

Figure 2.   Mean differences between maximal and minimal values of count profiles in non-corrected and attenuation corrected studies.

normal range of count distributions in myocardial SPET images is obtained. It can be hypothesized that attenuation correction therefore improves the differentiation between normal and impaired myocardial blood flow representation.

In none of the 10 patients with inferior wall infarction the inferior count deficit was overcompensated by attenuation correction. On the contrary, attenuation corrected images showed a more distinct delineation of the infarcted region well correlated with angiographic results. In non-corrected studies, however, such a clear-cut delineation between count deficits caused by attenuation or by real defects was not possible.

The quantitative assessment of the perfusion defect is significantly improved by attenuation correction. The segment of the profile courve corresponding to the region involved in the infarction is definitely more distant from the normal range than in the non-corrected images (Fig. 3).

A significant improvement of delineation of pathological count densities in inferior wall infarctions was obtained for the group of 10 patients investigated. The maximal distance of the individual count profiles from the normal range averaged 25.9 % in attenuation corrected studies, in NC studies, however, only 16.4 %. In one patient a small pathological defect in the inferoapical area which was verified by angiography was visible only in attenuation corrected , images, but could not be identified in the non-corrected study.

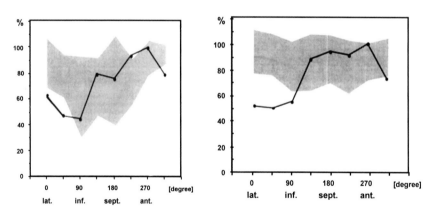

Figure 3.   Male patient after posterolateral wall infarction. Count rate profile in non-corrected (left) and attenuation corrected (right) studies in comparison to the normal range (mean ± twofold SD).

It is suggested that the accuracy of SPET for the prediction of RCA stenoses - unsatisfactory until now (4, 5) - will be improved by attenuation correction.

CONCLUSION

Non-corrected myocardial SPET studies show considerable systematic regional differences in count rate distributions of normal subjects due to attenuation effects. Attenuation corrected studies exhibited significantly smaller segmental differences in relative count rates. The relative count density increased significantly in inferolateral, inferior and inferoseptal segments. This effect of attenuation correction produces considerable narrowing of the width of normal range for the count rate distribution. First results suggest that diagnosis of RCA lesions will be improved by attenuation correction, but the diagnostic performance of both methods has to be clarified in further studies.

REFERENCES

1. Bailey DL, Hutton BF, Walter PJ. Improved SPECT using simultaneous emission and transmission tomography. J Nucl Med 1987;28:844-851.

2. Esquerre J-P, Coca FJ, Martinez SJ, Guiraud RF. Prone decubitus: a solution to inferior wall attenuation in thallium-201 myocardial tomography. J Nucl Med 1989;30:398-401.

3. Jaszczak RJ, Coleman RE, Whitehead FR. Physical factors affecting quantitative measurements using camera-based single photon emission computed tomography. IEEE Trans Nucl Sci 1981;28:69-80.

4. Kahn JK, McGhie I, Akers MS, et al. . Quantitative rotational tomography with 201 Tl and 99m Tc-2-methoxy-isobutyl. A direct comparison in normal individuals and patients with coronary artery disease. Circulation 1989;79:1282-1293.

5. Kiat H, Vantrain KF, Maddahi J, et al. . Development and prospective application of quantitative 2-day stress-rest Tc-99m methoxy isobutyl SPECT for the diagnosis of coronary artery disease. Am Heart J 1990;120:1255-1266.

6. Manglos SH, Thomas FD, Gagne GM, Hellwig BJ. Phantom study of breast tissue attenuation in myocardial imaging. J Nucl Med 1993;34:992-996.

7. Tan P, Bailey DL, Meikle SR, Eberl S, Fulton RR, Hutton BF. A scanning line source for simultaneous emission and transmission measurements in SPECT. J Nucl Med 1993;34:1752-1760.

Radioactive Isotopes in
Clinical Medicine and Research XXII
ed. by H. Bergmann, A. Kroiss and H. Sinzinger
© 1997 Birkhäuser Verlag Basel/Switzerland

18-FDG SINGLE PHOTON EMISSION COMPUTED TOMOGRAPHY IN HEART AND BRAIN SCINTIGRAPHY: INSTRUMENTATION AND PHYSICAL ASPECTS

C. Haas[1], E. Hillbrand[1], T. Hoch[1], H. Fritzsche[2]

[1]Department of Medical Physics, [2]Department of Nuclear Medicine
Landeskrankenhaus Feldkirch, Carinagasse 47, A-6800 Feldkirch, Austria

Summary: The physical properties of a conventional dual-head gamma camera system with particularly designed extra-high-energy collimators for the purpose of detecting radiation from positron emitters were investigated. The system sensitivity for F-18 was found to be 50.3 cpm / 37 kBq, which is 25 % of the sensitivity for Tc-99m with a high-resolution collimator. The FWHM of the line spread function for a source-collimator distance of 10 cm was measured to 12.0 mm in air. Reconstructed images of a SPECT phantom showed the necessity for a Compton correction in double-isotope studies with both F-18 and Tc-99m, which is performed by counting photons in a third energy window at 170 keV.

Introduction

Since the development of positron emission tomography scanners (PET), F-18-Fluoro-deoxyglucose (FDG) and other positron emitters have attained increasing importance in metabolic studies. Imaging annihilation photons (511 keV) of electron-positron-interactions with gamma cameras is a cheaper alternative to obtain diagnostic information on the glucose metabolism in addition to perfusion studies usually performed with Tc-99m (140 keV gamma ray energy).

In our department a conventional dual-head gamma camera system is in use, which is equipped with a pair of collimators especially designed for imaging 511 keV radiation. The system is clinically used for double-isotope studies with F-18-FDG together with Tc-99m-MIBI (heart scintigraphy) and Tc-99m-HMPAO (brain scintigraphy), respectively.

The aim of the measurements which we present was to evaluate the physical properties of our system in comparison with conventional SPECT scintigraphy as well as to optimize the acquisition and processing procedure to ensure high image quality.

Materials and Methods

The applied dual-head gamma camera has rectangular detectors with a size of 53 cm x 39 cm. The thickness of the NaI crystal is 0.95 cm, scintillations are detected with 59 photomultiplier tubes per head. According to the manufacturer's specifications the extra-high-energy collimators have hexagonal holes with a diameter of 3.4 mm. The septal thickness is 3.0 mm, the septal length 75 mm. All investigations were additionally performed with low-energy high-resolution collimators representing the conditions of standard Tc-99m scintigraphy. Previous measurements on the same type of camera system were performed with different collimators and a 1.27 cm NaI crystal (1), therefore the results cannot be directly compared.

System sensitivity was measured following the NEMA standard for performance measurements of scintillation cameras (2). Solutions of the nuclides Tc-99m and F-18, respectively, were put into a plastic cup with a diameter of 5 cm, which was positioned at the centre of the collimator surface. The thickness of the liquid layer was 3 mm to minimize the influence of scatter and self absorption. Counts were detected during 3 minutes (count rate approx. 1.5 kcts/s) in a 15 % analyzer window in the total field of view (TFOV) for a matrix size of 256 x 256. System sensitivity was determined as the ratio of detected counts per time unit to emission rate of photons. The activity of the solution was corrected for radioactive decay over the measurement period.

The planar spatial resolution was evaluated using a fillable line source of 650 mm length with an inner diameter of 0.75 mm. Planar images were recorded at source-collimator-distances from 6 to 20 cm in air and with a 6 cm scatter block of PMMA between source and detector. 200 line profiles were calculated across each image of the line source at different positions to reduce the influence of inhomogenities along the line source. A Gaussian fit was performed for each profile and finally the average profile for one acquisition was evaluated. As the line source is sufficiently thin, those profiles can be interpreted as the line spread function of the system. The halfwidth of the line spread function (FWHM) is a measure for the planar spatial resolution.

SPECT performance finally was investigated using a commercially available SPECT phantom. Six PMMA spheres representing cold lesions with diameters of 9.5, 12.7, 15.9, 19.1, 25.4 and 31.8 mm are mounted inside a cylindrical tank which can be filled with a nuclide solution. A circulation pump provides a uniform distribution of the radionuclide in the water tank. An activity of 200 MBq F-18 was used combined with activities of Tc-99m from 200 to 600 MBq. The reconstructed images were analyzed following a protocol based on the AAPM report #22 (3,4) and compared with regard to root-mean-square-noise (rms-noise) in a slice with uniform activity distribution and contrast in the area of the spheres.

Results and Discussion

System sensitivity: The results of the system sensitivity are summarized in Table 1. The value for F-18 with the extra-high-energy collimators was measured to 50.3 cpm / 37 kBq. This means a drop in sensitivity to 25 % compared to Tc-99m and the high-resolution collimators (197.6 cpm / 37 kBq). In case of double-isotope studies with the extra-high-energy collimators it is important that the sensitivity for Tc-99m (56.5 cpm / 37 kBq) is not much different from F-18.

Table 1: System sensitivity for Tc-99m and F-18

Isotope, Collimator	Absolute sensitivity cpm / 37 kBq	Relative sensitivity
Tc-99m, High resolution	197.9	1.00
Tc-99m, Extra-high-energy	56.5	0.29
F-18, Extra-high-energy	50.3	0.25

Planar spatial resolution: The increase of the FWHM of the line spread function in air with the source-collimator distance is shown in figure 1. The FWHM is lowest for Tc-99m with the high-resolution collimators and only slightly larger for Tc-99m with the extra-high-energy collimators up to a distance of 10 cm. The FWHM for F-18 is significantly higher in any case. The standard deviation for the FWHM values obtained by averaging over 200 profiles for each line source image is 3 %.

Under scatter conditions a general shift to higher FWHM values of about 10 % was observed for all configurations. For a source-collimator distance of 10 cm a FWHM of 13.3 mm was measured for F-18.

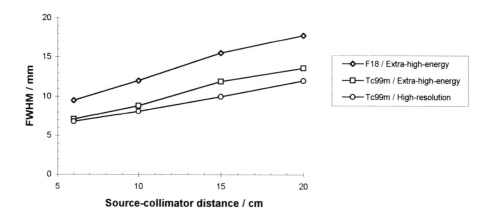

Figure 1: FWHM of the line spread function in air as a function of the source-detector distance

SPECT performance: The performance of the system for Tc-99m with the high-resolution collimators is characterized by a rms-noise of 3 % and an image contrast which permits to distinctly resolve the sphere with a diameter of 19.1 mm. Even the 15.4 mm sphere can be seen with a contrast of 0.2. Compared to that, the rms-noise for F-18 was found to be 5 %, which is not significantly worse and within the proposed range for clinical use (4). The contrast of 0.25 for the 19.1 mm sphere is not very good, whereas the contrast for the 25.4 mm sphere is about 0.35. Therefore cold structures to be evidently resolved in the reconstructed F-18-FDG slices need to have a size of approximately 25 mm.

Double-isotope phantom images (Tc-99m + F-18) showed a steady performance for F-18, but the noise and contrast values for the Tc-99m images were almost beyond the limit for clinical acceptance. This was obviously caused by Compton-scattered photons from the decay of F-18.

Therefore we implemented a scatter correction algorithm which before image reconstruction subtracts a fraction of 0.75 to 0.9 of scatter images pixel by pixel from the Tc-99m projection images. These scatter images are acquired by detecting scattered F-18 annihilation photons in a third energy window at 170 keV (15 %). The correction leads to a 50 % reduction of the rms-noise and a contrast increase of 20 to 30 % for the spheres.

The stated values were obtained for a Tc-99m to F-18 nuclide activity ratio of 2:1. The usage of less Tc-99m leads to images with higher noise and lower contrast because of the worse signal-to-background ratio. The application of more Tc-99m does not improve image quality significantly, but increases the radiation exposure to the patient.

Conclusion: The results show an expected lower performance of the gamma camera system with the extra-high-energy collimators compared to the standard low-energy high-resolution collimators. Nevertheless the values of the physical parameters count sensitivity, spatial resolution and SPECT performance are in a range, where a useful clinical application of the system is clearly possible. Bearing in mind the physical limits we regard the method as an important supplementation to the conventional methods of heart and brain scintigraphy with perfusion markers.

References

1. Schaefer A, Oberhausen E. Physical Performance of a Multispect 2 Gamma Camera for Imaging Postiron Emitters. Nucl-Med 1995; 34:40-46

2. The National Electrical Manufacturers Association (NEMA). Performance Measurements of Scintillation Cameras. NEMA standards publication No. NU 1-1980

3. American Association of Physicists in Medicine (AAPM). Rotating Scintillation Camera SPECT Acceptance Testing and Quality Control, AAPM Report No. 22. Published for the AAPM by the American Institute of Physics, New York 1987

4. Graham LS (Chairman), Fahey FH, Madsen MT, van Aswegen A, Yester MV. Quantitation of SPECT Performance: Report of Task Group 4, Nuclear Medicine Committee. Med Phys 1995; 22: 401-409

Radioactive Isotopes in
Clinical Medicine and Research XXII
ed. by H. Bergmann, A. Kroiss and H. Sinzinger
© 1997 Birkhäuser Verlag Basel/Switzerland

ITERATIVE RECONSTRUCTION IN PET ROUTINE

P. Schmidlin, M.E. Bellemann, J. Doll, G. Brix, W.J. Lorenz

Forschungsschwerpunkt Radiologie, Deutsches Krebsforschungszentrum Heidelberg,
Germany

SUMMARY: A single projection procedure with high overrelaxation for iterative reconstruction of PET images is described which is precise and rapid, and therefore suitable for practical use. The best values of overrelaxation are determined with typical data. An image needs bewtween three and eight iterative steps, depending on the requested precision. Results with phantoms and patients are shown and compared with maximum-likelihood EM.

INTRODUCTION

Iterative image reconstruction is theoretically well examined, but it is used seldom in clinical practice, mainly due to the long computation time needed for a satisfactory image.

In our PET unit, iterative reconstruction was implemented in 1986 (Schmidlin et al 1988) and several versions were routinely used since that time. It was shown that the use of subsets of the projections speeds iteration, because higher overrelaxation can be used.

MATERIALS AND METHODS

In a recent version, overrelaxation was optimized using modified maximum likelihood postulates. Overrelaxation was determined to achieve maximum gain of likelihood within one or two iterative steps. This procedure was used with single projection iteration.

Tab. 1. Procedures for optimisation of likelihood.

MAXIMUM GAIN OF LIKELIHOOD DURING ONE STEP	MAXIMUM GAIN OF LIKELIHOOD DURING TWO STEPS
	START:
set initial values	set initial values
set image to b(0)	reset image to b(0)
set n to 0	reset n to 0
	reset local ML etc.
NEXT APPROXIMATION:	NEXT APPROXIMATION:
set n → +1 (stop if n>limit)	set n → +1 (stop if n>limit)
NEXT z(n):	NEXT z(n):
calculate b(n) using z(n)	calculate b(n) using z(n)
calculate approximated projections, likelihood etc.	calculate approximated projections, likelihood etc.
	has zopt(n-1) been set ?
	yes: go to NEXT APPROXIMATION
	no:
L > ML ?	L > local ML ?
yes: set ML= L	yes: set local ML= L
set bopt = b(n)	
all values of z(n) examined ?	all values of z(n) examined ?
no: set new value for z(n)	no: set new value for z(n)
reset image to b(n-1)	reset image to b(n-1)
go to NEXT z(n)	go to NEXT z(n)
	local ML > global ML ?
set image to bopt	yes: set zbest = z(n-1)
go to NEXT APPROXIMATION	set global ML = local ML
Symbols:	all values of z(n-1) examined ?
n : approximation	yes: set zopt(n-1) = zbest
z(n) : overrelaxation	no: set new value for z(n-1)
zopt(n) : optimum z	
L : likelihood	go to START
ML : maximum likelihood	
b(n) : image (n-th approx)	
bopt : optimum image	

Tab. 1 shows the programs used for evaluation of the optimum overrelaxation values. Optimisation in one step was achieved in the following way: In each step a sequence of integer overrelaxation values was examined, and iteration was continued with the value which gave the highest likelihood in the step. For optimisation during two steps, two sequences of overrelaxation values were examined in two consecutive steps, and the value in the first step which gave the best results in the second step was chosen. Then the procedure was restarted from the beginning with the chosen optimum values.

For non-Poisson data, the maximum gain of likelihood was replaced by maximum decrease of a normalized mean square error. Otherwise the procedures were similar.

For routine, values are used which were extracted prevoiusly from typical data.

RESULTS AND DISCUSSION

The postulates yield high initial overrelaxation parameters which then drop quickly. The overrelaxations obtained with the two-step postulate are much higher in the beginning, leading to still more rapid convergence. Fig. 1 shows a result with non-Poisson PET data with high statistics, obtained with the two-step postulate. An image is visually ready after 3 steps. A high precision image is obtained with 6 to 8 steps. The image obtained with 6 steps is similar to an image obtained with about 170

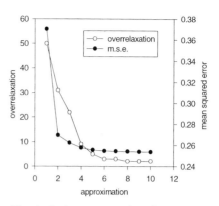

Fig. 1. Optimum overrelaxation parameters (two-step procedure) and normalized mean squared error of approximation 1 to 10 of a phantom measurement.

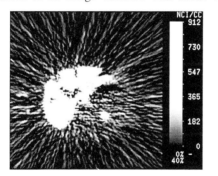
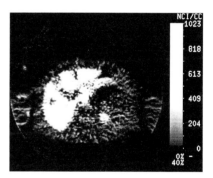

Fig. 2. Uptake of 5-[F-18]-fluorouracil in a metastatic liver, reconstructed with filtered back-projection (left) and with 8 iterative steps.

steps of ML-EM. Continuation of iteration does not alter the image.

Fig. 2 shows reconstructions of a metastatic liver with filtered back-projection and 8 iterative steps. The contrasts are similar, but the reconstructed image has no beam artefacts.

Fig. 3 shows the image of a recurrent colon carcimona in the neighbourhood of the bladder, using the same procedures. Iterative reconstruction produces finer noise structure. This may be modified by simple smoothing of the projections, as seen in the lower row.

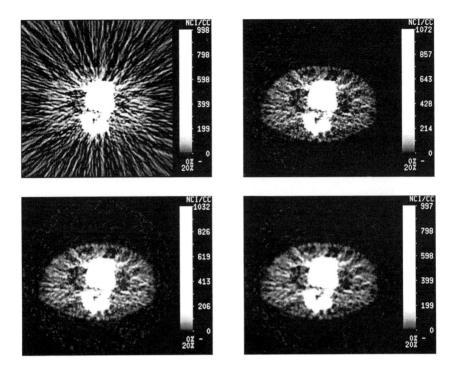

Fig. 3. Uptake of [F-18]-FDG in a recurrent colon carcinoma in the neighbourhood of the bladder, reconstructed with filtered backprojection (top left), and with 8 iterative steps, top right: without smoothing, bottom: smoothing of the projections with a 1-2-1-filter one time (left) and two times (right).

A procedure given by Herman and Meyer 1993, optimizing a relaxed multiplicative ART, corresponds to our one-step postulate, with qualitatively agreeing results.

The OS-EM procedure of Hudson and Larkin 1994 is also related to our procedure. They define an 'iteration level' which is the number of subsets of projections taken simultaneously. This iteration level is equivalent to a constant overrelaxation when comparing with our definitions. Our results show that this overrelaxation is too high for the final iterative steps and provokes additional noise in the image.

REFERENCES

Schmidlin P., Kübler W.K., Doll J., Strauss L.G., Ostertag H.: Image processing in whole body positron emission tomography. In: Schmidt, Csernay (edts), Nuklearmedizin, Schattauer Stuttgart-New York 1988, p. 84-87.

Herman G.T., Meyer L.B.: Algebraic reconstruction techniques can be made computationally efficient. IEEE-MI 12,600-609 (1993).

Hudson H.M., Larkin R.S.: Accelerated image reconstruction using ordered subsets of projection data. IEEE-MI 13,601-609 (1994).

Radioactive Isotopes in
Clinical Medicine and Research XXII
ed. by H. Bergmann, A. Kroiss and H. Sinzinger
© 1997 Birkhäuser Verlag Basel/Switzerland

QUANTITATIVE EVALUATION OF DYNAMIC RENAL STUDIES
USING FUZZY REGIONS OF INTEREST AND FUNCTIONAL FACTOR IMAGES

M.Šámal[1], C.C.Nimmon[2], K.E.Britton[2], H.Bergmann[3]

[1]Institute of Nuclear Medicine, First Faculty of Medicine, Charles University Prague,
Salmovská 3, CZ-120 00 Praha 2, Czech Republic,
[2]Department of Nuclear Medicine, St. Bartholomew's Hospital,
West Smithfield, London EC1A 7BE, United Kingdom,
[3]Ludwig Boltzmann Institute of Nuclear Medicine, and
Department of Biomedical Engineering and Physics, Vienna Univesity Hospital AKH,
Währinger Gürtel 18-20/4L, A-1090 Wien, Austria.

SUMMARY

New algorithms for application of factor analysis in dynamic renal scintigraphy are tested. The results are compared with quantitative diagnostic parameteres obtained by well established clinical routines. Test values of renal transit times correlate well with the reference ones but are significantly longer due to a relatively large extent of factor structures. Test values of relative renal uptake agree well with the reference values.

INTRODUCTION

Experimental application of factor analysis to a selected dynamic renal study usually provides a good separation of renal parenchyma from pelvic, vascular and background structures. However, attempts to apply the method in a routine clinical practice often fail indicating a need for more robust extraction of so called physiological factors. In general, the physiological factors can be enhanced in two ways: by improving an oblique rotation of factors, and by a modification of input data in order to simplify the analytic problem. Because it is unlikely to improve the so-phisticated rotation algorithm significantly in a short time, we have examined the methods for adjustment of the input data. The aim of our experiment was to suggest a realistic, robust and clinically useful algorithm for routine application of factor analysis in dynamic renal scintigra-phy.

MATERIALS AND METHODS

Factor analysis

Factor analysis of image sequences used in this study is described elsewhere (1). Our ap-proach to enhancement of physiological factors benefits from an old concept of data "masking" (2). In brief, many dynamic structures (factors) visualized in a scintigraphic data (as e.g. the re-nal vessels, parenchyma, or calyces) manifest themselves just for a short period of time or in a relatively small area of image matrix. Due to that, such factors usually form a small part of input data variance and their estimation is unreliable. Local application of factor analysis to the subset of input data results in better resolution and estimation of local factors. Full scale of locally ex-tracted factors then can be restored using the linear model of factor analysis and the respective subsets of input data. We suggest to use the local factor analysis to create "fuzzy" regions of in-terest and functional or parametric factor images.

Fuzzy regions of interest

Fuzzy regions of interest are optimized factor images of individual dynamic structures. They are obtained by a local application of factor analysis to several different data subsets in which the respective factors are locally strong. Thus, for instance, the fuzzy region of interest of the left renal parenchyma is obtained by factor analysis of a region over the left kidney at the short time interval in which the activity in renal parenchyma dominates over that in the renal pelvis and vessels. After extracting all the local factors from different data subsets, factor images of large structures are completed to the full scale of the matrix, while those of paired and small organs are just padded by zero pixel values in order to emphasize their local presence and differentiate the relative function. Local factor images are then stacked into the new file and used to calculate the corresponding time-activity curves (3).

Functional factor images

Functional factor images are extracted from a data subset selected in such a way that the resulting factors correspond to a well defined physiological function. Our intention was to construct a functional image of a renal uptake in order to provide a simple method for measurement of relative function of the left and right kidneys. Factor analysis has been performed in a large rectangular region of interest containing both kidneys at the shortest time interval between the peaks of the cardiac and parenchymal curves. Resulting factor images demonstrate the vascular structures (with decreasing intensity) and kidneys (with increasing intensity). In the latter image, the pixel values over the left and right kidneys reflect the relative renal uptake.

Evaluation of results

Time-activity curves from fuzzy regions of interest and the functional factor images have been constructed applying the factor analysis to 43 dynamic renal studies (99mTc-MAG3, 180 images 64x64 word in 10 second intervals) selected randomly from the clinical data base of the Department of Nuclear Medicine, St.Bartholomew's Hospital London. No regard has been given to pathology so that the analyzed sample contained the kidneys with a wide range of renal function from normal to absent. Transit times have been calculated using a matrix deconvolution algorithm. Relative renal function has been measured using the counts over the left and right kidneys in functional factor images of renal uptake.

Test values of the transit time and relative renal uptake have been compared with those provided by well established clinical procedures. Transit time measurement has been described by Britton and Nimmon (4). Relative renal function has been measured by integration of background-subtracted renal curves over the time interval defined with the help of the Patlak-Rutland plot. Because the very long transit times measured by the clinical procedure were truncated, the time interval for comparison of the whole-kidney transit times has been limited to 0-300 s and that of parenchymal transit times to 0-240 s. The relative renal uptake has been compared in a full range of 0-100 %. Pairs of reference and experimental values have been compared using a paired t-test and correlation coefficient. Occasional outliers have been discarded.

RESULTS

Comparison of transit times is given in Table 1. Test values of the whole-kidney transit time correlate well with the reference values, however, they are longer by more than half a minute on average. The correlation between the test and reference parenchymal transit times is relatively low but still statistically significant. The test values are 17 s longer on average. In comparison with the reference, both test values have greater variance.

Table 1. Comparison of transit-time values calculated using the time-activity curves from fuzzy regions of interest with those calculated using a standard clinical procedure.

	n	mean (s)	s.d. (s)	p-diff.	r	p-corr.
WKTT ref.	34	220	36			
WKTT test	34	256	46	<0.001	0.939	<0.001
PTT ref.	41	183	26			
PTT test	41	200	38	0.006	0.409	0.008

WKTT = whole-kidney transit time, PTT = parenchymal transit time, n = number of paired measurements, mean = arithmetic mean, s.d. = standard deviation of individual measurement, p-diff. = significance level of mean difference, r = paired correlation coefficient, p-corr. = significance level of paired correlation coefficient

Comparison of relative renal uptake is given in Table 2. Both the correlation between the test and reference values and the agreement of the mean values are very good. The quantitative information provided by both methods can be considered to be practically identical.

Table 2. Comparison of relative renal function values calculated using the functional factor images with those calculated using a standard clinical procedure.

	n	mean (%)	s.d. (%)	p-diff.	r	p-corr.
LK ref.	37	51.5	20.3			
LK test	37	50.9	19.8	0.142	0.992	<0.001

LK = left kidney relative uptake

DISCUSSION

The difference between the test and reference values of the whole-kidney transit time perhaps can be explained by the fact that the fuzzy structure of renal pelvis often involve also a part of a ureter. Thus the extent of the structure through which the transit time has been measured is probably bigger than in the case of the standard region.

Similarly, the difference between the test and reference values of the parenchymal transit time is likely due to the larger extent of parenchymal structure as defined by factor analysis in comparison with a narrow strip of a kidney cortex defined manually. Providing the reference values represent a golden standard, great variance of the test values demonstrates that in different individual kidneys, the factor analysis extracts different extent of renal parenchyma depending on the relation between the speed of activity flow through the kidney and the sampling frequency given by acquisition scheme.

In the experiment with functional factor images, we have often found that two factors are not enough to describe the activity changes in the selected time interval properly, and that the third factor is necessary to account for blood flow through the abdominal area. It has made the functional factor images of renal uptake even better than with two-factor analysis, however, the third factor was very variable showing different arterial and venous structures in different patients. This variance again reflects the discrepancy between the individual speed of involved physiological processes and the relatively low and constant frequency of its sampling. The outcome is that the contribution of the same physiological process (which is the crucial parameter for factor extraction) is different in a different data.

CONCLUSION

The experiment provides quantitative evidence that factor analysis using oblique rotation of factors is good enough for extracting the physiologically relevant information from dynamic scintigraphic data. Its routine clinical application seems to be feasible and useful, however, it should be tailored carefully to the specific clinical task, respecting the features of both the method and the measured physiological function.

ACKNOWLEDGEMENT

The work has been partially supported by the European Commission (COST B2 Short-term Scientific Mission Grant 1995), Austrian Ministry of Science and Research (project nr.GZ - 45.250 / 2-IV-6a / 92), and Granting Agency of the Czech Republic (project nr.312 / 94 / 0679).

REFERENCES

1. Šámal M, Kárný M, Zahálka D. Bayesian identification of a physiological model in dynamic scintigraphic data. In: Information Processing in Medical Imaging. Barrett HH, Gmitro AF, editors. New York: Springer, 1993: 422-437.

2. Šámal M, Sůrová H, Kárný M, Maříková E, Michalová K, Dienstbier Z. Enhancement of physiological factors in factor analysis of dynamic studies. Eur J Nucl Med 1986; 12: 280-283.

3. Martel A, Barber DC. A new approach to dynamic study analysis. In: Information Processing in Medical Imaging. Ortendahl DA, Llacer J, editors. New York: Wiley-Liss, 1991: 327-340.

4. Britton KS, Nimmon CC. The measurement of renal transit times by deconvolution analysis. In: Evaluation of Renal Function and Disease with Radionuclides. Blaufox MD, editor. Basel: Karger, 1989: 108-116.

Radioactive Isotopes in
Clinical Medicine and Research XXII
ed. by H. Bergmann, A. Kroiss and H. Sinzinger
© 1997 Birkhäuser Verlag Basel/Switzerland

IONISATION CHAMBER MEASUREMENTS OF I123 USING A COPPER FILTER

Thomson WH, Hesslewood SR, Hepplewhite J, Parker K and Perrin B.
City Hospital NHS Trust, Birmingham, B18 7QH, UK

SUMMARY: The low energy X-ray emissions of ^{123}I lead to large variations in activity measurements using an ionisation chamber. A copper filter 0.5mm thick removes these X-rays but only reduces the 159 keV emissions by 14%. However the ionisation chamber needs to be recalibrated for the copper filter attenuation. We outline a simple method using a measurement made on ^{99}Tc^m to determine the change in sensitivity of the ionisation chamber using the copper filter. With the copper filter, the variation of activity measurements when ^{123}I is in a syringe compared to those in a vial is reduced from 80% to 3%. The ratio of the manufacturers stated activity to measured activity was 102% and 111% for two manufacturers respectively.

INTRODUCTION

Activity measurements of ^{123}I in vials or syringes with an ionisation chamber often demonstrate large variations from expected values. The reason for these variations is that ^{123}I emits low energy X-rays in the range 27-32 keV, identical to those of ^{125}I, and the ionisation chamber is sensitive to these low energy emissions. In fact 62% of the activity reading of our ionisation chamber (Capintec ARC-120) is due to the X-rays. Although most calibrators have a calibration factor for ^{123}I this is likely to be for a particular type of vial. However the varying attenuation of different manufacturers' glass vials or of syringes leads to the observed variation in measurements.

It is possible to use the measurements of a particular manufacturer's vials as a continuous check on subsequent deliveries. This is shown in figure 1 where it can be seen that the vials of iodide consistently measured about 25% less than the stated activity whereas syringes measure about 27% higher than expected. The vials of MIBG were generally about 7% less than expected until shipment number 6. The latter measurement was 20% less than expected, leading to uncertainty regarding the true activity. In fact the manufacturer had changed the type of vial which led to the reduced activity measurement. As seen in figure 1 further deliveries were consistent with the lower observed percentage value of the new vial type.

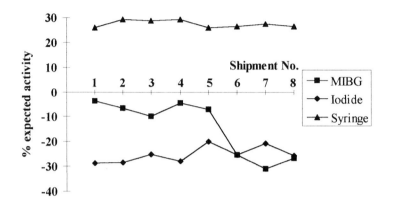

Figure 1. Measured activity of ^{123}I as a % of expected activity for two suppliers of iodide and MIBG and for syringe activities

Ideally the ionisation chamber measurement should be reliable no matter what type of vial or syringe is used. This can be achieved by filtering out the low energy X-rays and a procedure using a copper filter has already been described (1). Harris et al examined the requirements for a copper filter in detail. They employed a system of two filters, measurements using a gamma camera and the solution of three simultaneous equations. Although the latter approach provides a comprehensive analysis we present here a simpler method of implementing the use of a copper filter for ^{123}I measurements.

MATERIALS AND METHODS

Harris et al (1) showed that a copper filter of thickness 0.5mm reduces the X-rays by greater than 99% and a thicker filter than this is therefore unnecessary. This filter thickness only attenuates the 159keV gamma rays by about 14% and is therefore recommended. Copper sheet of

0.5mm thickness is readily available and a cylindrical container can be easily constructed using thinly soldered joints. A foam layer placed in the bottom of the copper can prevents any vial damage. Our filter is 17cm tall and 3.5cm in diameter and fits in the measuring cradle of the ionisation chamber.

The principal difficulty in implementing such a filter is obtaining the correction factor for the sensitivity of the chamber. As illustrated in figure 2 the situation is that of broad beam geometry and the apparent thickness of the copper filter in terms of its attenuation will be greater than the true thickness. Attenuation calculations based on the thickness of the copper filter are therefore not appropriate. This also means that measurements based on other detector systems or geometries could also be inappropriate.

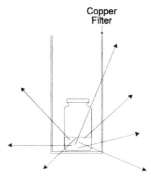

Copper
Filter

Figure 2. Geometry of a vial inside the copper filter. The lines denote gamma rays and show the increased path length compared to the thickness of the copper filter (no interactions are shown).

Fortunately the main gamma ray emissions of $^{99}Tc^m$ at 140 keV are similar in energy to the 159 keV of ^{123}I. Therefore a vial containing $^{99}Tc^m$ is measured in the ionisation chamber with and without the copper filter giving the broad beam attenuation of this geometry at 140 keV. For example, with our chamber and filter the ratio of the measured activity of a vial of $^{99}Tc^m$ with and without the copper filter was 0.856. Using this attenuation together with the value for the linear attenuation coefficient of copper at 140 kev (0.21 mm^{-1}) the apparent thickness (t_a) of the copper filter can be calculated. For example, for our filter the calculation is

$$\exp(-0.21 \times t_a) = 0.856 \text{ , giving } t_a = 0.74\text{mm} \qquad .....(1)$$

It can be seen therefore that the 0.5mm filter appears to have a thickness of 0.74mm for $^{99}Tc^m$ gamma rays. Using this calculated effective thickness and the linear attenuation coefficient of copper at 159 keV , $0.17mm^{-1}$, the attenuation of the 159keV emissions of ^{123}I can be calculated. For example, our filter gives $\exp(-0.17 \times 0.74) = 0.86$.

In order to calculate a new sensitivity factor for the ionisation chamber with the copper filter the decay scheme of ^{123}I must also be considered. Firstly the 159keV emissions occur in only 89% of decays. Also there are a range of higher energy gamma emissions in a small percentage of decays. The sensitivity factor of the ionisation chamber at the energy of each emission must be known in order to calculate the overall sensitivity for a particular radionuclide. For our ionisation chamber, a sensitivity value is obtained for each energy of emission and this is multiplied by the fractional emission per decay. The total sensitivity is then $= \sum_E$ sensitivity$_E$ x abundance$_E$.

The total sensitivity value is linked to a dialled factor on the chamber in order that the reading is expressed in MBq. In order to correct for the copper filter, at each energy the attenuation factor of the copper filter is obtained from the effective thickness value and the appropriate linear attenuation coefficient value for copper at that energy. Therefore with the copper filter the amended sensitivity factor of the chamber for ^{123}I is obtained from

$$\text{total sensitivity} = \sum_E \text{sensitivity}_E \times \text{abundance}_E \times \exp(-\mu_E.t_a) \qquad ......(2)$$

where μ_E is the linear attenuation at energy E and t_a is the calculated effective thickness. With this new value for the total sensitivity a new value for the dialled factor can be obtained.

Table 1. ratio of activity measurements of ^{123}I in a syringe to those in a vial with and without the use of a copper filter.

	ratio syringe/vial	range
without copper filter	1.79	(1.7 - 1.86)
with copper filter	1.03	(1.0 - 1.05)

The effectiveness of the copper filter can be seen in table 1. Whereas the syringe activity measurements are about 79% greater than the vial measurements without the copper filter, this reduces to 3% when the copper filter is used.

Using the copper filter together with the sensitivity factor calculated as in equation 2 the ratio of the measured activity to the manufacturers' stated stock activity is shown in Table 2. It can be seen that the measurements of stock activity supplied by manufacturer 1 are only 2% different from the stated activity whereas the stock measurements for manufacturer 2 are 11% greater than the stated value.

Table 2 ratio of the measured activity to the stated activity for two manufacturers products.

	measured/stated activity	range
Supplier 1	1.02	0.97 - 1.03
Supplier 2	1.11	1.08 - 1.14

DISCUSSION

The use of a copper filter to exclude the low energy X-ray emissions greatly improves the reliability of the measurements of ^{123}I, particularly with regard to the ratio of measured activity in vials and syringes (Table 1). However in order to obtain true activity values the change in sensitivity using the copper filter has to be calculated. The method described above relies on the fact that the observed attenuation effects measured at 140 keV with ^{99}Tc^{m} can be applied to the 159 keV emissions. At 140keV over 53% of the interactions with copper are Compton effect and at 159 keV 62% of the interactions are with the Compton effect. The parameter of the effective thickness calculated with ^{99}Tc^{m} will therefore be energy dependent. However measuring the effective thickness provides a more accurate estimate of the measurement geometry than simply using the measured thickness of the copper filter. In any event the attenuation of the 159 keV emissions with a 0.5mm copper filter is not great. Even a 10% change in the effective thickness used in the calculations of the sensitivity (0.81mm instead of 0.74mm) would result in a calculated total sensitivity factor only 1% lower.

The calculated effective thickness value for $^{99}Tc^m$ has also been applied to the low energy X-ray emissions and to the high energy emissions. The value of the effective thickness is likely to be different at these energies. However since the total contribution of these emissions to the ionisation chamber sensitivity using the 0.5mm copper filter is very small then the overall error in using this value is minimal. If sources are available, a more accurate estimate could be made with ^{125}I for the low energy X-rays and eg ^{131}I for the higher energies.

Table 1 shows that the filter effectively removes all variation due to ^{123}I being in different containers. The small 3% difference observed with the copper filter for activity in a vial compared to a syringe is due to attenuation and geometry differences for the 159 keV emission, as shown by the fact that the same value is obtained with $^{99}Tc^m$.

An alternative procedure could be to rely on the manufacturers' stated activity and obtain empirically the appropriate ionisation chamber setting which gives the correct activity value with the copper filter. However figure 1 shows that it is important that the vial type remains consistent. Also, as demonstrated in Table 1 the manufacturers may not themselves be totally consistent in terms of their stated activity. Clearly there would appear to be a discrepancy in one of the manufacturers' estimates of activity by about 10%. It is unclear which manufacturer is correct at this stage since our technique of calibrating the ionisation chamber, although calculated with reference to the known sensitivity of the chamber strictly requires independent validation against a secondary standard and this has not yet been carried out.

Application of our technique does require knowledge of the variation of sensitivity of the chamber with energy. For some ionisation chambers this may require contacting the manufacturer. We believe that the method outlined of evaluating the effective thickness using $^{99}Tc^m$ is straightforward and provides an independent evaluation of the effect of the copper filter.

References

1.   Harris CC, Jaszczak RJ, Greer KL, Briner WH, Coleman RE. Effect of characteristic
        X-Rays on Assay of I-123 by Dose Calibrator.   J Nucl Med 1984;25:1367-1370.

Radioactive Isotopes in
Clinical Medicine and Research XXII
ed. by H. Bergmann, A. Kroiss and H. Sinzinger
© 1997 Birkhäuser Verlag Basel/Switzerland

THE SEPARATION OF CHURCH AND STATE: HOW TO PROVIDE A CLEAN INTERFACE BETWEEN ACQUISITION AND PROCESSING.

Todd-Pokropek A, C. Hutton, J. Paredes.

Department of Medical Physics, University College London, and The Institute for Child Health, London, U.K.

SUMMARY

The boundary between the gamma camera, the acquisition system and the processing system is fuzzy. The gamma camera clearly requires control from the acquisition system for uniformity correction etc, and the camera and acquisition computer cannot really be separated. However, increasingly, it is desirable to be able to separate acquisition from processing, so that the processing computer can be replaced (having a much shorter life), and to be able to mix and match between different manufacturers. This is recognized in both the DICOM standard and Interfile. However experience shows that in particular in SPECT, raw data is difficult to transfer. As part of the COST B2 initiative, a preliminary specification of a clean interface for the transfer of all types of raw data between acquisition and processing has been prepared, together with indications of the constraints that this will impose, for example for centre of rotation correction during reconstruction. This is proposed as an extension to Interfile.

INTRODUCTION

Historically, gamma camera computer systems were not manufactured by the same companies manufacturing gamma cameras. However, over a period of time this changed, and the link between the computer and the camera became very tight and often very proprietary. The further development of such technology introduced the concept of networks and multiple acquisition of processing workstations. Nevertheless, the basic unit remained one where both acquisition and processing could be performed. This paper explores the need for ad the possibilities of achieving a clean separation of functions between Acquisition and Processing workstations.

There are significant commercial implications associated with such a division. Separation of acquisition and processing creates new market opportunities, and permits companies not involved in the instrumentation to bid for market share. What has become increasingly obvious is that processing systems have a much shorter life than acquisitions systems, as computer technology develops very rapidly, whereas gamma camera technology at the moment is essentially static. There is an important requirement that the clinical protocols used by a nuclear medicine service need to survive, such that results and normal ranges remain valid even when the processing system is replaced. There is a secondary desire for the Human Computer Interface to be standardised as the retraining of technical and clinical users to be competent on a new system is expensive and time consuming.

The hypothesis presented here is that the is potentially a significant advantage to defining a clear and clean interface between acquisition and processing, with the aim of making 'plus and play' matching of different systems possible such that processing system could be replaced easily with minimal disruption of a clinical service. However, to achieve such benefits implies work being undertaken in the area of standardization, not just of file transfer, but also of the user interface and clinical protocols employed.

THE COMPONENTS: THE FUNCTIONS OF AN ACQUISITION

When acquiring data, we can consider the functions of the system specific to acquisition. These would include:

   a) PScope mode- the setting up of the study

   b) Static/dynamic/gated acquisition- handling events and time in various clinical modes

   c) SPECT control- controlling the gantry and acquiring SPECT data

   d) Uniformity/energy/ spatial distortion/ scatter correction- performing and managing all the real time corrections that need to be performed in or near the detector.

It is also clear the various types of 'Smart acquisition' and a number of currently undefined new functions involving processing during acquisition likely to become available, examples might be motion correction, depth of interaction correction and PET coincidence. Thus it is also clear that no rigid specification of handling data during acquisition is likely to be acceptable.

SPECT acquisition presents specific problems due to the nature of the correction which are required. The same is not true in general for reconstructed data. There is a need for quantitative information (pixel size, attenuation and other corrections) to be available on the processing side of any interface. There may also be a need to extract information from the raw data unreconstructed data even after reconstruction. Thus the place of tomographic reconstruction is not clear: it could be considered as part of either the acquisition or processing software systems.

A processing system has the functions of performing the clinical analysis functions, display, acting as the interface to the patient administrative system, and also acting as the interface to the archiving system. In particular, information such as patient demographic information should be managed at this level, not at the acquisition level.

SPECT, COST B2 AND CURRENT STANDARDS

A problem has become apparent with work undertaken by COST B2 and other groups. Raw SPECT data transferred between different systems often gives very different results after reconstruction. Correction tables for example for the centre of rotation correction are very variable in form. Since we believe that there is a need for a clean separation between acquisition and processing, such problems must be addressed. In general the problem arises because corrections are performed as part of the reconstruction. The solution is to insist that all corrections for SPECT data should be performed prior to processing, and therefore that in input data stage can be defined for corrected data such that any reconstruction algorithm can handle such data. This is therefore an appropriate point at which to define an interface.

COST B2 has published and is still working of user requirements which include the specification of an 'ideal' computer system (1). Included in the concept of an ideal computer is that of plug and play between acquisition and processing. Both DICOM (2) and Interfile define file formats (3), but in practice they cannot handle raw (SPECT) data from certain manufacturers. The definitions involved need to be extended and generalized.

Standardisation has a component which might be called: Reglementation. However, making systems, user interfaces, reports and the definition of clinical values conform to standards should improve clinical efficiency. On the other hand, making systems too rigid will prevent the improvement of current instrumentation of procedures, and prevent the development of new tests.

REQUIREMENTS OF THE INTERFACE

It is clear that energy correction must be applied as part of acquisition as energy information or list mode data is require. Therefore ALL such corrections should be applied at acquisition level. Only corrected data should be passed to a processing workstation. This includes centre or rotation correction. Logically reconstruction should be part of acquisition (following the CT and MR model), since it is performed more easily at acquisition stag; all the needed information is available. But reconstruction is also as part of processing, and some manufacturers will still certainly want to reconstruct as part of their processing package. Some novel reconstruction techniques (iterative algorithms etc) will be developed as part of processing. Some processing techniques require (some of) the additional acquisition information for example positional, for example as part of an attenuation correction algorithm.

There are implications with respect to acquisition. There is a need to work at higher sampling rates since the corrections to be performed generally need fine sampling. However, new acquisition systems have less limitations with respect to sampling. Since processing should be performed on clean data, many more corrections are likely to be implemented

Thus additional information must be availed to be passed between acquisition and processing for example:

For each head/ device:

Positional information for each sample:

3.D position with respect to fixed position or axis and detector

Angle information in 3.D

Temporal information (inc. gating)

This requires just a set of additional tables which can be coded in DICOM form (extended Interfile)

Even if as recommended, centre of rotation corrected data is passed , various post processing techniques require detailed information about sampling. We may assume that the detector is 'stationary' as a function of initial sampling. However, collimator function is also likely to be required . A format must be chosen for example a general form would be as 3-d response map.

With respect to defining such an interface, the problems that need to be addressed include definition appropriate for:

Gated SPECT

Complex dynamic acquisitions

Temporal information for multi-phase acquisitions

3-D multi channel data

Multi-energy data

Other areas that need to be addressed include

> Other types of detectors (rings, coded aperture, configurable, etc.)
>
> Coincidence and handling of positrons
>
> Whole body variants (3 headed whole body, long spiral scans etc.)
>
> QA and setting up information

CONCLUSIONS: WHAT TO DO NOW

It is proposed that it is now appropriate to start to make detailed recommendations to CEN, ACR/NEMA and the EANM. We need to ensure that manufacturers will support such recommendations enthusiastically. However, they can also be included as part of equipment procurement.

Thus it is recommended to:

> Separate acquisition and processing
>
> Always pass only corrected data
>
> Pass (preferably) reconstructed data in SPECT
>
> Provide mechanisms for passing of additional tables containing full sampling information

and not least:

> Keep all 'patient database' functions at processing level.

REFERENCES:

1.   Todd-Pokropek A, Vauramo E, Cosgriff P, Sippo-Tujunen I and Britton K. User requirements for information systems in nuclear medicine. Nucl. Med. Commun. 1992; 13:299-305.

2.   Digital Imaging and Communications in Medicine Part 1 to 10. NEMA Standards Publication PS3.2 (199x)

3.   Todd-Pokropek A., Cradduck T.D. and Deconinck F. A file format for the exchange of nuclear medicine image data: a specification of Interfile version 3.3. Nucl. Med. Commun. 1992; 13:673-699.

Varia

Radioactive Isotopes in
Clinical Medicine and Research XXII
ed. by H. Bergmann, A. Kroiss and H. Sinzinger
© 1997 Birkhäuser Verlag Basel/Switzerland

COLONIC TRANSIT IN LACTULOSE AND POLYETHYLENE GLYCOL INDUCED OSMOTIC DIARRHEA

Hammer J, Hammer HF*, Lang K, Lipp R*, Kletter K[#], Gangl A

Universitätsklinik für Innere Medizin IV, Abteilung für Gastroenterologie und Hepatologie;
    AKH Wien, Austria
*Medizinische Universitätsklinik Graz; Austria
[#]Universitätsklinik für Nuklearmedizin; AKH Wien, Austria

ABSTRACT

INTRODUCTION: Colonic transit is accelerated in lactulose (LL) induced diarrhea; it is not clear whether this is simply due to an osmotic effect or is influenced by bacterial metabolism of LL. AIMS: To compare colonic transit induced by LL with that produced by PEG, an osmotically active, non metabolizable solute ("pure osmotic diarrhea"). METHODS: To cause similar severity of diarrhea (J Clin Invest 1989, 84:1056) 10 healthy volunteers (24±6 yrs, 3F, 7M) ingested 99 g/d LL and 7 subjects (26±4 yrs, 2F, 5M) ingested 59 g/d PEG 4000 in 3 divided doses for 3 consecutive days. On day 2 a delayed release capsule containing 1 gram of ^{111}In-labeled resin pellets (0.1 mCi) was ingested. Transit of the capsule was followed with gamma-camera imaging. Anterior and posterior images were taken 12 and 24 hours after the capsule had reached the cecum. Counts in the ascending (AC) and transverse (TC) colons were determined at 12 and 24 hr. The weighted average of counts in the colon at hour 24 (Geometric center (GC)) and cumulative counts (CC) appearing in stool were calculated as parameters of total colonic transit. RESULTS: Percent activity remaining in the AC and proximal colon (PC, sum of activity in AC and TC) at 12 and 24 hours, and total colonic transit are shown: mean±SEM, * p<0.05 and ^{ns} not significant vs PEG.

	stool weight	AC (%)		PC (%)		total colonic transit	
	(g/d)	12 hr	24 hr	12 hr	24 hr	GC	CC (%)
LL	513±71 ^{ns}	34±6 ^{ns}	27±5*	45±8 ^{ns}	36±6*	3.2±0.2*	38±8*
PEG	527±77	16±6	10±6	24±9	14±6	4.5±0.4	79±10

CONCLUSION: With comparable stool weights, LL diarrhea had slower right colonic and total colonic transit; products of bacterial metabolism (short chain fatty acids?) reduce the acceleration of transit caused by an increased colonic volume load.

INTRODUCTION

Osmotic diarrhea is caused by an accumulation of poorly absorbable, osmotically active substances in the gut lumen (1). In spite of the frequency of osmotic diarrhea in clinical practice, the pathophysiology of colonic transit during osmotic diarrhea has yet not been carefully looked at. Lactulose ingestion has been shown to hasten colonic transit (2). Lactulose is a carbohydrate that can not be absorbed in the small intestine and is metabolized in the colon by bacterial fermentation (3). The mechanisms whereby lactulose induces accelerated transit through the large intestine are unclear. It might be merely due to an increased fluid volume in the colonic lumen, but products of bacterial metabolism might also influence colonic transit. We aimed to compare colonic transit in lactulose induced diarrhea with polyethylene glycol (PEG)- induced diarrhea. PEG is an osmotically active, biologically inert, non-metabolizable solute which therefore serves as a model of pure osmotic diarrhea.

METHODS

Experimental osmotic diarrhea:

Lactulose induced diarrhea: 10 healthy volunteers (24±6 yrs, 3 women, 7 men) ingested 99 gram per day lactulose in 3 divided doses for three consecutive days.

PEG induced diarrhea: 7 healthy volunteers (26±4 yrs, 2 women, 5 men) ingested 59 g/ d PEG 4000 in 3 divided doses for 3 consecutive days.

The ingested amounts of lactulose and PEG were, based on previous experiments (3), chosen to induce similar severities of diarrhea in both study groups.

Study design:

Colonic transit was measured on day two. A delayed release capsule containing Indium-111 labeled resin pellets (4) were ingested in the morning of day two and gamma-camera images were taken 12 and 24 hours after ingestion of the capsule. Stools were collected for 24 hours on day 2 and stool weight was determined.

Data analysis:

A variable region of interest program (ROI) quantified radioactivity in the four colonic regions (figure 1): the ascending colon, transverse colon, descending colon, and rectosigmoid.

Proximal colonic transit was expressed as the percentage of counts in the ascending colon and in the proximal colon (ascending plus transverse colon) determined at hours 12 and 24.

Total colonic transit was expressed i) as the cumulative counts in stools 24 hours after ingestion of the capsule and ii) as the geometric center of isotopes, i.e. the weighted average of counts in the colon, at hour 24.

Calculating the geometric center (figure 1) each colonic region and the stools are assigned a rank number from 1 (ascending colon) to 5 (stool). To "weigh" the counts in the colonic compartments, the percentage of counts in each region is multiplied with the rank number in this region. The sum of these calculations gives the geometric center of counts, that is a number between 1 (when all counts are in the ascending colon) and 5 (when all counts are in the stool). A high geometric center at a given time therefore stands for fast colonic transit and vice versa.

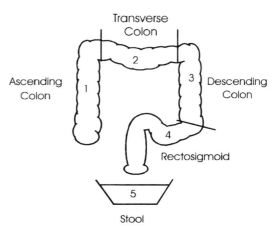

Figure 1

RESULTS

Severity of diarrhea was similar in both groups (figure 2) and stool weights were 527±77 g for PEG and 513±71 for the group receiving lactulose, respectively.

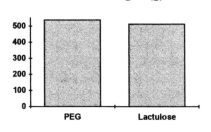

Figure 2

Right colonic transit (figures 3 and 4) was significantly faster in PEG-induced diarrhea. After

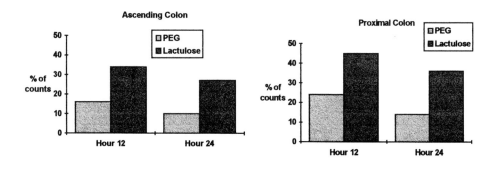

Figure 3   Figure 4

12 hours the percentage of counts in the ascending colon were 16±6% vs. 34±6% for PEG- and lactulose induced diarrhea, respectively (figure 3); after 24 hours percentage of counts in the ascending colon was 10±6%(PEG) and 27±5% (lactulose) (p<0.05). Similarly, percentage of counts in the proximal colon was 24±9% and 45±8% at hour 12, and 14±6% and 36±6% at hour 24 (p<0.05), for PEG and lactulose, respectively (figure 4).

Figure 5 demonstrates the significantly faster **total colonic transit** after ingestion of PEG compared to lactulose induced diarrhea. Geometric center at hour 24 was 4.5±0.4 for the group receiving PEG and 3.2±0.2 after lactulose ingestion (p<0.05). Cumulative counts in stools after 24 hours was 79±10% and 38±8% for PEG and lactulose (p<0.05), respectively (figure 5).

Figure 5
Total colonic
transit:

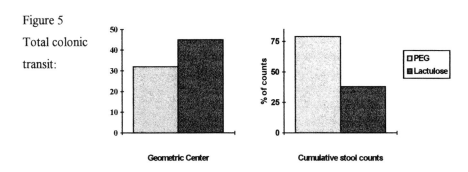

CONCLUSION AND SUMMARY

At comparable stool weights lactulose induced diarrhea had slower right colonic and total colonic transit compared to the model of pure osmotic diarrhea. We suggest that products of bacterial metabolism - maybe short chain fatty acids - reduce the acceleration of transit caused by an increased volume load.

These experiments show the effect of bacterial metabolism of lactulose to safeguard the human body to loose water: Although the osmotic load after ingestion of lactulose (275 mosm) was more than twofold the osmotic load after PEG ingestion (120 mosm) stool volumes were similar in both groups and colonic transit was even slower in lactulose induced diarrhea.

LITERATURE

1. KD Fine, GJ Krejs, JS Fordtran: Diarrhea. p290 - 316. In "Gastrointestinal Disease, Pathophysiology, Diagnosis, Management", MH Sleisinger, JS Fordtran (editors), 4th edition, 1989

2. J Hammer, HF Hammer, RW Lipp, RE Stauber, A Gangl, GJ Krejs: Colonic transit and its role in carbohydrate salvage capacity in lactulose induced diarrhea. Gastroenterology, 1993; 104, 251

3. HF Hammer, CA Santa Ana, LR Schiller, JS Fordtran: Studies of osmotic diarrhea induced in normal subjects by ingestion of polyethylene glycol and lactulose. J Clin Invest, 1989; 84, 1056-1062

4. M Proano, M Camilleri, SF Phillips, ML Brown, GM Thomforde: Transit of solids through the human colon: regional quantification in the unprepared bowel. Am J Physiol, 1990; 258, G856-862

Radioactive Isotopes in
Clinical Medicine and Research XXII
ed. by H. Bergmann, A. Kroiss and H. Sinzinger
© 1997 Birkhäuser Verlag Basel/Switzerland

CLINICAL VALUE OF LUNG PERFUSION SCINTIGRAPHY IN INFANTS WITH CONGENITAL CARDIO-PULMONARY DISEASE

P. Theissen, M. Dietlein,
M. Schmidt, U. Menniken*, H. Schicha

Clinic for Nuclear Medicine
*Dept. of Paediatric Cardiology
University of Cologne
D-50924 Cologne, Germany

SUMMARY

The value of lung perfusion scintigraphy with Technetium-MAA was studied in 95 infants and children (mean age 4.0 years) with a variety of congenital cardio-pulmonary anomalies. The majority of the patients underwent palliative or corrective surgery. In 137 perfusion scans tracer distribution over the lungs, as well as the systemic circulation, and right-to-left-shunts were calculated. Compared to cardiac catheterization and clinical follow-up findings the frequencies of answering the clinical question and of providing additional information was evaluated. The results showed that the clinical question could be answered in 92% and that in about 72% the value of the examinations could be improved because of additional information.

INTRODUCTION

Perfusion scintigraphy of the lungs is a routine method in the diagnosis of acquired lung disease in adults, mainly in pulmonary embolism. But also in congenital cardio-pulmonary anomalies it can provide functional information about distribution of lung perfusion, perfusion of the systemic circulation, and shunts. More recently, such information becomes of increasing relevance because a growing number of children with cardio-pulmonary anomalies can be treated surgically by correction or palliative procedures. Therefore, complete diagnostic information about morphological and functional aspects is essential not only pre-operatively but also post-operatively and for a non-invasive follow-up. Lung perfusion scintigraphy is non-invasive, works without higher radiation doses and is as well quick and quantifiable also in infants. Therefore, it seems to be of value in the diagnostic in patients with congenital cardio-pulmonary diseases. With respect to the value of this clinically usefull method no reports with larger patient groups exist.

Therefore, the purpose of the recent study was to answer the following questions: Is routine lung perfusion scintigraphy of clinical relevance in congenital cardio-pulmonal disease in childhood, especially in the advent of high-sophisticated methods as magnetic resonance imaging? How often does lung perfusion scintigraphy provide additional information to clinical symptoms and cardiac catheterization ? How often and especially in which anomalies does lung perfusion scintigraphy provide aid for decision-making concerning the diagnostical and therapeutical procedure ?

PATIENTS AND METHODS

Ninty-five children (58 male and 37 female) have been examined. Their age ranged between 7 days and 16 years with a mean age of 4.0 ± 4.3 years. Grouping the patients by age table 1. shows that the majority of the patients were younger than 5 years.

Table 1. Patients groups by age

< 1 year	n = 32	5 - 10 years	n = 18
1 - 5 years	n = 32	> 10 years	n = 13

Seventy-two of the children underwent different types of corrective or palliative surgical procedures (s. table 2.). All children had a pre- and post-operative cardiac catheterization. The variety of the main diagnoses and the surgical procedures of the children included in the recent study is summarized in table 2..

Table 2. Main diagnoses and surgical procedures

n	Main Disease	n	Correction / Palliative OP
25	Pulmonary atresia	37	Total correction / closure
13	Single ventricle	36	Palliative shunts
11	Misconnection of pulmonary veins	13	Banding of pulmonary artery
11	Tetralogy of Fallot	6	Switch operation
8	Transposition of great arteries	2	Modified Fontane operation
6	Ventricular septal defect (VSD)	1	Resection of lung sequester
6	Periph. pulmonary stenosis, hypoplast. pulmonary arteries		
4	Atrial septal defect		
3	Tricuspid atresia		
3	Hemitruncus		
2	Single atrium		
2	Anatom. changes of the lungs		
1	Patent ductus arteriosus		

In the 95 patients 137 lung perfusion scintigrams have been performed. Sixty-four patients underwent only a single examination. A second group of 31 patients underwent multiple examinations. This patient group consisted of 19 patients with pre- and post-operative control examinations, 2 patients with pre-operative follow-up examinations, and 10 patients with post-operative follow-up examinations only. ^{99m}Tc-MAA was administered intravenously with an activity dosage depending on body weight (according to the values recommended by the EANM paediatric task group). The number of particles was limited between 20,000 and 30,000. The tracer distribution over the lungs was assessed qualitatively and quantitatively. For quantitative assessment irregulare regions of interest were applied over the lungs (right / left lung ratio) and for the systemic circulation over the head, the proximal extremities, and the body stem. The amount of a right-to-left-shunt was calculated.

Based on these assessments of the single scintigrams the diagnostic aid of the lung perfusion scintigraphy in congenital cardio-pulmonary diseases was proven by the questions mentioned below, which had to be answered for every examination. It was assessed by a paediatric cardiologist and a nuclear medicine physicist, whether these questions could be answered sufficiently or not and whether information in addition to answering the clinical questions could be provided. The scintigraphic results were compared to the findings of cardiac catherterization (CC) and to those of the further clinical follow-up examinations. To explain how the question for additional information was judged the example of one patient with a VSD and an atresia of the right pulmonary artery is presented: The clinical question was answered by showing the relative amount of perfusion of the right lung and the distribution of the tracer within both lungs. The additional information consisted in specifying the part of the systemic perfusion which supplies the right lung.

For the (primary) single examinations the questions were as follows:

- Pre-operative distribution of lung perfusion, size of R/L-shunt

- Pre-operative determination of the type and localization of a palliative aorto-pulmonary shunt

- Assessment of the effect of a peripheral pulmonary artery (PA) stenosis

- Effect of circumscript changes of lung morphology

- Evaluation of lung perfusion in case of an atypical connection of the lung vessels

- Reduction of O_2-saturation after PA-banding and palliative aorto-pulmonary shunt operation

- Post-operative complications concerning lung perfusion

- Post-operative question: Which lung or part of the lung did profit from a correction resp. aorto-pulmonary shunt operation ?

For the pre- and post-operative follow-up examinations the following questions should be answered regarding the assessment of the outcome of operation:

- In comparison to the pre-operation: Efficiency of correction or palliative shunt operation. - Improvement of the lung perfusion (amount of tracer accumulation in the lungs compared to shunt reduction resp. radionuclide up-take within the systemic circulation).

- Compared to the pre-operation: Which lung or part of the lung did profit from the correction procedures resp. from palliative shunt operation ?

- Reduction or removal of R/L-shunt ?

- Normalized lung inflow after correction of abnormal pulmonary vessel connections.

RESULTS

Table 3. summarizing the results of the (primary) single examinations in all patients allows the conclusion that the clinical question could be answered in about 92% of the patients and that additional information was achieved by lung perfusion scintigraphy in more than two thirds of the examined children.

Table 3. Results of single examinations in all patients grouped by diagnoses

No. of patients	Clinical question	Additional information	Main diagnoses
25	23	22	Pulmonary atresia
13	11	10	Single ventricle
11	11	11	Tetralogy of Fallot
11	10	6	Misconnection pulmonary veins
8	7	5	Transposition great arteries
6	6	3	Ventricular septal defect
6	6	6	Periph. pulmonary stenosis, hypoplast. pulmonary arteries
6	6	1	Atrial septal defect, single atrium
3	2	2	Hemitruncus
3	3	0	Tricuspid atresia
2	2	2	Anatom. changes of the lungs
1	0	0	Patent ductus arteriosus
95	87 (91.6 %)	68 (71.6 %)	

The highest percentages answering the clinical question occurred in complex anomalies with different types of surgigal procedures.

As shown in table 4. the pre- and post-operative scintigrams after palliative shunt or correction operation could also answere the clinical question in most patients. A good accordance with catheterization findings in the assessment of the surgical outcome was achieved as well.

Table 4. Results of pre-/post-operative follow-up

n	Clinical question	Accordance with CC	Operation	Diagnoses
11	10	10	Palliative aorto-pulmonary shunt	Pulmonary atresia / stenosis Tetralogy of Fallot Single ventricle Periph. pulmonary stenosis Hypopl. pulmonary artery
8	6	7	Correction operation	Tetralogy of Fallot Transposition of great arteries Misconnection pulmonary veins Single atrium

DISCUSSION

Although perfusion scintigraphy of the lungs with albumine particles is not only an easy and quickly to perform but also a quantifiable method, its value for complementary information in addition to echocardiography and cardiac catheterization seems to be underestimated. In contrast to observations in primary congenital lung diseases (1) only a few authors report results of perfusion scintigraphy of the lungs in patients with congenital cardio-pulmonary diseases (1,2,3,4,5). In accordance with these authors the catheterization data confirm the results of the scintigraphic examinations also in the recent study. Moreover, the high ratios of answering the clinical questions and providing the clincan with additional information indicate the diagnostic value of lung perfusion scintigraphy. Only minor efforts are given in simple congenital anomalies. But in complex cardio-pulmonary changes especially in such with anomalies of the lung morphology, with anomalous pulmonary blood supply, anomalous pulmonary venous return, and/or shunts this method seems to be valuable with respect to decison-making in the diagnostical and therapeutical procedure. Therefore, lung perfusion scintigraphy can aid in setting up the indication for an intervention or re-operation in case of occurrence or worsening of a pulmonary (re-)stenosis or stenoses after Fontan-procedure or aorto-pulmonary shunts (2). The shunt calculation should be done carefully and if possible from regions over the lungs and over the head and the body stem including the proximal extremities (1,6). If necessary (e.g. modified Fontan-OP with intraatrial tunnel), an examination after injection from the arm and the leg should be performed. For special questions this examination technique can be combined with radionuclide ventriculography or ventilation scintigraphy (1,3).

Because lung perfusion scintigraphy also in infants and children is a simple, reliable, and quantifiable method, it should be used more widely in cases with appropriate clinical question and for decision-making before re-catheterization or re-operation in first instance in complex anomalies with shunts and/or anomalies of pulmonary veins or arteries or post-operative shunts or conduits.

REFERENCES

1. Treves ST, Harris GBC. Chapter 17 Lung. In: Pediatric Nuclear Medicine. Traves ST ed. New York Springer 1985: 289 - 330
2. Meins S, Luhmer I, Kotzerke J, Hundeshagen H. Einsatz der Lungenszintigraphie im Kindesalter bei Fallot-Tetralogie und Pulmonalatresie mit Ventrikelseptumdefekt. Nucl. Med 1993; 32:A34
3. Dowdle SC, Human DG, Mann MD. Pulmonary Ventilation and Perfusion Abnormalities and Ventilation Perfusion Imbalance in Children with Pulmonary Atresia or Extreme Tetralogy of Fallot. J Nucl Med 1990; 31:1276-1279
4. Chen JTT, Robinson AE, Goodrich JK. Uneven distribution of pulmonary blood flow between left and right lungs in isolated valvular pulmonic stenosis. AJR 1969; 107:343-50
5. Mishkin F, Knote J. Radioisotope scanning of the lungs in patients with systemic-pulmonary anastomosis. AJR 1968; 102:267-73
6. Waters W. Lunge. In: Nuklearmedizin. Schicha H. ed. Stuttgart: Schattauer 1995

Radioactive Isotopes in
Clinical Medicine and Research XXII
ed. by H. Bergmann, A. Kroiss and H. Sinzinger
© 1997 Birkhäuser Verlag Basel/Switzerland

ASSESSMENT OF MEDIASTINAL INVOLVEMENT IN LUNG CANCER WITH [99mTc]-SESTAMIBI SPET

A. Chiti, G. Grasselli, L. Maffioli, M. Infante*, M. Incarbone*, E. Bombardieri.

Nuclear Medicine Division and *Thoracic Surgery Division
Istituto Nazionale per lo Studio e la Cura dei Tumori, Via Venezian 1, I-20133, Milano, ITALY

SUMMARY: We evaluated the role of [99mTc]-hexakis-2-methoxy-isobutyl-isonitrile (MIBI) SPET in lung cancer staging. 47 patients (mean age 63.3 years) with clinical and radiological suspicion of lung cancer, were enrolled in this study. All patients underwent, among the other staging procedures, CT scan and MIBI SPET of the thorax. In 36 patients a histological diagnosis was made and mediastinal lymph node involvement was demonstrated in 11. Using pathology staging as the standard MIBI SPET showed a sensitivity of 91% and a specificity of 84% while CT scan gave a sensitivity of 73% and a specificity of 60%. The MIBI SPET results were better than those of CT scan also when considering positive and negative predictive values and accuracy.

INTRODUCTION

The stage of lung cancer at the time of surgery is the most important determinant for prognosis and therapeutic strategy. Accurate imaging of primary lung cancer can be obtained with transmission computed tomography (CT) and magnetic resonance (MR) imaging, whereas the preoperative assessment of mediastinal lymph nodes with radiological procedures is still a matter of debate. In fact, the disadvantage of these imaging techniques is that the only useful criterion for determining metastatic involvement of mediastinal lymph nodes is based on the evaluation of their size (1,2). At present, the most accurate technique is doubtless mediastinoscopy, which is a surgical, invasive procedure.

The aim of this study is to assess the diagnostic contribution of SPET to the staging of lung cancer, so that mediastinoscopy can be avoided with no decrease in sensitivity.

METHODS

Forty-seven patients, 44 males and 3 females, mean age 63.3 years, range 49-82, with clinical and radiological suspicion of lung cancer were enrolled in the study. The staging procedures included: plain film X-ray and CT scan of the thorax, fiberoptic bronchoscopy with biopsy, pulmonary function tests, preoperative cardiological examination, arterial blood analysis, routine laboratory tests and SPET. Of the whole patient series, 31 subjects underwent thoracic surgery and 5 patients were submitted to mediastinoscopy with sampling of mediastinal nodes. A total of 36 patients (34 males and 2 females, mean age 63.3 years, range 49-82) were finally evaluated for mediastinal involvement. The thoracic surgery techniques were lobectomy or pneumonectomy, depending on the locoregional extension of the disease. Nine patients were not operated because the extension of their disease precluded surgical treatment. Two patients were not submitted to surgery after clinical and instrumental demonstration of the phlogistic nature of their disease.

All patients gave their informed consent before entering the study. They were injected with 740-925 MBq of MIBI. Scintigraphic acquisition started 25 minutes after tracer administration. Data from the first 38 patients were acquired using a Toshiba GCA-901A single head gamma camera.

The remaining images were acquired using a Toshiba GCA-7200A dual head gamma camera. Acquisition were performed using low energy, high resolution, parallel hole collimators. The acquisition parameters were: 60 frames over 360°, 30 s per frame, matrix 64×64, zoom 1.5. All images were processed on the Toshiba GCA-7200A console. The data were visually evaluated by two experienced nuclear medicine physicians with knowledge of the CT results and blinded to the pathological findings. CT scan of the thorax was performed after i.v. injection of non-ionic iodinated contrast medium with a window for the lung parenchyma and a window for the mediastinum. Transaxial slices of 8 mm without overlap were reconstructed and evaluated by experienced radiologists.

RESULTS

Of the 47 patients we studied, eleven were not operated due to the extensive disease or presence of distant metastases and excluded from the final evaluation. So, we studied 39 lung lesions in the 36 patients evaluated. Seventeen patients had adenocarcinomas, 12 squamous cell carcinomas and 2 small cell lung cancer. One patient had a lung carcinoid, 1 multiple lung amartochondromas and 1 had a metastasis from gastric cancer. Five patients turned out to suffer from non-neoplastic lung diseases, including 1 lung fibrosis, 1 abscess bronchiolitis 1 pachy-pleuritis and 2 phlogistic lesions. In this series, 1 patient had 2 tumors, an adenocarcinoma and a squamous cell carcinoma, 1 had bilateral adenocarcinomas and another had a bifocal squamous cell carcinoma. Mediastinal node involvement was pathologically demonstrated in 11 of the 36 patients (31%) and all the 5 mediastinoscopies were positive (Figure 1).

Results of MIBI SPET and CT scan in mediastinal imaging are summarized in Table 1, while Table 2 illustrates our results in the primary tumor evaluation.

Table 1. CT scan and MIBI in the evaluation of mediastinal node involvement

	CT scan	MIBI
Sensitivity	73% (8/11)	91% (10/11)
Specificity	60% (15/25)	84% (21/25)
Positive Predictive Value	44% (8/18)	71% (10/14)
Negative Predictive Value	83% (15/18)	95% (21/22)
Accuracy	64% (23/36)	86% (31/36)

Table 2. Results of MIBI SPET in 39 primary lung lesions evaluated in 36 patients

Sensitivity	85% (29/34)
Specificity	100% (5/5)
Positive Predictive Value	100% (29/29)
Negative Predictive Value	50% (5/10)
Accuracy	87% (34/39)

DISCUSSION

CT and MR imaging are certainly superior to other diagnostic procedures in the detection of primary lung tumors. Mediastinal involvement is a critical issue both for therapeutic decision making and prognosis assessment (3,4). Mediastinoscopy is the most accurate staging technique for the evaluation of nodal involvement. It is generally acknowledged that lymph node enlargement on CT requires histological confirmation by mediastinoscopy or an alternative tech-nique, particularly if the demonstration of nodal metastases would preclude surgical resection (5).

Radiological procedures, such as CT or MR imaging, are commonly used for this purpose but are flawed by their low sensitivity (6,7).

The oncological application of MIBI is gaining interest among clinicians. Some authors have reported data on MIBI in bronchogenic carcinoma that seem very similar to the results obtained with ^{201}Tl (8,9,10). When the primary lesion is investigated, the lack of specificity and the high myocardial uptake of both tracers lead to discouraging results. Moreover, in our opinion it is not necessary to evaluate the primary lesion with techniques other than CT or MR imaging. This approach will only be interesting if new radiopharmaceuticals that are able to distinguish different tumor types will become available.

Recently, two papers have been published that report on the evaluation of mediastinal involvement with MIBI. LeBouthillier et al. (11) studied 26 patients and concluded that MIBI could be a useful tool in the evaluation of negative hilar and mediastinal lymph node regions, so that mediastinoscopy could be safely omitted. Aktoloun et al. (12) reported data from 38 patients with lung cancer studied with CT scan and planar MIBI acquisition. They concluded that MIBI can be employed for the staging of lung cancer patients, for the evaluation of mediastinal involvement and in follow-up, to distinguish residual or recurrent disease from post-radiotherapy necrosis.

In our series, it must be emphasized that data were matched with the final histological staging, which is crucial for a correct analysis of a new imaging technique. Our findings demonstrated that MIBI SPET was superior to CT scan in evaluating mediastinal node metastases from lung cancer.

We found a sensitivity and specificity for CT in our patients similar to those reported in the literature (9). It has been reported that SPET gives no additional information with respect to planar imaging (12). This is a quite controversial statement since SPET is generally considered as having a superior resolution, which is why we preferred to acquire only SPET images, and thus avoid patients to be submitted to time consuming acquisitions.

CONCLUSION

On the basis of our results, we can conclude that MIBI SPET is a sensitive, non-invasive method to assess mediastinal involvement in the preoperative staging of lung cancer and its diagnostic accuracy is better than that of CT scan. This technique, performed in combination with CT and/or MR imaging, in selected patients can safely overcome invasive staging procedures such as mediastinoscopy.

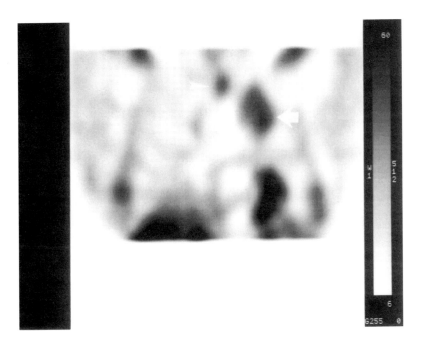

Figure 1. Coronal slice showing a left upper lobe tumor (arrow) and a large adenopathy in the upper mediastinum (arrowhead). This patient had a positive mediastinoscopy and the tumor was assessed as being an adenocarcinoma.

REFERENCES

1. Libschitz HI, McKenna RJ. Mediastinal lymph node size in lung cancer. *Am J Roentgenol* 1984; 143:715-718.

2. Genereux GP, Howie JL. Normal mediastinal lymph node size and number. CT and anatomic study. *Am J Roentgenol* 1984; 142:1095-1100.

3. Ginsberg RJ, Kris MG, Armstrong JG. Non-small cell lung cancer. In: De Vita VT, Hellman S, Rosenberg SA eds. *Cancer: principles and practice of oncology*, 4th edition. Philadelphia: JB Lippincott Co; 1993:673-723.

4. Kayser K, Buzelbruk H, Probst G, et al. Retrospective and prospective tumor staging evaluating prognostic factors in operated bronchus carcinoma patients. *Cancer* 1987; 59:355-361.

5. Laurent F, Drouillard J, Dorcier F, et al. Bronchogenic carcinoma staging: CT vs MR imaging. Assessment with surgery. *Eur J Cardiothorac Surg* 1988; 2:31-36.

6. McCloud TC, Bourgouin PM, Greenberg RW, et al. Bronchogenic carcinoma: analysis of staging in the mediastinum with CT by correlative lymph node mapping and sampling. *Radiology 1992; 182:319-323.*

7. Rubin E, Sanders C, Harvey JC, Beattie EJ. Diagnostic imaging and staging of primary lung cancer. *Seminars in Surgical Oncology* 1993; 9:85-91.

8. Hassan IM, Sahweil A, Constantinides C, et al. Uptake and kinetics of Tc-99m-hexakis 2-methoxy isobutyl isonitrile in benign and malignant lesions in the lungs. *Clin Nucl Med* 1989; 14:333-340.

9. Muller ST, Reiner C, Paas M, et al. Tc-99m-MIBI and Tl-201 uptake in bronchial carcinoma. *J Nucl Med* 1989; 30:845.

10. Muller ST, Guth-Taugelides B, Creutzig H. Imaging of malignant tumors with Tc-99m-MIBI SPECT. *J Nucl Med* 1987; 28:562.

11. LeBouthillier G, Taillefer R, Lambert R, et al. Detection of primary lung cancer with Tc-99m-SestaMIBI. *J Nucl Med* 1993; 34:140p

12. Aktolun C, Bayhan H, Pabuccu Y, Bilgic H, Acar H, Koylu R. Assessment of tumor necrosis and detection of mediastinal lymph node metastasis in bronchial carcinoma with technetium-99m sestamibi imaging: comparison with CT scan. *Eur J Nucl Med* 1994; 21:973-979.

Radioactive Isotopes in
Clinical Medicine and Research XXII
ed. by H. Bergmann, A. Kroiss and H. Sinzinger
© 1997 Birkhäuser Verlag Basel/Switzerland

BONE SCANNING IN PREOPERATIVE DECISION–MAKING IN HEMIMANDIBULAR ELONGATION

K.H. Bohuslavizki, A. Kerscher, W. Brenner, B. Fleiner, H. Wolf, C. Sippel,
S. Tinnemeyer, U. Teichert, M. Clausen and E. Henze

Clinics of Nuclear Medicine and Oral Surgery, Christian-Albrechts-Universitiy,
Arnold-Heller-Str. 9, 24105 Kiel, Germany

SUMMARY: To evaluate the usefullness of bone scanning in hemimandibular elongation (HE) 22 patients underwent bone scanning prior to surgery. Activity of growth was quantified by calculating a L/R ratio. Correcting osteotomy (CO) was performed in patients showing L/R < 1.10, and patients with L/R > 1.10 underwent condylectomy (CE). 20 patients showed L/R < 1.10. In 13 of them a CO was performed without any relapse. 2 patients showed marked unilateral increased uptake. In one patient bone scan was not considered, and CO was performed with subsequent recurrence of laterognathia. The other patient underwent CE without any relapse. In conclusion, bone scanning has significant clinical value in preoperative decision-making in HE.

INTRODUCTION

Hemimandibular elongation is characterized by persistent unilateral growth of the mandibular bone (1) resulting in laterognathia (2). Usually growth is ceasing spontanously. When growth has stopped correcting osteotomy can be performed. In case of persistent growth and progressive facial asymmetry the growth center should be removed by condylectomy. However, growth activity can not be assessed by conventional radiological procedures.

Therefore, it was the purpose of this study to define the pathophysiological status of patients suffering from hemimandibular elongazion and to evaluate the clinical impact of bone scanning in preoperative decision-making.

MATERIALS AND METHODS

Bone scans were performed in 22 patients suffering from hemimandibular elongation. There were 8 male and 14 female patients ranging in age from 15 to 35 years. Anterior and lateral views of the skull were obtained 3 hrs after i.v. injection of 450-650 MBq Tc-99m-MDP. A L/R ratio was calculated from irregular ROI´s located at the mandibular condylus of each side after correction for background activity. L/R was defined to be symmetric (<1.05), borderline asymmetric (1.05–1.10) or clearly asymmetric (>1.10) as suggested by various authors (3-7). Consequently, in patients showing L/R < 1.10 correcting osteotomy was performed, and patients with L/R > 1.10 underwent condylectomy (8).

RESULTS

In 16 out of 22 patients L/R-ratio was <1.05 indicating symmetric growth of both mandibular bones. Mean L/R-ratio was 1.009 ± 0.004. 4 of 22 patients showed borderline asymmetry with a L/R-ratio of 1.079 ± 0.009. Of these 20 patients 13 underwent correcting osteotomy in various surgical methods. During a follow-up period of 5 years no relapse occured. One patient with a L/R-ratio of 1.008 is shown in Figure 1.

Two patients exhibited a marked asymmetric growth with L/R-ratios of 1.65 and 2.47, respectively. In the latter patient (see Fig. 2) with rapidly progressive laterognathia condylectomy was performed. As the growth zone was removed no relapse occured during the next 3 years. In the patient with a L/R-ratio of 1.65 correcting osteotomy was performed. Again, this patient developped a laterognathia within 6 months postoperatively.

DISCUSSION

Hemimandibular elongation is characterized by a persistent growth of the mandibulo-condylar region resulting in a laterognathia. When bone growth spontanously ceases surgical correction will yield stabil results, and when surgical correction is desired despite bone growth persists the surgeon has to assure that he removes the active growth zone. Therefore, it is mandatory for the surgeon to by aware of the growth state of the mandibulo-condylar growth zone in order to chose the appropriate surgical procedure. However, conventional radiological procedures are not able to provide this information. On the other hand, bone scintigraphy represents the activity of bone meatbolism. Therefore, bone scanning was suggested to help in diseases in which treatment options differ with a varying degree of bone growth (6, 9). This holds true for hemimandibular elongation.

The surgical manouever chosen was concordant with the results of bone scintigraphy in all but one patients who underwent surgery. In one patient a clearly asymmetric growth was demonstrated by a L/R-ratio of 2.65. Consequently, the growth zone was removed by condylectomy. In the follow-up of 3 years no relapse occured. In the other patients symmetric or borderline asymmetric growth was demonstrated. Consequently, correcting osteotomy was performed, and none of them relapsed.

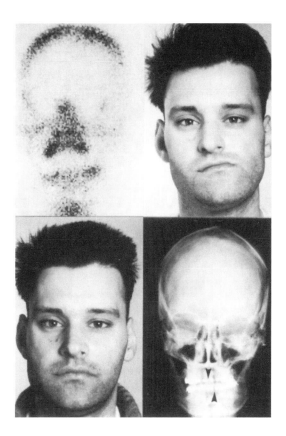

Fig. 1: 26 year old patient with left-sided latherognathia (right upper) as demonstrated in conventional a.p. radiograph of the skull (right lower). Observe, symmetric tracer uptake in the anterior view of the bone scan (left upper). Consequently, 6 months after correcting oseteotomy yielded stabil results (left lower).

The surgical manouever chosen was discordant with the result of bone scintigraphy in 1 patient. Despite the clearly elevated L/R-ratio of 1.65 indicating persistent active growth correcting osteotomy was performed in this patient rather than the appropriate procedure, i.e. condylectomy.

Bone scintigraphy was performed in planar technique in this study. Therefore, L/R-ratios were calculated from anterior images. However, bone scintigraphy can not differentiate between persistent growth and degenerative processes in the mandibulo-condylar region. Therefore, in every patient conventional radiographs were obtained to exclude degenerative processes. No degenerative processes were shown in our patients as could be expected from their young age.

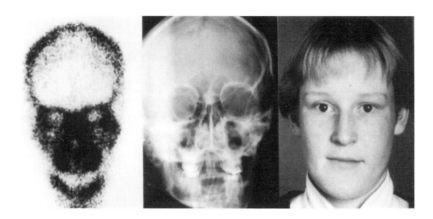

Fig. 2: 16 year old patient with right-sided latherognathia (right) as demonstrated more clearly in a conventional a.p. radiograph of the skull (middle). Observe, clearly asymmetric tracer uptake with a R/L-ratio of 2.47 (left). Consequently, growth zone was removed by condylectomy, and no relapse occured within a follow-up period of 3 years.

From our data we may suggest the following procedure in patients with hemimandibular elongation:

- In case of symmetric tracer uptake in both mandibulo-condylar regions correcting osteotomy may be performed.
- In case of borderline asymmetry of tracer uptake bone scan should be repeated after 6 months.
- In case of clearly asymmetric tracer uptake bone scan should be repeated after an observation period of 1 year if clinically tolerable. If surgical intervention cannot be delayed the growth zone should be removed by condylectomy.

CONCLUSIONS

With respect to clearly defined diagnostic criteria bone scanning has significant clinical value for treatment planning in hemimandibular elongation by quantification of pathological bone growth.

REFERENCES

1. Wangerin K. Einzeitige bimaxilläre Korrektur extremer Fehlbisse. Vorbehandlung, Planung und Operationsmethode mit funktionsstabiler Fixierung im Ober- und Unterkiefer. Dtsch Z Mund Kiefer Gesichtschir 1990; **14:** 424–431.

2. Obwegeser HL, Makek MS. Hemimandibular hyperplasia – hemimandibular elongation. J Maxillofac Surg 1986; **14:** 183–208.

3. Beirne OR, Leake DL. Technetium-99m pyrophosphate uptake in a case of unilateral condylar hyperplasia. J Oral Surg 1980; **38:** 385–386.

4. Kaban LB, Cisneros GJ, Heyman S, Treves S. Assessment of mandibular growth by skeletal scintigraphy. J Oral Maxillofac Surg 1982; **40:** 18–22.

5. Matteson SR, Proffit WR, Terry BC, Staab EV, Burkes EJ. Bone scanning with 99m-technetium phosphate to assess condylar hyperplasia. Report of two cases. Oral Surg Oral Med Oral Pathol 1985; **60:** 356–367.

6. Murray IPC, Ford JC. Tc-99m medronate scintigraphy in mandibular condylar hyperplasia. Clin Nucl Med 1982; **7:** 474–475.

7. Norman JEDB, Painter DM. Hyperplasia of the mandibular condyle. J Maxillofac Surg 1980; **8:** 161–175.

8. Paulus G, Hirschfelder U, Feistel H. Computergestützte quantitative Skelettszintigraphie bei der Therapieplanung der kondylären Hyperplasie. Fortschr Kiefer Gesichtschir 1986; **32:** 180–181.

9. Steinhäuser EW. Kondylektomie oder korrektive Osteotomie bei der kondylären Hyperplasie. Fortschr Kiefer Gesichtschir 1980; **25:** 132–135.

Free Papers

Radioactive Isotopes in
Clinical Medicine and Research XXII
ed. by H. Bergmann, A. Kroiss and H. Sinzinger
© 1997 Birkhäuser Verlag Basel/Switzerland

Copper-67 labeled mAb chCE7 as a potential therapeutic agent for neuroblastoma: improved biodistributions of copper-67-chCE7 F(ab')2

I. Novak-Hofer, K. Zimmermann, H. Amstutz[#], H. Maecke[+], U. Doerr[*], H. Bihl[*], A. Haldemann[$], P. A. Schubiger
Radiopharmacy Division, Paul Scherrer Institute, CH-5232 Villigen, [#]ZLB, Swiss Red Cross Berne, Depts. of Nuclear Medicine, [$]Inselspital, Berne, [*]Katharinenhospital Stuttgart and [+]Kantonsspital, Basel.

Introduction:

Neuroblastoma relapses associated with bone marrow infiltrations are considered a favorable therapeutic setting for radioimmunotherapy (RIT), because access of radiolabeled, tumor specific monoclonal antibodies (mAbs) is much better than in solid tumors. MAb chCE7 is a chimeric antibody directed against a neuroblastoma associated cell surface glycoprotein, which is internalized into its target cells (1) and first clinical results with ^{123}I and ^{131}I-labeled chCE7 have shown that it is taken up rapidly and strongly into bone marrow infiltrations (2,3). We plan to evaluate mAb chCE7 for RIT applications in such cases.

Antibody conjugates chelating beta-particle emitting radionuclides such as for instance ^{90}Y, ^{186}Re, ^{67}Cu, are thought to bring a therapeutic advantage over ^{131}I-labeled preparations used at the present time and in particular reduced emission of gamma radiation is expected to lower dose limiting toxicity. We have chosen ^{67}Cu because it is a potential therapeutic nuclide with a mean beta emission of 141 keV similar to ^{131}I but with a much reduced gamma component (182 keV, 60% compared with over 80% in the case of ^{131}I) and has a half life of 2.6 days, which is well suited to the biokinetics of antibodies. For labeling of mAb chCE7 and its F(ab')2 fragments macrocyclic amine ligands which form copper complexes of high in vivo stability are used and labeling with ^{67}Cu produced in house at PSI can be achieved by efficient and convenient procedures (4).

As mAb chCE7 is internalized into neuroblastoma cells and degraded intracellularly in lysosomes we investigated the metabolism of ^{67}Cu-chCE7 at the level of tumor cells in culture (5) and found that cellular retention of its terminal degradation product leads to prolonged association of radioactivity with tumor cells in contrast to the rapid release of metabolites arising from radioiodinated chCE7.

The use of antibody fragments is frequently evoked in RIT concepts, because of their more rapid clearance from the circulation and consequently lower toxicity compared with intact mAbs (6). As ^{67}Cu-chCE7 F(ab')2 was also found to be internalized, we investigated its biodistributions in nude mice bearing neuroblastoma xenografts in order to find out if rapid clearance from the blood combined with prolonged retention of radioactivity in tumor cells could lead to an additional therapeutic benefit. Rapid tumor uptake and good tumor/blood ratios were found, but as observed in other systems using F(ab')2 fragments with metallic radionuclides including ^{67}Cu and ^{64}Cu (7,8,9) high levels of radioactivity were found to accumulate in the kidneys.

In order to delineate some factors contributing to this effect, we analyzed the time course of appearance of ^{67}Cu-labeled metabolites in the kidney and identified the nature of the principal degradation products. We also tested the effect on biodistributions in neuroblastoma-bearing nude mice of changing the cationic CPTA ligand used for ^{67}Cu labeling to a novel anionic, more hydrophilic ligand (DO3A). Using this new copper chelator led to a four-fold reduction of radioactivity present in the kidneys and a concomittant four-fold increase in tumor-bound radioactivity.

Materials and Methods:

Materials: MAb chCE7 was purified from tissue culture supernatants as described previously (5) and F(ab')2 fragment was prepared by digestion with immobilised pepsin using a kit from Pierce according to the manufacturer's protocol for human IgG1. F(ab')2 fragments were purified by FPLC gelfiltration chromatography with Superose 6 and purity of preparations was checked with SDS-PAGE.

The bifunctional copper ligand CPTA (4-(1,4,8,11-tetraazacyclotetradec-1-yl)methyl benzoic acid tetrahydrochloride)was custom synthetized and the bifunctional copper ligand DO3A (1-(p-amino benzyl)-1,4,7,10-tetraazacyclodecane 4,7,10- triacetate) as well as the lysine conjugate of CPTA were synthetized as described previously (9).

^{67}Cu was produced in house at the Paul Scherrer Institute (10).

The human neuroblastoma cell line SKN-AS was cultured as described (1) and was used for cell binding assays for quality control of labeled immunoconjugates and for generating subcutaneous tumors in nude mice.

Methods:

Radiocopper labeling: MAb chCE7 and its F(ab')2 fragment were derivatized with the N-hydroxysuccinimide ester of the CPTA ligand and labeled with ^{67}Cu as described (5). For labeling via the DO3A ligand, the ligand was activated with thiophosgene, its isothiocyanate derivative was coupled to chCE7 F(ab')2 fragments and ^{67}Cu labeling was performed as described (9).Specific activity of labeled immunoconjugates ranged between 0.5 and 1.0 µCi/µg Immunoreactivity of ^{67}Cu-labeled preparations was measured with a cell binding assay (1) and was found to range between 80-100%.

^{67}Cu activity was measured in a gamma counter using a 160-210 keV energy setting.

Analysis of tissue extracts by HPLC and SDS-PAGE: At the indicated time points after injection of ^{67}Cu-labeled immunoconjugates (10 µg, 5-10 µCi) into the tail vein of nude mice, kidneys were removed, extracts were prepared and analyzed by SDS-PAGE and reverse phase HPLC as described (9).

Measurement of chCE7 F(ab')2 biodistributions: Adult female nude mice (strain ICR-ZH nu/nu) from the University of Zuerich were inoculated with $5 \cdot 10^6$ SKN-AS human neuroblastoma cells on each flank and were used after 14 days when tumor weight was 200-600 mg. Groups of 3 animals were injected with ^{67}Cu-CPTA -or ^{67}Cu-DO3A-chCE7 F(ab')2 (5 µCi, 8 µg) into tail veins. At the indicated time points animals were sacrificed, tumor, blood and the indicated organs were removed, rinsed in saline and counted in a gamma counter. The percent injected dose was determined by measuring in parallel a diluted aliquot of the injected solutions.

Results and Discussion:

Low molecular weight metabolites appearing after injection of ^{67}Cu-chCE7 and ^{67}Cu-chCE7 F(ab')2 fragments in nude mice bearing neuroblastoma xenografts:

When cellular uptake and degradation of ^{67}Cu-chCE7 in the SKN-AS human neuroblastoma cell line was studied, a low MW degradation product was found to accumulate intracellularly (5). Extracts from SKN-AS cells were analyzed after 24h of internalization and degradation by reverse phase HPLC and a principal peak of radioactivity was detected with the same retention time as a standard consisting of the lysine adduct of the ^{67}Cu-CPTA complex (Fig.1A). Although extracts were treated with EDTA prior to separation in order to chelate any "loosely" bound ^{67}Cu no peak corresponding to the ^{67}Cu-EDTA standard was found to be present, and there was also no evidence of a degradation product consisting of the ^{67}Cu-CPTA complex without attachement of a terminal amino acid. Low MW degradation products were analyzed by the same procedure in SKN-AS tumor xenografts (Fig.1B) and in the liver (Fig.1C) of nude mice 24h after injection of ^{67}Cu-chCE7 and were also found to consist mainly of the lysine-^{67}Cu-CPTA complex. Two minor degradation products with retention times of 6min and 19.5min could not be identified so far. Injection of ^{67}Cu-chCE7 F(ab')2 fragments into tumor bearing mice leads to rapid and strong accumulation of radioactivity in the kidneys (Table 1A). HPLC analysis of kidney extracts 2h after injection (Fig. 1D) showed that the low MW radioactivity present in the kidneys consists of the lysine-^{67}Cu-CPTA metabolite. The results indicate that this metabolite is the principal low MW degradation product of ^{67}Cu -chCE7 and its F(ab')2 fragment.

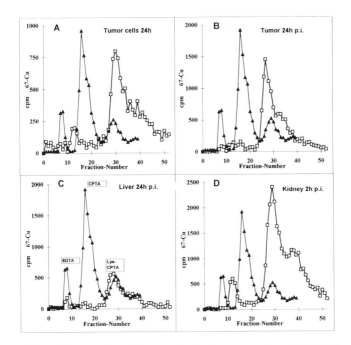

Figure 1: Separation of tumor cell and tissue extracts by reverse phase HPLC after injection of ^{67}Cu-chCE7 F(ab')$_2$ (D) and ^{67}Cu-chCE7 (A,B,C)

Time course of appearance of degradation products in the kidney of mice after injection of ^{67}Cu-chCE7 F(ab')$_2$:

It is known that although the kidney plays no role in the catabolism of intact IgG, IgG fragments such as L-chains or Bence-Jones proteins are actively catabolized in the kidney. In the case of ^{67}Cu-chCE7 F(ab')$_2$ fragments which are,with a MW of 100 000, theoretically above the cut off of the glomerular filter, it is not clear whether they enter the kidney and are degraded in the glomeruli or proximal tubule cells, followed by readsorption of amino acid-linked metabolites, or whether smaller fragments enter the kidney and are subject to glomerular filtration.In order to address this question we analyzed kidney extracts early after injection of ^{67}Cu-chCE7 F(ab')$_2$, Fig.2 shows an electronic autoradiograph of an SDS-gel separating kidney extracts prepared 15min, 30min, 1h and 2h post injection . At the earliest time points ^{67}Cu-chCE7 F(ab')$_2$ fragments (MW 100 kD), fragments with a MW of 35kD and smaller fragments migrating with the dye front and below were detected. From these data it appears that early after injection F(ab')$_2$ fragments are present in the kidney, however degradation into smaller fragments and the main lysine-^{67}Cu-CPTA metabolite proceeds very rapidly.

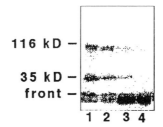

Figure 2: Autoradiograph of an SDS-gel separating kidney extracts after 15 min (1), 30 min (2), 1h (3) and 2h (4) post injection of ^{67}Cu-chCE7 F(ab')$_2$. Numbers on the left indicate MWs in Kilodalton.

We conclude that at least some ^{67}Cu-F(ab')$_2$ enters the kidney, is degraded in glomeruli or proximal tubule cells and the terminal degradation product which contains the lysine residue over which the chelator is coupled to the F(ab')$_2$ accumulates in renal tissue, possibly because its reuptake is facilitated by the positively charged nature of the lysine-CPTA-copper complex. Several different strategies have been adopted to overcome both rapid catabolism and accumulation of radiometal - labeled metabolites in the kidney, including the construction of "stabilized" F(ab')$_2$ fragments with a thioether linkage repacing the interchain disulfide bridge, the pharmacological blocking of kidney reuptake of radiometal labeled metabolites, the introduction of cleavable linkers between mAb and metal complex,or the adaption of anionic metal complexes with decreased kidney uptake.

Biodistributions of chCE7 F(ab')$_2$ labeled with a ^{67}Cu-DO3A complex:

MAb chCE7 was derivatized with the DO3A ligand a 4N-macrocycle similar to CPTA but bearing 3 carboxylic groups , labeled with ^{67}Cu and its biodistributions in nude mice bearing neuroblastoma xenografts were measured. Results in table 1B indicate that radioactivity present in the kidneys was reduced significantly (about four-fold) compared with ^{67}Cu-CPTA-chCE7 F(ab')$_2$ (Table1A) .

Other differences in biodistributions between the two copper ligands include a slower clearance from the blood of ^{67}Cu-DO3A-chCE7 F(ab')$_2$ and possibly as a conseqence of higher blood levels at 48h post injection about four-fold higher tumor levels with ^{67}Cu-DO3A-chCE7 F(ab')$_2$.

Table 1A: Uptake of ^{67}Cu-CPTA-labeled chCE7 F(ab')$_2$ fragments in neuroblastoma xenografts over a period of 48h. Data are means +/- s.d. of three animals and are expressed in % ID/g tissue.

Tissue	4	8	2 4	4 8
Tumour	7.1 +/- 2.3	9.0 +/- 1.7	5.5 +/- 0.7	2.5 +/- 0.9
Blood	1.7 +/- 0.3	0.7 +/- 0.1	0.4 +/- 0.0	0.4 +/-0.0
Heart	2.4 +/- 0.8	1.8 +/- 0.3	1.5 +/- 0.2	0.3 +/- 0.1
Liver	6.0 +/- 0.7	6.4 +/- 2.0	5.8 +/- 0.7	5.5 +/- 0.9
Spleen	6.6 +/- 1.1	8.7 +/- 5.4	7.2 +/- 1.1	4.9 +/- 1.2
Kidney	138.2 +/- 25.7	97.8 +/- 5.7	87.9 +/-8.4	60.0 +/-7.4
Stomach	0.4 +/- 0.1	0.8 +/- 0.1	0.9 +/- 0.2	1.0 +/- 0.2
Bowel	0.9 +/- 0.2	1.3 +/- 0.4	1.5 +/- 0.2	1.3 +/- 0.2
Muscle	0.5 +/- 0.1	0.4 +/- 0.1	0.4 +/- 0.1	0,3 +/- 0.0

Table 1B: Uptake of ^{67}Cu-DO3A-labeled chCE7 F(ab')$_2$ fragments in neuroblastoma xenografts over a period of 48h. Data are means +/- s.d. of three animals and are expressed in % ID/g tissue.

Tissue	4	8	2 4	4 8
Tumour	8.8 +/- 1.3	11.4 +/- 2.0	8.9 +/- 2.4	10.2 +/- 1.9
Blood	18.1 +/- 0.8	8.7 +/- 1.3	1.4 +/- 0.6	0.8 +/- 0.1
Heart	8.2 +/- 1.9	4.8 +/- 0.4	2.6 +/- 0.3	2.1 +/- 0.3
Liver	10.1 +/- 0.9	10.3 +/- 0.4	11.4 +/- 3.2	7.5 +/- 0.7
Spleen	7.0 +/- 1.7	6.2 +/- 1.0	5.3 +/- 0.1	3.6 +/- 0.2
Kidney	32.5 +/- 4.9	30.5 +/- 0.4	21.5 +/- 0.5	14.1 +/- 3.0
Stomach	1.0 +/- 0.2	1.3 +/- 0.6	0.5 +/- 0.2	0.5 +/- 0.1
Bowel	2.2 +/- 0.4	2.0 +/- 0.5	1.5 +/- 0.4	1.7 +/- 0.1
Muscle	1.5 +/- 0.2	1.1 +/- 0.1	0.8 +/- 0.2	0.7 +/- 0.0

Our results indicate that biodistributions of ^{67}Cu-labeled chCE7 F(ab')$_2$ fragments are improved significantly by the adaption of an anionic, more hydrophilic copper chelator. Despite these improvements a further reduction of radioactivity accumulating in the kidneys is necessary in order to envisage therapeutic application . It is to be expected that further insight into the multiple factors which govern kidney retention of radiometal-labeled metabolites will eventually lead to the design of improved antibody-fragment - or peptide -derived tumor seeking substances labeled with therapeutic nuclides.

References:

(1) Novak-Hofer,I.,Amstutz,H.P., Haldemann,A., Blaser,K., Morgenthaler,J.J., Blaeuenstein,P., and Schubiger,P.A. (1992) Radioimmunolocalization of neuroblastoma xenografts with chimeric antibody chCE7. J.Nucl.Med.33, 231-236.

(2) Doerr,U., Haldemann,A.R., Leibundgut,K., Novak-Hofer,I., Amstutz,H., Wagner,H.P., Schubiger,P.A.Morgenthaler, J.J., Roesler,H., Schilling,F., Kscielniak,E.,Treuner,J.,and 3 3 3 Bihl,H. (1993) First clinical results with the chimeric antibody chCE7 in neuroblastoma. Targeting features and biodistribution data. Eur.J.Nucl.Med.20,858.

(3) Haldemann,A.R.,Leibundgut,K., Doerr,U., Novak-Hofer,I., Amstutz,H.P., Wagner,H.P., Treuner,J., Bihl,H., Roesler,H. (1994) Radioimmunszintigraphie mit dem chimaeren Antikoerper CE7: erste klinische Erfahrungen. SGMR, 81. Jahresversammlung.

(4) Smith-Jones,P.M.,Fridrich,R.,Kaden,T.A.,Novak-Hofer,I.,Siebold,K.,Tschudin,D.,and Maecke,H. (1991) Antibody labeling with copper-67 using the bifunctional macrocycle 4-(1,4,8,11-tetraazacyclotetradec-1-yl)methyl) benzoic acid. Bioconjugate Chem.2,415-421.

(5) Novak-Hofer,I.,Amstutz,H.P., Maecke,H.R., Schwarzbach,R., Zimmermann,K., Morgenthaler,J.J., and Schubiger,P.A. (1995) Cellular processing of copper-67-labeled monoclonal antibody chCE7 by human neuroblastoma cells. Cancer Res.,55,46-50.

(6) Buchegger,F.,Pellegrin,A.,Delaloye,B.,Bischof-Delaloye,A., and Mach,J.P.(1990) Iodine-131-labeled mAbF(ab')2 fragments are more efficient and less toxic than intact antiCEA antibodies in radioimmunotherapy of large human colon carcinoma grafted in nude mice. J.Nucl.Med. 31, 1035-1044.

(7) Smith,A., Alberto,R., Blaeuenstein,P., Novak-Hofer,I., Maecke,H., and Schubiger,P.A. (1993) Preclinical evaluation of [67]Cu-labeled intact and fragmented anti-colon carcinoma monoclonal antibody MAb35. Cancer Res. 53, 5727-5733.

(8) Anderson,C.J., Schwarz,S.W., Connett,J.M., Cutler,P.D., Guo,L.W.,Wu,L., Germain,C.J., Philpott,G.W., Zinn, K.R., Greiner,D.P., Meares,C.F., and Welch,M.,J. (1995) Preparation, biodistribution and dosimetry of copper-64-labeled anti-colorectal carcinoma antibody fragments 1A3-F(ab')2. J.Nucl.Med.36, 850-858.

(9) Novak-Hofer,I., Zimmermann,K., Maecke,H.R., Amstutz,H.P., Carrel,F., and Schubiger,P.A. (1996) Tumor uptake and metabolism of copper-67-labeled monoclonal antibody chCE7 in nude mice bearing neuroblastoma xenografts. J.Nucl.Med., in press.

(10) Schwarzbach,R., Zimmermann,K., Blaeuenstein,P., Smith,A., and Schubiger,P.A. (1995) Developement of a simple and selective separation of [67]Cu from irradiated zinc for use in antibody labeling: A comparison of methods. Appl.Radiat.Isot.5, 329-336.

Radioactive Isotopes in
Clinical Medicine and Research XXII
ed. by H. Bergmann, A. Kroiss and H. Sinzinger
© 1997 Birkhäuser Verlag Basel/Switzerland

FINAL EVALUATION OF A PROSPECTIVE CLINICAL COMPARATIVE TRIAL OF 111IN-LABELED POLYCLONAL HUMAN IGG (HIG) SCINTIGRAPHY VS. ULTRASONOGRAPHY IN 100 PATIENTS WITH CAROTID ARTERY DISEASE.

Margarida Rodrigues*, H. Kritz and H. Sinzinger.

Department of Nuclear Medicine, University of Vienna, and Rehabilitation Center "Engelsbad-Melanie", Baden, Austria.

SUMMARY: The treatment of choice of atherosclerosis is the prevention of lesional formation at the earliest stage possible rather than reparative treatment of late vascular changes. Thus, early non-invasive diagnostic techniques could severely improve the practical managing of the disease. Human immunoglobulin G (HIG) is bound to Fc-receptors which are present at the surface of the macrophages. In this prospective study, the value of ^{111}In-labeled polyclonal HIG scintigraphy was investigated and compared with ultrasonography in one hundred patients with carotid artery disease.

Anterior scintigraphic images of the neck were obtained after i.v. injection of 500 µCi ^{111}In-HIG. Real time two-dimensional B-mode ultrasonography of the left and the right carotid arteries was performed as well.

Focal increased uptake of ^{111}In-HIG in the carotid arteries was found in 61 patients. No significant correlation between scintigraphy and ultrasonography was found. HIG-scintigraphy is not promising for early detection and assessment of the extent of atherosclerosis.

INTRODUCTION

Current non-invasive radiological and nuclear medicine techniques are of limited value for the early diagnosis of atherosclerotic lesions. There has been thus a great hope and a growing interest for the evaluation of metabolic changes in the arterial wall and in elucidating functional aspects of atherosclerosis at a rather early stage of the disease with radioisotopic techniques.

One of the earliest events during atherogenesis is the adherence of circulating monocytes to the intact endothelial lining of the artery, followed by migration across the endothelial barrier, and accumulation of monocyte-derived macrophages in the subendothelial space of the vessel wall (1, 2) where they may become loaded with cholesterol and are transformed to foam cells (3). Both non-specific immunoglobulin G and Fc fragments bound to Fc-receptors which are present in great number at the surface of the macrophages (4, 5).

In a recent experimental preliminary study (6), we have reported that ^{111}In-human polyclonal immunoglobulin G (HIG) allowed to identify atheromatous lesions, seeming to be promising for providing useful data and valuable information concerning metabolic aspects of atherosclerosis. We therefore assessed the value of scintigraphy with ^{111}In-HIG for diagnosis and evaluation of the stage and the clinical extent of carotid artery disease in humans. A comparative prospective study between ^{111}In-HIG-scintigraphy and ultrasonography of the carotid arteries was performed.

* Dr. Margarida Rodrigues is on leave from the Oncology Hospital, Lisbon, Portugal.

MATERIAL AND METHODS
Patients

One hundred patients (61 males, 39 females; mean age: 60.6±7.5 years) with ultrasonographically detected carotid artery lesions were studied. All patients suffered from hypercholesterolemia (total cholesterol (CH), 271±49 mg/dl; LDL-CH, 165±47 mg/dl; HDL-CH, 53.6±24 mg/dl; CH/ HDL ratio, 5.8±2.6).

111In-labeled HIG

111In-labeled HIG was obtained from Dr. P. Angelberger, Department of Chemistry, Research Center, Seibersdorf, Austria. Briefly, nonspecific intact polyclonal HIG (Sandoglobulin, Sandoz AG, Nürnberg, Germany) was radiolabeled with 111In using diethyleneaminepentaacetic anhydride (DTPA) .

Scintigraphic studies

Scintigraphic anterior images of the neck (acquired for 10 minutes) were obtained at 30 minutes and 4 hours post-injection of 500 µCi 111In-HIG, using a large field-of-view gamma-camera with a parallel-hole, medium-energy collimator. Acquisition was recorded in a 256x256 matrix. Both the 173 KeV and 247 KeV 111In gamma peaks with symmetric 20% windows were used.

Ultrasonographic studies

All patients underwent ultrasonographic studies within 1 to 5 days of the scintigraphic study. A real time two-dimensional B-Mode ultrasonography of the left and the right carotid arteries was performed using a 10 MHz linear array transducer.

The examinations were done in supine position and included approximately 5 cm of the common artery, the carotid bulbus, and 1 cm of the internal and external arteries. The regions were scanned both longitudinally and transversally. The precise method for measuring and recording was partly adopted from Wendelhag et al. (7) and the Asymptomatic Carotid Artery Plaques Study (8).

To summarize the ultrasonographic data, and for comparison with scintigraphic findings, a simplified classification scheme of lesions was used applying a six grades scale (Table 1).

Table 1 - <u>Simplified six grades ultrasonographic classification</u>

Classe 1: No lesions. Homogenous layers of the carotid wall

Classe 2: Slight to medium inhomogenicity (fragmentation) of the inner wall layer

Classe 3: Severe inhomogenicity (granulation) of the inner layer with increased echogenic areas. Mean wall thickness < 1.0

Classe 4: Mean wall thickness > 1.0 mm and/or plaques below 25% of the lumen

Classe 5: Plaques between 25% and 75% of the lumen diameter

Classe 6: Hemodynamic relevant stenosis with a plaque size exceeding 75% of the lumen diameter

Statistical evaluation

Values are presented as mean ± standard deviation.

Calculation for significance was performed by Student's t-test for paired data. Values were considered significant when p<0.01.

RESULTS

Ultrasonography of the carotid arterial wall detected wall thickening in all the 100 patients ($\leq$1mm, 22 patients; >1mm, 78 patients) and plaques in 72/100 patients. In the left carotid artery, 33 patients were in ultrasonographic stage $\leq$3 and 67 patients in stage >3. In the right carotid artery, 36 patients were in stage $\leq$3 and 64 patients in the stage >3.

Scintigraphic imaging of the carotid arteries provided increased focal uptake of ^{111}In-HIG in 61 patients (Figure 1) and no abnormal uptake of ^{111}In-HIG in the other 39 patients.

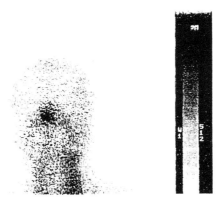

Figure 1 - Increased ^{111}In-HIG uptake in the left carotid artery.

There was no significant correlation between the scintigraphic findings and the ultrasonographic data (Figure 2).

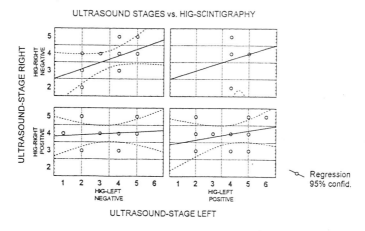

Figure 2 - Correlation between scintigraphic- and ultrasonographic data.

DISCUSSION

In human atherogenesis three major pathogenetic events, i.e. (parietal) thrombus formation, lipid infiltration (cholesterol and in particular low-density lipoproteins (LDL)) and cellular proliferation are centrally involved (9). No technique allowing non-invasive measures on severity, extent, composition and complications of atherosclerosis is available yet. The radiolabeling of autologous platelets, LDL and monocytes offers the promising approach to identify the kinetics and local metabolic fate of these compounds in-vivo in man (9, 10). The use of radiolabeled platelets allows the identification of arterial lesion sites showing an enhanced thrombogenicity and a platelet trapping which is also reflected by shortened platelet survival (9, 11). Scintigraphy with radiolabeled platelets reflects the activity of the disease and the number of platelets involved, but not the stage or the extent of the lesion. Radiolabeled LDL have been found long ago to behave like native LDL and have thereafter been successfully used to study LDL-accumulation in vascular tissue in experimental animals (10). LDL are a useful tool to identify the quality of surface lining (normal, re- or deendothelialization) as well as the amount of foam cells. However, only lipid lesions demonstrate a relevant LDL-retention, while advanced lesions such as fibrous plaques, for example, show almost no uptake at all. Preliminary studies (12) with radiolabeled autologous monocytes have shown that monocytes are attracted to vascular lesions rich in monocytes. These nuclear medicine techniques are thus of valuable information concerning metabolic aspects of atherosclerosis, while they are far away from providing information on the extent of the disease. Therefore, they may be not of help in the future for late stage disease monitoring.

In New Zealand white rabbits after de - endothelialization of the abdominal aorta by a modified Baumgartner technique according to Tschopp et al. (13), it was demonstrated that ^{111}In-labeled, nonspecific, polyclonal IgG (each molecule of which contains a Fc subunit) and Fc fragments accumulate in atherosclerotic lesions in sufficient concentrations to allow consistent external imaging (14). The highest uptake of IgG was found in the healing edges of the regenerating endothelium but not in de - endothelialized areas (14). In Watanabe Heritable Hyperlipidemic rabbits, Dormans et al (15) failed to detect early atherosclerotic lesions by 111In-HIG scintigraphy, despite clear differences in incorporation of the tracer in situ.

It was suggested that ^{111}In-IgG uptake may be caused by inflammatory reaction at the site of injury independently of atheromatous plaque formation (13). Increased vascular permeability and other non-specific mechanisms related to the inflammatory process could play an important role in the mechanism of IgG uptake (10). Demacker et al. (3) found, however, that polyclonal IgG and, specifically, Fc fragments, indeed are preferentially bound to atherosclerotic lesions, most particularly in young lesions in which the foam cell is most abundant. Recent research (13) in animals has shown that ^{111}In-IgG accumulation can be found both in arteries with active atheroma formation and in arteries with endothelial injury but without atheroma formation. Atherosclerotic lesions preferentially localize at sites of hemodynamic stress, namely where the major arteries branch or are curved (15). Around such ramifications, the number of IgG - positive endothelial cells is much higher (approximately 10 times) than in areas remote from these branches (16). It was observed that injured endothelial cells also contained intracellular IgG (15). These data provide a base for detection of early atherosclerosis with HIG-scintigraphy.

In our previous experimental study (6) there was evidence that HIG clearly is unspecific, being related to lipids and macrophages. It seemed that ^{111}In-HIG scintigraphy would be promising to provide useful data and metabolic information concerning atherogenesis. However, the imperfect nature of animal models of atherosclerosis makes extrapolation to human atherosclerosis imaging difficult (14). Human imaging studies were thus necessary for the correct evaluation of the value and indications of HIG-scintigraphy for the study of atherosclerotic lesions in humans. In this prospective study, HIG-scintigraphy did not, however, correlate to the stage and the clinical extent of the disease, as indicated by ultrasonography. Furthermore, higher uptake of ^{111}In-HIG was seen in patients with more advanced stage of the disease. Thus, ^{111}In-HIG is not yet the promising imaging agent for the non-invasive early detection of atherosclerotic lesions, serial assessment of the presence and extent of the disease and treatment monitoring of atherosclerosis in the future.

ACKNOWLEDGMENTS
The authors appreciate the collaboration of Dr. M. Wenger and the technical assistance of Judith Bednar, Ingrid Blazek, Susanne Granegger and Bettina Mosing.

REFERENCES
1. Gerrity RG. The role of the monocyte in atherogenesis. Am J Pathol 1981;103: 181-190.

2. Steinberg D, Parthasarathy S, Carew TE et al. Beyond cholesterol. Modifications of low-density lipoprotein that increase its atherogenicity. N Engl J Med 1989; 320: 915-924.

3. Demacker PNM, Dormans TPJ, Koenders EB and Corstens FHM. Evaluation of indium-polyclonal immunoglobulin G to quantitate atherosclerosis in Watanable heritable hyperlipidemic rabbits with scintigraphy: effect of age and treatment with antioxidants or ethinylestradiol. J Nucl Med 1993; 34: 1316-1321.

4. Fischman AJ, Rubin RH, White JA et al. Localization of Fc fragments of nonspecific polyclonal IgG at focal sites of inflammation. J Nucl Med 1990; 31: 1199-1205.

5. Fowler S, Shio H and Haley NJ.Characterization of lipid-loaden aortic cells from cholesterol - fed rabbits. I. Investigation of macrophage-like properties of aortic populations. Lab Invest 1979; 41: 372-378.

6. Rodrigues M, Kritz H, Wenger M and Sinzinger H. [111]Indium polyclonal human immunoglobulin G in human and experimental atherosclerosis. In: Radioactive Isotopes in Clinical Medicine and Research, Advances in Pharmacological Sciences. H. Bergmann and H. Sinzinger (eds.), Birkhäuser Verlag, Basel, 1995; 329 - - 334.

7. Wendelhag I, Gustavson T, Suurküla M et al. Ultrasound measurements of wall thickness in the carotid artery. Fundamental principles and description of a computerized analysing system. Clin Physiol 1992; 11, 1001; 565.

8. ACAPS Group. Rationale and design for the asymtomatic carotid artery plaque study (ACAPS) control. Clin Trials 1992; 13: 293 - 314.

9. Sinzinger H and Virgolini I. Radioisotopic imaging of human atherosclerosis. Progress in Angiology 1991; 323-325.

10. Sinzinger H and Virgolini I. Nuclear medicine and atherosclerosis. Eur J Nucl Med 1990; 17: 160-178.

11. Fritz E, Ludwig H, Scheithauer W and Sinzinger H. Shortened platelet half-life in multiple myeloma. Blood 1986; 68: 514 - 520.

12. Virgolini I, Fitscha P and Sinzinger H. Imaging of autologous [111]In - labelled monocytes in patients with arteriosclerosis. Circulation 1990; 82: 517.

13. Tschopp TB, Baumgartner HR, Silberbauer K and Sinzinger H. Platelet adhesion and platelet thrombus formation on subendothelium of human arteries and veins exposed to following blood in vitro. A comparison with rabbit aorta. Haemostasis 1979; 8: 19-29.

14. Fischman AJ, Rubin RH, Khwa BA et al. Radionuclide imaging of experimental atherosclerosis with nonspecific polyclonal immunoglobulin G. J Nucl Med 1989; 30: 1095-1100.

15. Petterson K, Björk H and Bondjers G. Endothelial integrity and injury in atherogenesis. Transplantation Procceedings 1993; 25: 2054-2056.

16. Pettersson K, Bejne B, Björk H et al. Endothelial injury in atherogenesis. Circ Res 1990; 67: 1027-1029.

Radioactive Isotopes in
Clinical Medicine and Research XXII
ed. by H. Bergmann, A. Kroiss and H. Sinzinger
© 1997 Birkhäuser Verlag Basel/Switzerland

CORRELATION ON SPECT AND CT IMAGES IN BRAIN TUMOR RADIOIMMUNOTHERAPY

G. Giorgetti, Lazzari S., Sarti G.

Health and Medical Physics Dpt, Bufalini Hosp. Cesena – Italy

SUMMARY: A particular methodology of CT and DTPA SPECT image correlation as been applyed to identify the advantages that this kind of technique brings to radioimmunotherapy in brain gliomas. Several improvements reveal to be possible if we implement image fusion; these improvements are therefore illustrated.

INTRODUCTION

The implementation of image fusion techniques implies several kinds of problems that goes from the digital image acquisition and elaboration, the superimposition algorithm and the detection of anatomical referring points to the therapeutical and diagnostical applicability. To this pourpose, our physician and medics has studied separately some cases and then they have compared they result to point out possible advantages in this situations:

- 99mTc-DTPA SPECT shows in particular the facial bone; when the lesion is particularly near to it, it is difficult to distinguish it from a recurrence.

- A recurrence is distinguishable first in SPECT and, after some days, in CT; it is possible that a zone that is seen as perfused is interpreted as BAT (brain adjacent tissue); to know where the perfused region is exactly located maybe resolutive in this cases.

- The dosimetric calculation model suppose that during the therapy, the radioisotope is uniformly distributed in all the lesion; sometimes, if the shape is particularly complex maybe that some parts of the hole are not perfused; this could be detected with the superimposition.

- To establish if a lesion is increasing or decreasing during the follow-up is not always so easy. To correlate two subsequent SPECT images maybe helpful in determining the cronological evolution of the lesion.

MATERIAL AND METHODS

SPECT images which anticipate treatment planning are made with a GE STARCAM 4000 with 64 acquisition of about 30 seconds with 99mTc DTPA, double window at 140 KeV 20% with scatter and attenuation correction, while image ricostruction in slices of 64x64 pixel is done with back projection algorithm and butterworth and ramp filters.

CT images come from a scanner Siemens SOMATOM and have been extracted with an analogic to digital converter from the screen image.

CT images come from a scanner Siemens SOMATOM and have been extracted with an analogic to digital converter from the screen image.

The images we have obtained in this way have been subsequently translated in one byte per pixel raw data files with a C program.

Raw data files are transferred to a Silicon Graphics Indy workstation with Irix 5.3 as OS. The image fusion program has been developed by the Montreal Neurological Institute. It is named "MNI_Register" and use a least square algorithm based on anatomical markers signed on the images. In this way, no anatomical markers have to be put on the patient during the image acquisition and no particular protocol has to be created to agree the different departments of the hospital.

In agreement with the medical images experts of our equipes we agreed a set of points suitable for DTPA SPECT and CT superimposition, they are: the facial bone, the eyes, longitudinal sinus, the summit of the brain, sphenoid alas and tentorium.

RESULTS

The results are well showed and explained in the following figures and captions, so let's take a look at them.

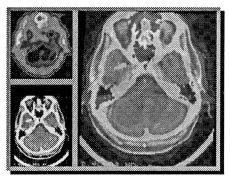 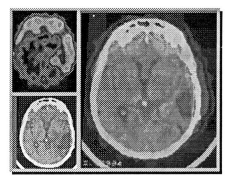

Figure 1 - This is a case of radioimmunotherapy that follow the surgical removal of a brain glioma. We see in the left side of the brain the lesion (black in the CT) and the catheter (white in CT) near the sphenoidic ala. Even if the perfused zone highlight by the SPECT image near the lesion may be thought as a recurrence, we see in the superimposed image that it correspond to the left sphenoidic ala itself.

Figure 2 - Like fig. 1 with the lesion in the right side. We see the skull more perfused where it has been removed and also two points highlighted in SPECT image. We see in the superimposed image that one correspond to the right ventricle (that has been covered with a particular biological tissue to avoid perfusion) and the other, less visible in SPECT, that lies in the border of the lesion; a subsequent CT exam has revealed it to be a recurrence.

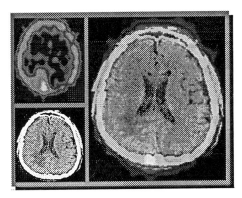

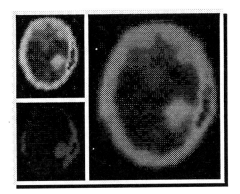

Figure 3 - (poor CT image quality is due to the scanning-from-the-film acquisition). In this case, we clearly see in the superimposed image that the 99mTc-DTPA has not perfused all the lesion shown in black in the CT image. This could compromise the dosimetric calculations, if they consider all the lesion to be uniformly perfused.

Figure 4 - This are DTPA SPECT images of the same patient taken during a radioimmunotherapy, one following the other after three month. Where the two lesions correspond we see the superimposed image colored in cyan (green plus blue) and where they don't (lower zone) the blue color prevails. If the images were correctly normalized the skull would appear cyan too.

CONCLUSION

As already introduced, the aim of this work is only to extablish possibly ways to apply image fusion in intralesional I131 therapy in brain tumor and to predict the directions that this methodic can get in this field. We think that the further progress can be described in this way:

- An object detection protocol that join the knowledge of the medical imaging expert and the computer and which can take advantage from the multimodality image to recognize lesion from object normally perfused by DTPA; we can also think to the use or even creation of an atlas.

- An instrument which can correlate succeding SPECT images during patient follow-up, that can also interactively extimate the dimension of the lesion as an helpful instrument for the time evolution evaluation of the lesion.

- The program we currently use for dosimetry suppose the cavity unfirmly perfused; it can be improved as we can detect the correct distribution of the radioisotope. We'll try to correlate CT with I131 images; the problem rise as what we see in the I131 image is only the lesion and no other possible anatomical marker.

ACKNOWLEDGEMENTS

We cannot take this work to the end if we hadn't received the help of some people that we would like to thanks. They are

Dr A. Evans, Dr D. Mc Donald from Montreal Neurological Institute that freely furnished us their precious software package "MNI_Register"

Dr A. Schenone, Dr M. Gambaro from IST Genova that suggest us how to realize image correlation

Dr P. Riva, Dr G. Franceschi, Dr G. Moscatelli from the Nuclear Medicine dpt of Bufalini Hospital that help us in understanding the anatomical significance of the medical images

All our colleagues that are involved in the Health and Medical Physics dpt daily work, their patience and collaboration permit us to achieve this results although their name won't be mentioned anywhere.

REFERENCES

1. J. C. Liehn et al. Superimposition of computed tomography and single photon emission tomography immunoscintigraphic images in the pelvis: validation in patients with colorectal or ovarian carcinoma recurrence. European journal of nuclear medicine (1992) 19:186-194.

2. H. Loats. CT and SPECT image registration and fusion for spatial localization of metastatic processes using radiolabeled monoclonals. The journal of nuclear medicine vol. 34 no 3 mar 1993.

3. K. F. Foral et al. CT-SPECT fusion plus conjugate views for determining dosimetry in iodine-131-monoclonal antibody therapy of lymphohoma patients. The journal of nuclear medicine vol. 35 no 10 oct 1994.

Radioactive Isotopes in
Clinical Medicine and Research XXII
ed. by H. Bergmann, A. Kroiss and H. Sinzinger
© 1997 Birkhäuser Verlag Basel/Switzerland

PLANAR AND SPECT IMAGING IN THALLIUM MYOCARDIAL SCINTIGRAPHY

Eva Strobl-Jäger, E. Pollross, F. Eghbalian and M. Klicpera

Rehabilitation center Hochegg, Austria

SUMMARY: To compare planar and subsequent Spect images retrospectively in 127 thallium myocardial perfusion studies, planar and Spect-studies were read in separate batches in a completely blinded fashion. The results for each study were interpreted as either normal (N), reversible (R) or irreversible (I) defect or mixture (Mix) of R and I. Precise concordance was 65% (45 N, 5 R, 12 I and 21 Mix). When categorizing N vs. abnormal, the agreement was 84%. Out of 27 patients with angiography, 23 had a pathologic angiogram, 20 of which were true positive both by planar and Spect. In 2 patients the diseased artery was localized only in the Spect studies; one patient was false negative both by planar and Spect. 4 patients without sign. coronary stenosis (one after myocardial infarction and dilatation) were assigned correctly.

INTRODUCTION

In the the past 2 decades, exercise thallium-201 perfusion scintigraphy has gained wide acceptance in the detection and localization of coronary artery disease (CAD,1). In spite of the development of new Tc-99-labeled perfusion agents (2,3) with more favorable physical characteristics, thallium-201 has remained unique for its ability of redistribution to detect viable ischemic myocardium. Several studies reported Spect imaging to have superior sensitivity to detect CAD as compared to planar imaging (1,2). In our cardiac center we have continued to use both methods in a part of our patients. The aim of this retrospective study was to re-evaluate planar and tomographic cardiac imaging separately and compare the results to the angiographic data available.

PATIENTS

127 patients (100 males, 27 females; age range 36 - 76 years) with known or suspected CAD were examined. 70 patients had a previous myocardial infarction, 17 had undergone bypass surgery.

PROTOCOL

All patients were examined after an overnight fast. Betablockers were paused for 3 days. All other antianginal medication was discontinued for 12 hours, except in 11 symptomatic patients.

Exercise bycicle testing was performed according to standard protocol in 108 patients. Endpoints were physical exhaustion, the development of symptoms or severe alterations of the ECG. Pharmacologic vasodilation with dipyridamole (0.5 mg/kg) plus medium exercise to achieve a heart rate of 115/min was used as an alternative in 19 patients with lack of training or motivation. At peak exercise, 1.2 to 3.2 mCi of thallium-201 (0.03 mCi/kg) was injected and the patient was encouraged to exercise for an additional minute.

Planar imaging was started within 5 minutes after injection on a Siemens ZLC camera. Cardiac images were acquired in the anterior, 45° and 70° LAO projection. Subsequently, tomographic images were performed on an Elscint APEX SP4 camera, 30 images being acquired at 6° intervals over an 180° arc. Planar and Spect redistribution images were obtained 4 hours after exercise.

In 27 patients, coronary angiography was performed in our cardiac centre. Coronary stenosis of 70% or more was considered as a significant lesion.

INTERPRETATION

Planar and Spect studies were read and evaluated retrospectively in separate batches in a completely blinded fashion, without knowledge of the clinical data or the outcome of the corresponding study. An interpretation was made for each patient based on one of four possible categories: normal (N), ischemia (R-reversible defect), scar (I-irreversible defect), or mixture (Mix) of fixed and reversible defect.

Septal, anterior or apical defects were related to disease of the left anterior descending coronary artery (LAD), inferior defects to the right coronary artery and lateral defects to the circumflex coronary artery.

RESULTS

Precise concordance in respect to the four categories was observed in 45 normal scans, further in 5 patients with reversible, 12 with irreversible patterns and 21 with mixed defects; overall agreement was 65%. When comparing normal versus abnormal scans, the agreement was 84%.

Table 1.

PLANAR IMAGES

		N	R	I	Mix	Total
S						
P	N	45	2*	2	2	51
E	R	4	5	0	2	11
C	I	6	0	12	14*	32
T	Mix	4	4	4	21	33
	Total	59	11	18	39	127

* due to early redistribution of thallium-201, some of the reversible defects were expected to be missed in the Spect-studies.

In angiography, 4 of the 27 patients examined were without sign. coronary stenosis. 3 of them had normal planar and Spect images, whereas the 4th patient - who had undergone successful dilatation of the LAD after a myocardial

infarction - had abnormal scans suggesting LAD-disease.
(However, while planar images detected the scar correctly,
Spect-studies suggested a mixted defect). One patient with a
2-vessel disease had normal planar and Spect images.
In 20 patients with abnormal planar and Spect-studies CAD
could be confirmed by angiography. In 2 patients with
inadequate exercise 2 of 3 diseased vessels were localized
correctly in the tomographic studies only.

Table 2.

ANALYSIS OF ANGIOGRAPHIC DATA

27 patients	angiography	
	N	Abn
planar/ SPECT		
N / N	3	1
Abn / Abn	1*	20
N / Abn	0	2**
Abn / N	0	0

*pat after MCI and successful PTCA
**pts. with inadeqate exercise

Table 3.

CORRECT LOCALIZATION OF PATHOLOGIC VESSELS BY PLANAR + SPECT

| | | | PLANAR | | | SPECT | | |
n	patients	n vessels	TP	FP	FN	TP	FP	FN
11	1-VD	11	9	1	1	10	1	0
9	2-VD	18	8	0	10	9	0	9
3	3-VD	12	3	-	9	3	-	9

CONCLUSION
Though Spect was performed with a delay after the planar
studies, the different modes of imaging relate closely to
each other as well as to our angiographic data.

REFERENCES

1. Mahmarian JJ and Verani MS. Exercise thallium-201 perfusion scintigraphy in the assessment of coronary artery disease. Am J Cardiol 1991; 67:2D-11D.

2. Kiat H, Maddahi J, Roy LT et al. Comparison of technetium 99mmethoxy isonitrile and thallium 201 for evaluation of coronary artery disease by planar and tomographic methods. Am Heart J 1989; 117:1-11.

3. Maddahi J, Kiat H, Van Train KF et al. myocardial perfusion imaging with technetium-99m sestamibi SPECT in the evaluation of coronary artery disease. Am J Card 1990; 66: 55E-62E.

Therapy

Radioactive Isotopes in
Clinical Medicine and Research XXII
ed. by H. Bergmann, A. Kroiss and H. Sinzinger
© 1997 Birkhäuser Verlag Basel/Switzerland

RADIOIMMUNOTHERAPY OF CEA-EXPRESSING CANCERS:
CLINICAL RESULTS WITH AN ^{131}I-LABELED ANTI-CEA MONOCLONAL IgG₁

T.M. Behr, R.M. Sharkey, M.E. Juweid, R.M. Dunn, R.C. Vagg, L.C. Swayne, J.A. Siegel,
and D.M. Goldenberg

Garden State Cancer Center at the Center for Molecular Medicine and Immunology,
1 Bruce Street, Newark, NJ 07103-2763, USA

SUMMARY: Fifty-seven patients with CEA-expressing tumors in very advanced stages were treated with 44-268 mCi of the ^{131}I-labeled murine anti-CEA monoclonal antibody NP-4. Differences in pharmacokinetics were found between different types of CEA-producing tumors: colorectal cancer patients cleared the antibody significantly faster from blood and whole-body than all other cancer types. The red marrow was the only dose-limiting organ; the severity of myelotoxicity was strongly related to the the red marrow dose and the pretreatment (chemotherapy or external beam radiation). Tumor doses ranged from 2 to 218 cGy/mCi. Anti-tumor effects were seen in 12 out of 35 assessable patients (1 partial remission, 4 minor/ mixed responses, 7 stabilizations of previously rapidly progressing disease).

INTRODUCTION

CEA-expressing adenocarcinomas belong to the most frequent types of cancer (1). Although there have been advances in the surgical management of primary tumors, the major cause of cancer mortality is disease relapsing at distant sites (1). The three conventional treatment strategies (surgery, external beam radiation, and chemotherapy) are only of limited value in the management of metastatic disease. The aim of this study was to determine in a phase-I/II clinical trial the pharmacokinetics, dosimetry, toxicity, as well as anti-tumor activity of the ^{131}I-labeled murine anti-CEA IgG₁ monoclonal antibody, NP-4 (2).

MATERIALS AND METHODS

A total of 57 patients with CEA-expressing tumors, mostly in very advanced stages, were treated (e.g., 29 colorectal, 9 lung, 7 pancreas, 6 breast, 4 medullary thyroid cancer patients). The patients underwent a diagnostic study (1-3 mg IgG, 8-30 mCi) to assess tumor targeting and to estimate dosimetry, followed by the therapeutic dose (4-23 mg, 44-268 mCi), based upon the radiation dose to the red marrow (3). Imaging was performed from 4 to 240 h post injection (planar and SPECT). Blood and whole-body clearance were determined from blood sampling and whole-body scanning, respectively.

Radiation doses were calculated according to the MIRD scheme (3). Plasma samples were analyzed by high-pressure size-exclusion chromatography on a GF-250 column (DuPont, Wilmington, DE), as described in more detail elsewhere (2,4).

Responses were graded as follows:

1. *Complete remission* - absence of clinically detectable disease, with complete normalization of serum tumor marker (CEA) levels for at least 1 month.
2. *Partial remission* - at least 50% reduction in the sum of the perpendicular diameter of measurable disease without appearance of new lesions and without increase in size of any lesion, for at least 1 month.
3. *Minor/mixed response* - less than 50% reduction in sum of the the perpendicular diameters of measurable lesions without increase in size of any lesion; or: reduction of tumor marker (CEA) serum levels by at least 50% for 1 month or longer without increase in size of any lesion for at least 1 month.
4. *Stabilization of disease* - no increase in the size of measurable lesions and no appearance of new lesions for at least 3 months in patients with rapidly progressing disease before therapy, who had failed chemo- and/or external radiotherapy.
5. *Progression* - greater than 25% increase in measurable disease and/or any new metastasis on treatment.

RESULTS

All fifty-seven patients in this study presented in advanced metastatic stages of their disease, and most were heavily pretreated with chemotherapy and/or radiation. These conventional treatment regimens had either failed or were abandoned because of severe side-effects.

Pharmacokinetics

Influence of human anti-mouse antibodies (HAMA)

As a consequence of their first therapeutic antibody injection, all but two out of 32 assessable patients developed human anti-mouse responses. HAMA titers typically began to rise three to four weeks after the therapeutic injection, reaching their apogee after 4 to 7 weeks, sooner if there was previous exposure to mouse proteins. Consequently, all but three patients had elevated HAMA titers at the time of retreatment (14/20 retreated patients had titers above 300). At HAMA titers below 300, no effect on the clearance rates of the antibody from the blood and whole-body was apparent, whereas with titers above this threshold a rapidly increasing plasma and whole-body clearance rate was observed, which was reflected by decreasing red marrow and whole-body doses. In early scans, enhanced uptake of the formed complexes was seen in the liver, spleen, and bone marrow. Later images showed increased uptake in the thyroid, stomach, salivary glands, and bowel, suggesting liberation of free iodide.

Influence of circulating antigen

Circulating CEA, as well as the type of CEA-expressing cancer, had a marked influence on the pharmacokinetics of NP-4 IgG. Over a similar range of circulating plasma CEA, colorectal cancer patients cleared the antibody significantly faster from blood and whole-body than all other types of CEA-producing cancer (blood-$T^{\frac{1}{2}}$ 21.4 $\pm$ 11.1 h versus 35.8 $\pm$ 13.2 h; p < 0.01). Similar differences between colorectal cancer and other CEA-expressing tumors were observed also in the whole-body half-lives (61.9 $\pm$ 39.9 h versus 96.1 $\pm$ 48.2 h for colorectal versus other tumor types; p < 0.01). Typically, a high liver uptake was seen in early scans in these rapidly-clearing colorectal cancer patients, with subsequent metabolic release of free iodine. In contrast to the rapid metabolic breakdown caused by HAMA, no enhanced bone marrow or splenic uptake was observed in these patients.

An especially rapid clearance of the injected antibody was seen in colorectal cancer patients having large liver metastases. There seemed to be a correlation between liver function parameters and blood clearance: an inverse correlation was found in colorectal cancer patients between the plasma half-life of NP-4 and the serum levels of both, AP and GOT, and the biokinetics of NP-4.

Dosimetry

Red marrow and whole-body doses

Red marrow doses ranged from 45 to 706 cGy, and whole-body doses from 31 to 344 cGy. Consistent with the shorter blood and whole-body half-lives, the radiation doses to red marrow and whole-body were significantly lower in HAMA-negative patients with colorectal than with other types of cancer (2.2 $\pm$ 1.1 vs. 3.5 $\pm$ 0.7 cGy/mCi for the red marrow, p < 0.001; and 0.6 $\pm$ 0.3 vs. 0.9 $\pm$ 0.2 cGy/mCi for the whole-body, p < 0.001). Patients with elevated HAMA (titers $\geq$ 300) had significantly decreased blood and whole-body half-lives, thus red marrow and whole-body doses. At HAMA titers above 1000, all red marrow doses were below 1.0 cGy/mCi, and the whole-body doses were below 0.3 cGy/mCi.

Tumor targeting and dosimetry

Overall, more than 85 percent of lesions known from conventional imaging methods (CT, MRI, ultrasonography, etc.) were visualized by the antibody scans. A strong dependence of antibody uptake in the CEA-expressing tumor lesions upon tumor size was observed. There was a linear correlation between the tumor mass and the decadic logarithm of the tumor uptake in percent of injected dose per gram (r=-0.95) or the logarithm of the tumor dose in cGy/mCi (dose range 2 - 218 cGy/mCi; r=-0.74). Interestingly, three lesions smaller than 2 grams had uptake values of as much as 0.95% of the injected dose/g, corresponding to a tumor dose of up to 217.8 cGy/mCi. Accordingly, tumor-to-red marrow ratios varied between 1.1 in a 163-g and 80.7 in a 1-g liver metastasis (mean $\pm$ SD, 11.3 $\pm$ 20.4), and the tumor-to-whole-body ratios were between 2.0 and 726.0 (mean $\pm$ SD, 74.8 $\pm$ 177.2).

Toxicity

The red marrow was the only dose-limiting organ. Figure 1 summarizes the results of the analysis of the red marrow toxicities seen in 44 assessable patients in correlation to the actually observed red marrow doses. In a total of 14 asessable patients without any previous chemo- or radiotherapy, no white blood cell toxicity greater than grade 2 was observed despite red marrow doses up to 613 cGy. In more heavily pretreated patients, severe leukocyte toxicities (grade 3 and 4) occurred at red marrow doses over 300 cGy, and platelet toxicities were seen even at doses below 200 cGy. All patients with grade 4 toxicities had prior irradiation of more than 10 percent of the bone marrow and/or chemotherapy within the last 6 months before radioimmunotherapy, and all of them had, additionally, multiple bone metastases (three lung cancer and one breast cancer patient). The presence of bone or bone marrow metastases was identified as an additional important risk factor for the development of red marrow toxicity. Generally, patients who were pretreated with mitomycin and/or cisplatinum tended to have very severe bone marrow toxicities after radioimmuno-therapy.

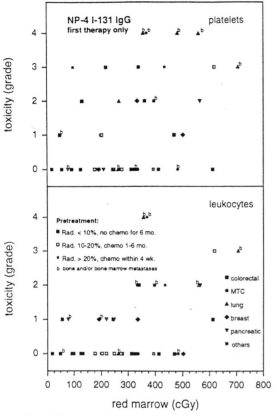

Fig. 1 *Myelotoxcity in relation to radiation dose and pretreatment.*

Typically, white blood cell and platelet counts began to drop, platelets usually preceeding leukocytes, two to three weeks after radio-immunotherapy, reaching their nadir four to seven weeks after the RAIT injection. The time to recovery was typically nine to eleven weeks post-radioantibody injection. In the case of retreatment, the toxicities observed were additionally dependent upon HAMA titers (the higher the HAMA, the lower the red marrow does, thus the less the red marrow toxicity), the time that elapsed between the prior treatment and the retreatment injection (the shorter the time, the higher the toxicity), as well as the time between the recovery of previous marrow toxicity and the subsequent radioimmunotherapy (the shorter the time, the higher the toxicity).

Anti-tumor effects

Anti-tumor effects were seen in 12/35 assessable patients. Among them was one partial remission, four mixed/minor responses, and seven patients showing a marked stabilization of previously rapidly-progressing disease. Figure 2 shows patient #589, who was a 66-year-old man with a primary pancreatic cancer and liver metastases. Chemotherapy with 5-fluorouracil, mitomycin, adriamycin, and strepto-zotocin had failed. The patient was treated with 146.2 mCi ^{131}I-NP-4 IgG. In the 3-month follow-up CT scan, a significant (> 50 percent) decrease in the size of the liver metastases was observed. One month later, they had disappeared completely (Fig. 2), whereas the pancreatic primary was stable over the whole post-treatment observation period (partial remission). The patient died 17 months after the therapy of en-docarditis of an aortic valve replacement. Figure 3 shows the treatment response of multiple small lung metastases of a 66-year old woman with cancer of the left lung (patient #775). She was treated with 100 and 105 mCi ^{131}I-NP-4 IgG three months apart. Two months after the second therapy, multiple small lung lesions could not be demonstrated any longer in CT, and the plasma CEA had dropped by 85%.

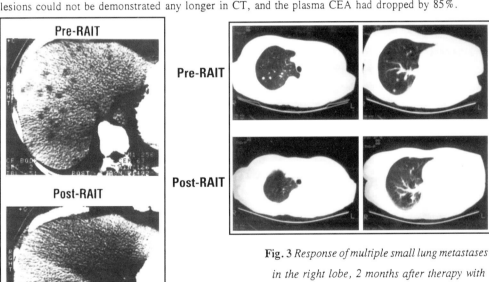

Fig. 3 *Response of multiple small lung metastases in the right lobe, 2 months after therapy with 100 and 105 mCi ^{131}I-NP-4 IgG, 3 months apart.*

Fig. 2 *Complete disappearance of liver metastases of a pancreatric primary, 4 months after therapy with 146 mCi ^{131}I-NP-4 IgG.*

Most of the anti-tumor effects were seen in lesions smaller than 3 cm in diameter and interestingly, all but one of the objective anti-tumor effects were seen in patients with cumulative red marrow doses of more than 400 cGy, and even in the disease-stabilization group, four out of seven patients had cumulated red marrow doses above this level.

DISCUSSION

These results suggest that prior chemotherapy or external beam radiation is an important risk factor for the development of hematological toxicity in radioimmunotherapy, and that higher radiation doses may be delivered to tumors of patients without prior therapy compromising the bone marrow reserve.

As we could show earlier for other anti-CEA MAbs, their clearance rate is influenced by complexation with circulating antigen. A fundamental difference between colorectal cancer and all other tumor types was found (5). Over a similar range of plasma CEA, colorectal cancer patients cleared the antibody significantly faster than did patients with other CEA-expressing malignancies. Microheterogeneities in the chemical structure of the CEA produced by different cancer types are probably responsible for the differences in clearance rates (5). CEA receptor-mediated clearance of the CEA-MAb complexes is likely, since these complexes tended toward a rapid clearance only in colorectal cancer patients; other murine (e.g., anti-mucin) MAbs show completely normal kinetics in these patients (5). Whether elevated liver function parameters are causally related to this rapid clearance or are just epiphenomena of a common underlying cause must remain speculative at this time. The different and, in the individual case, unpredictable clearance rates suggest the necessity of a dosimetry-based treatment planning rather than mCi/m² dosing.

Encouraging is the fact that some objective responses were observed in 12 out of 35 assessable patients, despite the fact that most of them had failed standard or even high-dose chemotherapy. Small tumors seem to be more suitable for radioimmunotherapy because of their favorable dosimetry. However, in order to achieve better therapeutic results in patients with bulky disease, the application of higher, potentially myeloablative doses is indicated.

REFERENCES

1. DeVita VT, S Hellman S, Rosenberg SA (eds.), Cancer - Principles & Practice of Oncology (4th ed.). Philadelphia: J.B. Lippincott, 1993.
2. Sharkey RM, Goldenberg DM, Goldenberg H, Lee RF, Ballance C, Pawlyk D, Varga D, Hansen HJ. Murine monoclonal antibodies against carcinoembryonic antigen: immunological, pharmacokinetic, and targeting properties in humans. Cancer Res 1990; 50: 2823-2831.
3. Dunn RM, Juweid ME, Behr TM, Siegel JA, Sharkey RM, Goldenberg DM. An automated internal dosimetry scheme for radiolabeled antibodies. Med Phys 1995; 22: 1549-1550.
4. Behr TM, Sharkey RM, Juweid ME, Dunn RM, Ying Z, Zhang CH, Siegel JA, Goldenberg DM. Variables influencing tumor dosimtery in radioimmunotherapy of CEA-expressing cancers with anti-CEA and anti-mucin monoclonal antibodies. J Nucl Med (submitted for publication).
5. Behr TM, Sharkey RM, Juweid ME, Dunn RM, Ying Z, Zhang CH, Siegel JA, Gold DV, Goldenberg DM. Factors influencing the pharmacokinetics, dosimetry and diagnostic accuracy of radioimmunodetection and radioimmunotherapy of CEA-expressing tumors. Cancer Res (submitted for publication).

Radioactive Isotopes in
Clinical Medicine and Research XXII
ed. by H. Bergmann, A. Kroiss and H. Sinzinger
© 1997 Birkhäuser Verlag Basel/Switzerland

ADVANCED PROSTATE CANCER THERAPY WITH YTTRIUM-90 CITRATE

S.K. Shukla[1,2], C. Cipriani[1], G. Argirò[1], G. Atzei[1], F. Boccardi[1], S. Boemi[1],
R. Cusumano[3], L. Ossicini[2]

[1]) Servizio di Medicina Nucleare, Ospedale S. Eugenio, Roma; [2]) Istituto di Cromatografia,
C.N.R., Roma; [3]) Clinica Urologica, Aurelia Hosp., Roma, Italy

SUMMARY

The systemic therapy of advanced prostate cancer, which progressed in spite of radical prostectomy, external radiation therapy, hormonal management, chemotherapy, and metastron therapy, has been achieved with i.v. injection of prostate cancer-affine yttrium-90 citrate solution, containing both cationic and anionic species. The total-body Bremsstrahlung imaging technique, introduced by us, has shown the concentration of the radionuclide both in the primary prostate cancer and in the bone metastases which had been seen a week earlier on bone scan with Tc-99m-MDP. The myelodepression caused by repeated injection of the radionuclide is the side-effect to be avoided. Other Y-90 prostate cancer-affine radiopharmaceuticals free from this disadvantage are under investigation.

INTRODUCTION

Prostate cancer incidence and death rate caused by it are increasing in all countries of the world.[1-3] Already at presentation, more than 50% patients have advanced cancer and about 25% have bone metastases.[2] Surgery (often redical prostatectomy), radiation therapy, hormonal management and chemotherpy are first treatments administered. When these therapies do not arrest the progress of the disease and the patient is in very poor state of health with intense bone metastases pain, he is referred to nuclear medicine departments for radionuclide pain palliation therapy[3] with Sr-89 chloride, Re-186-HEDP, Sm-153-EDTMP, or P-32-phosphates. Several whole issues of journals have been devoted to review the results obtained with these radiopharmaceuticals.[4-7] Our experience and also those of others have shown that although these radiopharmaceuticals temporarily cause pain palliation, the disease advances as seen by the patients conditions and his bone scintigrams posttherapy. After long experience with radionuclidic pain palliation in different cancer bone metastasis patients injected with Sr-89 chloride or Re-186-HEDP, Prof. G.S. Limouris[8] has shown recently that the combination radionuclidic therapy with sodium medronate--Sr-89-chloride--Re-186-HEDP, given in that order at the interval of 1 week, is more effective in pain palliation and causes less mylotoxicity than single radionuclide therapy. The combination therapy has also so far been unable to cure the patient completely and the disease progresses. Pain palliation has also been tried with yttrium-90 citrate solutions[9] by Kutzner and others. The composition of the Y-90 citrate solution has been poorly defined and in the patients myelotoxicity has been reported. We have shown earlier that advanced prostate cancer, resistant to other therapy modalities, could be cured with Y-90 solutions containing both cationic and anionic species, which respectively concentrate in primary cancer and in the bone metastasis of prostate cancer patient.[10] We have treated so far 32 patients with our Y-90 solution. All these patients had undergone radical prostatectomy, hormonal therapy, radiation therapy and in some cases also chemotherapy. In some cases we could show the concentration of the radionuclide in the prostate cancer biopsy specimen. The case reported here has been the first patient who came to us before surgery because he had very diffused bone metastases as seen in Fig. 1. Thus, we have been able to show now that Y-90 citrate species from prostate cancer-affine formulation concentrate not only in the bone metastases but also in the primary cancer which is responsible for the cure of the patients reported earlier.[10]

MATERIALS AND METHODS

Prostate cancer-affine Y-90 citrate solution was synthesized from commercially available Y-90 chloride or Y-90 citrate solution. The nature and stability of the Y-90 species in the radiopharmaceutical solution was examined always by chromatography and electrophoresis. To examine the affinity of the radionuclide for bone metastases and primary cancer only 37 Mbq of the radiopharmaceutical was injected intravenously. Total-body distribution of the radionuclide was studied 3, 24, 48 h postinjection by anterior and posterior imaging of Y-90 Bremsstrahlung scintigraphy with a gamma-camera, fitted with an ultra-high-sensitivity collimator and with the window set at Y-90 Bremsstrahlung spectrum peak, 72.7 KeV.

Prostate cancer patients from different urology departments of Rome are sent to us for radionuclide therapy because other therapies had failed. Most of them are in very bad condition having intense pain, are immobile, and carry permanent urinary catheter.

Before radionuclide therapy we make a total-body bone scintigraphy in order to be able to see the effect of the radionuclide therapy on the metastases. The patient's judgement of pain, urine elimination and well being, his PSA and PAP values, and posttherapy bone scintigrams are the test of our radionuclide therapy effect.

MED. NUCLEARE S.EUGENIO

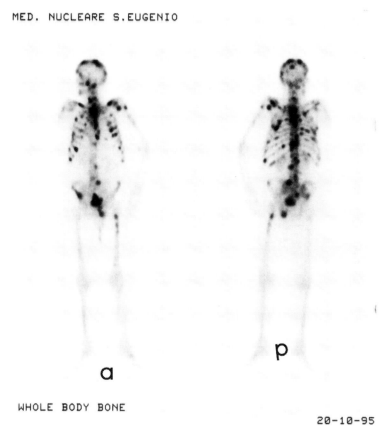

a

WHOLE BODY BONE

20-10-95

Figure 1. Widely diffused bone metastases in a prostate cancer patient seen with Tc-99m-MDP total-body scintigraphy i week before Y-90 citrate therapy.
(a) anterior view, (b) posterior view.

RESULTS

Bone scintigram done one week before the administration of our Y-90 citrate solution to the patient is shown in Fig. 1, which shows highly diffused bone metastases in the whole skeleton. The uptake of Y-90 in bone lesions and in the primary prostate cancer is shown in anterior and posterior segmentary Y-90 scintigrams shown in Figs. 2 and 3 respectively. Only big bone metastases could be clearly seen on Y-90 scintigrams. The uptake in the primary cancer is intense. The radionuclide binds strongly in bone metastases and in the primary cancer which permits repeated scintigraphic examination for more than 10 days p.i.

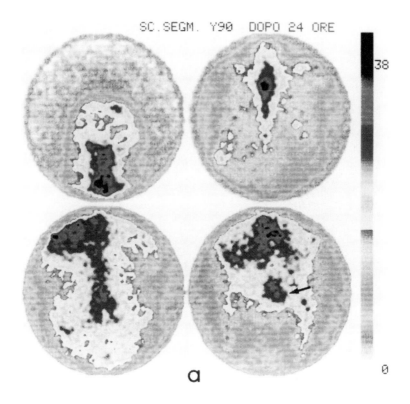

SC.SEGM. Y90 DOPO 24 ORE

Fig. 2. Anterior segmentary scintigram of the patient in Fig. 1 injected with Y-90 citrate, showing the concentration of the radionuclide in bone metastases and in the prostate cancer (arrow).

Pain relief is observed with Y-90 citrate within 24 h p.i.; and within a week the patient gains benefit in mobility. By repeated injection the patient was free of the disease as seen by PAP and PSA values. Two patients out of 32 so far treated with Y-90 citrate did not respond to the therapy.

Platelet depression in most patients was observed on repeated therapy. After the observation the therapy was discontinued and the platelet counts slowly regained the normal value.

Strangely, platelet depression in dogs was not observed after the therapy with Y-90 citrate solution.

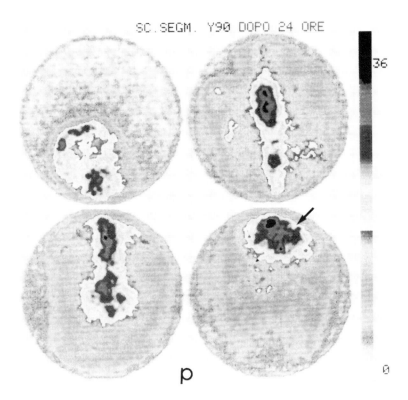

SC.SEGM. Y90 DOPO 24 ORE

Figure 3. Posterior segmentary scintigram of the patient in Fig. 1, injected with Y-90 citrate, showing the concentration of the radionuclide in bone metastases and in the prostate cancer (arrow).

DISCUSSION

The very favourable physical properties of Y-90 for systemic therapy of advanced cancer has been repeatedly stressed by many authors. We have shown that its unique position in the Periodic Table makes it biochemically very attractive for the synthesis of radiopharmaceuticals containing simultaneously cationic, neutral and anionic species. By choosing a suitable ligand the biochemical properties of the radionuclide could be tailored to the therapeutic need. As reported in the present case, the radionuclide then concentrates both in the primary and secondary tumours and thus cures the patient.

The platelet depression observed with Y-90-citrate has led us to investigate the biological properties of Y-90 complexes with other ligands, the antiprostate cancer properties of which are under study.

CONCLUSION

Y-90 citrato complex solution, containing stable cationic and anionic Y-90 species in the solution, is prostae cancer and its bone metastases-affine, for its use not only as a bone metastases pain palliation but also for the cure of the cancer patient. The platelet depression on repeated administration of the radiopharmaceutical has to be avoided.

[1] Coffey DS. Prostate Cancer. Cancer 1993; 71: 880-886.

[2] Bos SD. An overview of current clinical experience with Sr-89 (Metastron). Prostate Suppl. 1994; 5: 23-26.

[3] Garnick MB. The dilemma of prostate cancer. Sci Am 1994; 270 April: 52-59.

[4] Semin Nucl Med 1971; 1 (4).

[5] Semin Nucl Med 1979; 9 (2).

[6] Semin Nucl Med 1992; 22 (1).

[7] Semin Oncol Suppl 2 1993; 20.

[8] Limouris GS, Toubanakis S, Shukla SK, Saturaka A, Vlahos L. Prostate osseous metastases: Evaluation of the combined application of sodium pamidronate/Sr-89-chloride/Re-186-HEDP. Eur J Nucl Med 1996, 23: S15.

[9] Kutzner J, Hahn K, Grimm W, Rösler HP, Eckmann M, Bender S. Yttrium-90-Citrat zur Schmerztherapie bei Knochenmetastasen. Nuc-Compact 1990, 21: 128-132.

[10] Shukla SK, Cipriani C, Argirò G, Atzei G, Boemi S, Boccardi F, Schomäker K, Limouris GS, Baziotis N, Ossicini L, Fanali S, Cristalli M, Caponecchi G. in: Radionuclides for Therapy: Current Status and Future Aspects. Limouris GS, Shukla SK, editors, Athens: Mediterra Publishers, 1993: 47-51.

Radioactive Isotopes in
Clinical Medicine and Research XXII
ed. by H. Bergmann, A. Kroiss and H. Sinzinger
© 1997 Birkhäuser Verlag Basel/Switzerland

PROSTATE OSSEOUS METASTASES : EVALUATION OF THE COMBINED APPLICATION OF DISODIUM PAMIDRONATE / ^{89}Sr-CHLORIDE / ^{186}Re-HEDP

Limouris GS [a], Toubanakis N [a], Shukla SK [b], Manetou A [c], Stavraka A [a], Vlahos L[a]

[a] Radiology Dept, Nuclear Medicine Section, Areteion Univ Hospital, Athens, Hellas ; [b] C.N.R. Institute of Chromatography, Rome, Italy; [c] Nuclear Medicine Department, NIMTS Hospital, Athens, Hellas

SUMMARY

The moderate response, following the therapeutic i.v. application of ^{186}Re-HEDP in 29 patients treated in our Hospital for painful bone metastases [3,5] and the world-wide reservedness upon the efficacy of the radionuclidic palliative application, prompted us to investigate the possible causes of this non-satisfactory response.

We studied the pathology of the metastatic lesions [1, 3, 5] and we reached the conclusion that when the histologic structure of the bone metastases is mixed, therapy with either ^{89}Sr chloride or ^{186}Re-HEDP does not affect the lytic activity because both tracers accumulate into the blastic sites. So, a pure anti-osteolytic agent, Disodium Pamidronate, was used in combination with the osteoblastic-seeking agents ^{89}Sr chloride/^{186}Re-HEDP.

We report the preliminary results of 7 patients with multiple bone metastases due to prostate cancer. In parallel to the combined 148 ± 15 MBq ^{89}Sr chloride/1400 ± 100 MBq ^{186}Re-HEDP [Amersham Internat plc, Backinghamshire/Mallinckrodt Medical BV, Petten], Disodium Pamidronate = Aredia [Giba-Geigy Ltd, Basel] was given via i.v. infusion in a total monthly amount of 120 mg, for three months. The efficacy of the treatment was assessed by (i) a pain and performance questionnaire that the patients were asked to complete daily, (ii) a bone density comparison performed on MRI images, before and 12 weeks after the administration of ^{89}Sr chloride/^{186}Re-HEDP.

Twenty days after treatment, the patients experienced an obvious pain improvement. Four out of 7 expressed flare syndrome. A definite decrease of platelet count and no. of polymorphonuclear white blood cells was observed up to the fourth week following treatment with ^{89}Sr chloride/^{186}Re-HEDP.

Combined therapy appears to be very promising for the palliation of painful bone metastases. As compared to therapy with either ^{89}Sr chloride or ^{186}Re-HEDP alone, it seems to be more complete due to the diffent pharmacokinetics of the tracers.

INTRODUCTION

Skeleton is a frequent metastatic site for many epithlial *(carcinomas)* but a less frequent one for mesenchymal *(sarcomas)* tumours [5]. The pathoanatomic disturbance caused could be: (a) clastic or lytic lesions *(bone destruction)*, (b) blastic or sclerotic lesions *(bone formation)* or (c) mixed lesions *(= lytic lesion surrounded by sclerotic halo)*.

The current management of patients with skeletal metastases is directed towards pain palliation as cure is yet an unrealistic aim. Local or systemic are the available treatment modalities. External beam radiotherapy is the treatment of choice for localized metastatic bone pain; however relief may not be evident for two weeks.Chemotherapy, endocrine therapy and bone-seeking isotopes consist systemic therapies having direct or indirect actions [5].

The aim of our study is to evaluate the combined application of disodium pamidronate, strontium-89 and rhenium-186-HEDP in mixed osseous metastases. We report a new therapeutic scheme based on the histology differencies of the osseous metastases and the different kinetics of the applied pharmaceuticals [6, 7, 8, 9]. It is well known that the majority of prostate osseous metastases are mixed. Both strontium-89 and rhenium-186-HEDP, exclusively accumulate in osteoblastic lesions by active diffusion and chemisorption respectively with probably no effect on the clastic activity of the lesion; thus the monotherapy with radionuclides remains incomplete. On the other hand, disodium pamidronate is a bi-phosphonate, potent inhibitor of osteoclastic bone resorption, not inhibiting bone formation.

PATIENTS AND METHODS

Seven patients with painful mixed osseous metastases, due to prostate cancer (aged 67 to 75 yr) radiographically and scintigraphically confirmed, were enrolled into this study. All had failed to respond to at least one previous local or systemic treatment. Eligibility criteria are shown in Table 1.

The trial was performed in three phases (Appendix I). During the first phase 45 mg disodium pamidronate (Aredia, Ciba-Geigy Ltd, Basel-Switzerland) in 250 ml of normal saline was given as an i.v. infusion over 120 min, once every two days, three times a month, for three months. Episodes of phlebitis at the site of infusion were not noticed. The week following pamidronate application, 148 ± 15 MBq of Sr-89 chloride (Metastron, Amersham Internat plc, Backinghamshire) were i.v. administred. During the third phase 1400 ± 100 MBq of Re-186-HEDP (Mallinckrodt Medical BV, Petten) was intravenously applied.

Biochemical tests were performed every two weeks and included platelet counts, absolute polymorphonuclear white blood cells count, blood creatinine, bone isoenzyme alkaline phosphatase and serum osteocalcin (the latter two are markers of bone formation) as well as overnight fasting urine hydroxyproline and urine calcium to creatinine molar ratio (all three are markers of bone resorption).

---

1. Multiple bone metastases as documented by the bone imaging (radiographic and radioisotopic scan)

2. Documented pain score secondary to bone metastases) of at least 4

3. Estimated life expectancy of at least six months

4. Adequate hematological function as evidenced by two blood counts prior to study entry with platelet count $\geq 150.000/mm^3$, an absolute polymorphonuclear cell count $\geq 2.500/mm^3$ and a Hb ≥ 10 gr% without previous transfusion

5. A Karnofsky perfomance score ≥ 45

6. Patients who had received local irradiation to painful metastatic sites enrolled in the trial fourty days after the end of the radiotherapy

7. Informed consent

Table 1. Eligibility criteria

Pain severity is rated:

   none = 0

   mild = 1

   moderate = 2

   severe = 3

                                   Pain score = pain severity x pain frequency

Pain frequency is rated:

   no pain = 0

   occasional (less than daily) = 1

   intermittent (at least once a day) = 2

   constant (most of the time) = 3

Table 2. Assessment of the pain score

Plain radiograph, radionuclide imaging ($^{99}Tc^m$-MDP), and nuclear magnetic resonance images were used as objective evidence of response and were performed before and after three to eight months of the i.v. therapeutic application.

Subjective clinical assessments were made using pain and mobility scores; these began immediately before treatment and were recorded monthly thereafter. Pain was assessed on a 6-point analogue scale (Table 2) and mobility by the Karnofsky performance score.

Most metastases, however, primarily involve the cancellous bone while cortical destruction occurs at a later stage. It is for this reason that conventional radiology is relatively insensitive both for bone metastases detection as well as for the recognition of early response to treatment. The process in lytic bony metastases starts with sclerosis around periphery of the lesion which gradually moves in towards the centre until the whole area becomes sclerotic. However, the healing process can be misdiagnosed as radiographs may be interpreted as showing disease progression (a previously unnoticed lytic deposition becomes obvious due to its healing sclerotic rim and, however incorrectly described as a new lesion). Consequently conventional radiographs identify marked disease progression but their value in assessing an early response to treatment is limited.

In contradiction alterations before and after therapy can be easily monitored by MRI. In order to avoid interpreting contradictions it seems very useful to compare cortical and cancellous density changes and to distinguish sclerosis due to natural process of remodelling and sclerosis due to the manifestation of active metastatic disease.

Changes in mean gray-scale values from magnetic resonance images of the diseased bone were used to evaluate the progress of the disease. Regions of interest (ROIs) that outlined osteoblastic, osteolytic and normal bone were drawn on each image. The gray-scale values of random points within the ROIs were manually measured with the use of an X-Rite densitometer. The mean gray-scale values of diseased bone were normalised against that of normal bone in images to be compared. Subsequently, t-test was performed and the changes in optical, or bone density were determined.

RESULTS

There was a statistically significant decrease (p<0.001) in both the pain score and the analgesic requirements. A significant (p<0.001)) decrease in osteoclastic activity, as measured by the calcium/creatinine and hydroxyproline/creatinine ratios was noticed six to seven weeks after treatment. A statistically significant decrease in ostoblastic activity was also observed, as measured by the serum alkaline phosphatase. Transient fever or local reaction at the injection site was not noticed. All seven patients showed objective evidence of bone healing. In all, sclerotic areas appeared in sites of osteolytic lesions and decreased intensity of the radionuclide accumulation was noticed. Densitometrically, in three cases an improvement was noticed only in the osteosclerotic areas. No significant change in regions of osteolysis was recorded.

DISCUSSION/CONCLUSION

The moderate response, following a therapeutic i.v. application of Renium-186-HEDP, in 29 patients with painful osseous metastases (Limouris et al, unpublished results) and the still worldwide reservedness upon the efficacy of radionuclidic palliative application[2], prompted us to investigate the possible causes of this non-satisfactory response with the purpose to improve the therapeutic scheme. We considered the pathology of the metastatic lesions and the influence of the extent of the co-existance of osteolytic within the osteosclerotic areas. It has been showed, and should be kept in mind, that osseous metastatic pain is generated by both osteoblastic and osteolytic activity [2]. On the other hand the suitability of the dosology proposed in other reports or by us could be not secured .

We examined the co-existence of lytic-sclerotic lesions (mixed osseous metastases) and we delineated the border between clastic and blastic activity upon preselected ROIs in conventional radiographs and MRI images. In all examined cases osteolysis appeared by simple inspection as dark spots or extented areas surrounded by an osteoblastic rim. With the aid of an X-Rite densitometer we fixed the bountaries between lytic and sclerotic areas, calculated the mean gray-scale values within each of these areas and compared them to the values obtained after therapy.

In this study the efficacy of a combined application of disodium pamidronate [4, 5, 6] (a substance with a pure anti-osteolytic activity), strontium-85 and rhenium-186 HEDP [3,7] (both radiopharmaceuticals, exclusively accumulated in ostoblastic sites by chemisorption) to manage the pain in patients with osseous metastases has been established.

Based upon the different pharmacokinetics of the two osteoblast-seeking radiopharmaceuticals with similar ranges in bone (0.9 mm for Re-186 and 1.0 mm for Sr-89), we expect to increase radiotoxicity in order to enhence the therapeutic effect. The slight platelet and polymorphonuclear decrease, observed about 4 weeks after the i.v. application compared to that of the group of 29 patients previously treated with Re-186 alone in our section, was not of statistical significance.

The application of disodium pamidronate was performed in high dose and (120 mg) into a short time

APPENDIX I: Study design

				FIRST PHASE	SECOND PHASE		THIRD PHASE	
1st week	Mo	45 mg	i.v. infusion of pamidronate					
	We	45 mg						
	Fri	30 mg						
2nd week					We 148±15 MBq	i.v. injection of Sr-89 chloride		
3d week							Thu 1400±10²MBq	i.v. injection of Re-186-HEDP
4th week				*Free of treatment*				
5th and 9th week	Mo	45 mg	i.v. infusion of pamidronate etc.					
	We	45 mg						
	Fri	30 mg						

interval (5 days !) and preceded both the strontium-85 and rhenium-186-HEDP administration and repeated one month after the start of the therapeutic scheme and for the forthcoming three months.

We must underline that the small number of patients reported does not allow to draw precise conclusions. Nevertheless these preliminary results can serve as the vaulting bar for the application of new, more complete and effective therapeutic schemes and send the message to establish more individualized treatments. The question of whether the skeletal retention of pamidronate, strontium-85 and rhenium-186-HEDP have any long term detrimental effect on osseous metastasis is obviously of great importance in view of a prospective use in cancer patients for a longer term survival.

REFERENCES

1. Bos SD. An overview of current clinical experience with strontium-89 (Metastron). Prostate (suppl) 1994; 5: 23-6.

2. Edwards GK, Santoro J, Tayler AJ. Use of bone scintigraphy to select patients with multiple myeloma for treatment with strontium-89. J Nucl Med 1994; 35(12): 1992-3.

3. Guerrieri P, Madoni S, Parisi S, Fusco V, Oriolo V, Rendina G, Paleani-Vettori PG. Bone formation markers and pain palliation in bone metastases treated with strontium-89. Am J Clin Oncol 1994; 17(1): 77-9.

4. Klerk de JM, van-het Chip AD, Zonnenberg BA, van Dijk A, Stokkel MP, Han SH, Blijham GH, Rijk PP. Evaluation of thrombocytopenia in patients treated with rhenium-186-HEDP; guidelines for individual dosage recommendations. J Nucl Med 1994; 35(9): 1423-8.

5. Porter AT, Ben-Josef E, Davis L. Systemic administration of new therapeutic radioisotopes, including phosphorus, strontium, samarium and rhenium. Curr Opin Oncol 1994; 6(6): 607-10.

6. Porter AT, Davis LP. Systemic radionuclide therapy of bone metastases with strontium-89. Oncology-Huntigt 1994; 8(2): 93-6.

7. Samaratunga RC, Thomas SR, Hinnefeld JD, von Kuster LC, Hyams DM, Moulton JS, Sperling MI, Maxon HR. A Monte Carlo simulation model for radiation dose to metastatic skeletal tumor from rhenium-186 (Sn)-HEDP. J Nucl Med 1995; 36(2): 336-50.

8. Serafini AN. Current status of systemic intravenous radiopharmaceuticals for the treatment of painful metastatic bone disease. Int J Radiat Oncol Biol Phys 1994; 30(5): 1187-94.

9. Taylor AJ. Strontium 89 for the palliation of bone pain due to metastatic disease. J Nucl Med 1994; 35 (12): 2054.

Radioactive Isotopes in
Clinical Medicine and Research XXII
ed. by H. Bergmann, A. Kroiss and H. Sinzinger
© 1997 Birkhäuser Verlag Basel/Switzerland

RESULTS OF PET DOSIMETRY IN THE TREATMENT OF THYROTOXICOSIS BY [131]I

B.E Pratt, M.A.Flower, V.R.McCready, C.L Harmer and R.J.Ott
Royal Marsden (NHS) Trust, Sutton, Surrey, UK.

Summary: Despite its long history, there are many different approaches to the treatment of thyrotoxicosis with radioiodine. Our aim in this study is to increase the probability of achieving a euthyroid state with a single administration of [131]I. The parameters, uptake, effective half-life and volume, needed to calculate the activity of radioiodine for treatment and the subsequent radiation dose achieved, are determined from a [124]I tracer study and PET scanning. Preliminary results suggest that using this regime there is an increase in the number of patients becoming euthyroid after a single treatment as compared to those who received a fixed activity of radioiodine.

Introduction

Hyperthyroidism is a relatively common disease and is a disease which affects females predominantly. The treatment choices lie between medical treatment with antithyroid drugs, surgery or radioiodine. The two most common causes of hyperthyroidism, Graves' disease and toxic nodular goitre (Larkin, 1985), are also associated with increased trapping of iodide by the thyroid.

Radioiodine therapy provides a hazard free, easy to perform method of treating patients with hyperthyroidism. It has been in use for over 50 years and has been shown to be safe and free from the more serious side effects associated with the administration of antithyroid drugs such as agranulocytosis and hepatic dysfunction. Opinions differ as to what is the correct use of radioiodine: while some clinicians prefer to give a dose aimed at thyroid ablation followed by hormone replacement others give one or more relatively small doses of radioiodine, monitoring the patient until they become euthyroid. The advantage of this low dose treatment is that the onset of hypothyroidism is often averted, or delayed for several years. However, the patient may require many visits to the doctor/clinic over some years and it can take several months to achieve the euthyroid state. An alternative method is to try to tailor the dose to achieve euthyroidism without the necessity for hormone supplement or further radioiodine. Whatever method is adopted there remains the problem of the development of long-term hypothyroidism which occurs at a rate of about 4% per year. It can be argued that since hypothyroidism is inevitable, ablation and hormone supplement is the optimum treatment but, given the choice, most patients will opt for any technique which will increase the probability of rendering them euthyroid without the need for lifetime medication.

The aim of this study was to increase the probability of achieving euthyroidism as quickly as possible, using a single administration of radioiodine.

In a previous study we treated 63 patients with Graves' disease using a protocol in which 75MBq ^{131}I was administered as a fixed activity and this was repeated at 6 monthly intervals until the patient became euthyroid. During this study we measured the functioning thyroid volume using positron emission tomography (PET) and [124]I. This value, together with the uptake and half-life measurements, were used to estimated the radiation dose delivered to the thyroid gland. Results of that study showed that for patients with Graves' disease, most become euthyroid within twelve months of receiving a radiation dose to the thyroid of between 40Gy and 80Gy (Flower et al, 1994). A protocol has since been introduced where the aim is to give a radiation dose of 50_5Gy to the thyroid, and to wait at least 12 months before considering retreatment with radioiodine.

Patient Material and Methods

Forty-two patients (34 female: 8 male; age range 21-81 years) have been treated using the 50Gy protocol. All patients were hyperthyroid clinically and biochemically and none had had previous radioiodine treatment. Patients who were taking anti-thyroid medication were ask to stop the drug for four days prior to the radioiodine administration. All the patients were followed-up at 2 monthly intervals with thyroid function tests and maintained on antithyroid drugs if necessary. Twenty-six of these patients have been followed-up for more than twelve months.

The radioiodine protocol is as follows: on Day 0 the patient received a tracer dose (15MBq) of ^{124}I, a positron-emitting isotope with a half-life of 4.16 days. Thyroid uptake measurements were then carried out at various times from 2 hours to 5 Days. From these measurements the "maximum" uptake of radioiodine by the thyroid and the effective half-life were obtained. Twenty-four hours after the administration of the ^{124}I a PET scan of the thyroid was performed from which the functioning mass of the gland was assessed (Ott al, 1987). The activity of ^{131}I to be administered is calculated using:

$$A^{131} = \frac{50 \times V}{k \times U_{max}^{124} \times T_{eff}^{131}} \tag{1}$$

Where U_{max}^{124} = maximum uptake of ^{131}I, T_{eff}^{131} = effective half-life (in hours),

A^{131} = activity of ^{131}I to be administered (in MBq), V = the volume of the thyroid, k = 0.037g

Gy MBq^{-1} h^{-1}

The therapy dose of ^{131}I was given on Day 5. Twenty-fours following the administration of the ^{131}I a further uptake measurement is made.

The radiation dose received by the thyroid was estimated using:

$$D = \frac{k \times U^{131} \times T_{eff}^{131} \times A^{131}}{V} \tag{2}$$

Where U^{131} = uptake at 24 hours of ^{131}I. Equations (1) and (2) are derived from the MIRD scheme (Loevinger et al, 1991) for the estimation of internal radiation dose.

Results

Using the above protocol, the activities administered ranged from 32-297MBq and the dose delivered to the thyroid gland ranged from 39.7-70.4Gy. The results presented are from the twenty six patients who have been treated using the 50Gy protocol and followed up for twelve months or more. These are compared with the results from the 75MBq dose-response study (Table 1). The percentage of patients becoming euthyroid within 12 months has increased from

Status at 12 months after a single ^{131}I treatment	75MBq Protocol	50Gy Protocol
Euthyroid	14/63 (22%)	14/26 (54%)
Hyperthyroid	46/63 (73%)	11/26 (42%)
Hypothyroid	3/63 (5%)	1/26 (4%)

Table 1 Comparison of results, at 12 months, for patients in the two treatment groups

22% to 54%, while the percentage of patients remaining hyperthyroid has decreased from 73% to 42%. There was no significant difference in the percentage of patients becoming hypothyroid.

The time to become euthyroid was also compared for the two treatment groups (figure 1) This ranged from two months to eighteen months for the 50Gy treatment protocol and from two to fifteen months for the 75MBq protocol. Thus there is a large spread in the time to become euthyroid with a slight trend towards it taking longer in the 50Gy group. The fraction of patients who became euthyroid in less than six months has decreased from 0.52 to 0.43 as the prescription changed from a fixed 75MBq activity to a thyroid dose of 50Gy.

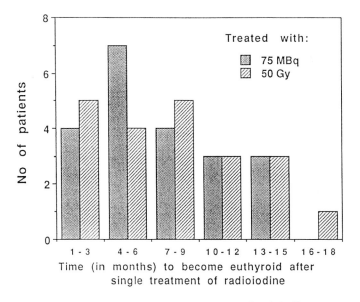

Figure 1 Time to become euthyroid after a single treatment of radioiodine.

Discussion

Opinions differ on the best approach to the treatment of hyperthyroidism. However, when consulted, patients invariably opt for a protocol which offers a chance of achieving euthyroidism without the need for life-long medication despite the fact that this might require repeated therapy with extra hospital visits. Our results show that, at least in the short term, it is possible to increase the number of patients being rendered euthyroid with a single administration of radioactivity.

It has been shown that the major factor in calculating the correct dose is the thyroid volume measurement (Flower, 1994). In this study we have used the MUP-PET system to measure the functional thyroid volume. Ultrasound is more widely available but a preliminary study in our laboratory, the ultrasound measurement of volume was usually larger than the PET assessed functional volume, especially for enlarged glands (Crawford, 1996). Thus it is difficult to translate the dosimetry from one clinic to another. However with the methods described above we feel that we are making progress in improving our treatment protocol for patients suffering from thyrotoxicosis and achieving the highest probability of rendering the patient euthyroid. We are correlating the ultrasound measurements with the PET study with a view to making the fixed dose protocol more cost effective.

Conclusions

The 50Gy study has achieved our first objective of reducing the incidence of hyperthyroidism and increasing the probability of becoming euthyroid while not increasing the incidence of hypothyoidism.

We have also confirmed the findings of the earlier dose-response study that retreatment at 6 months is in many cases too soon.

References
1. Larkins R.G. (1985) A Practical Approach to Endocrine Disorders. Williams & Williams Adis PTY LTD

2. Flower M.A., Al-Saadi A., Harmer C.L., McCready V.R, Ott R.J. (1994) Dose-response study on thyrotoxic patients undergoing positron emission tomography and radioiodine therapy. European Journal of Nuclear Medicine 21: 531-536

3. Ott R.J., Batty V, Webb S., Flower M.A., Leach M.O., Clack R., Marsden P.K., McCready V.R., Bateman J.E., Sharma H., Smith A. (1987) Measurement of   Radiation dose to the thyroid using positron emission tomography. British Journal of   Radiology 1987:245-251

4. Loevinger R., Budinger T.T., Watson E.E. (1991)MIRD primer for absorbed dose calculation, New York: Society of Nuclear Medicine

5. Crawford D.C, Pratt B.E, Hill C, Flower M.A, Moskovic E, McCready V.R, and Harmer C.L. Volume measurement of thyroid tissue in Graves' disease: comparison between volume estimates obtained using B-mode ultrasonography and positron emission tomography. To be submitted to Br. J. Radiology

Radiopharmacology

Radioactive Isotopes in
Clinical Medicine and Research XXII
ed. by H. Bergmann, A. Kroiss and H. Sinzinger
© 1997 Birkhäuser Verlag Basel/Switzerland

RADIOPHARMACEUTICAL DEVELOPMENT OF ^{123}I-(+)-3-IODO-MK 801 FOR NMDA-RECEPTOR SCINTIGRAPHY.

P. Angelberger, T. Brücke[1], H. Kvaternik, T. Wanek

Abt. Radiopharmaka, Forschungszentrum Seibersdorf A-2444,
[1] Univ. Klin. f. Neurologie, AKH Wien A-1090, Austria

SUMMARY: ^{125}I-(+)-3-iodo-MK 801 exhibited high affinity for the NMDA-receptor in-vitro, thus we aimed to develop the ^{123}I-analog as a potential in-vivo tracer. 3-trimethyl-silyl-MK-801 was used as precursor for electrophilic iodo-desilylation but no ^{123}I-MK 801 was formed in ordinary aqueous acid conditions. In non-aqueous trifluoro-acetic acid using chloramine-T as oxidant up to 60 % ^{123}I-MK 801 was obtained within 5 min at 25 °C. It was isolated from the reaction mixture by preparative HPLC. Specific activity was ~ 10^3 Ci/mmol, Radiochemical purity, determined by analytical HPLC and TLC was > 97 % and remained stable for > 20 hours. In-vivo distribution in tissues and brain regions of rats 4 hrs p.i. showed highest concentration in frontal cortex at 0.1 % dose/g, reflecting NMDA-receptor distribution.

INTRODUCTION

The N-Methyl-D-Aspartic acid (NMDA)-receptor is widely distributed in mammalian brain with highest density in cerebral cortex and has the function of a ligand-gated ion-channel. The neurotransmitter L-glutamate and related agonists bind and promote the opening of an ion-channel which permits entry of sodium and calcium ions into target cells. However in a target cell with normal resting membrane potential the ion-channel is blocked by Mg^{++} and this block is only removed when the target cell is depolarized by activation of other synaptic inputs. This "conditional" nature of NMDA-receptors may explain their postulated role in learning and memory.

NMDA receptors have been implicated in neuronal degeneration as in Alzheimer disease and in neuronal death as in ischemic insult (1).

(5 R,10S)-(+)-5-methyl-10,11-dihydro,5H-dibenzo[a,d]cyclohepten-5,10-imine (MK 801) is a non-competitive antagonist of the NMDA-receptor which acts by occupying a site within the ion-channel distinct from the Mg^{++}-site. It exerts a neuroprotective effect and may have therapeutic potential in ischemia and neurodegenerative diseases.

There has been considerable interest in labeled MK 801 as a radio-ligand to study NMDA-receptors. Most of the research to date has been performed as in-vitro binding studies using ^{3}H- and ^{125}I-(+)-3-iodo-MK 801 (^{125}I-MK 801) which exhibited high affinity for the NMDA-receptor (2, 3). ^{123}I-MK 801 may enable in-vivo imaging of the distribution, concentration and functional state of NMDA-receptors. The aim of this work was to develop ^{123}I-MK 801 as a potential radiopharmaceutical for NMDA-receptor scintigraphy.

MATERIALS AND METHODS

(+)-3-trimethylsilyl-MK 801 (TMS-MK 801) was obtained commercially as precursor for electrophilic iodo-desilylation in analogy to iodo-destannylation (4) (Fig. 1).

(+)-3-iodo-MK 801 (^{127}I-MK 801) was purchased as standard for ^{123}I-MK 801.

N.c.a. ^{123}I-NaI in 0.02M NaOH, ~ 300 µCi/µl, was obtained in highest radionuclidic purity from Forschungszentrum Karlsruhe, BRD.

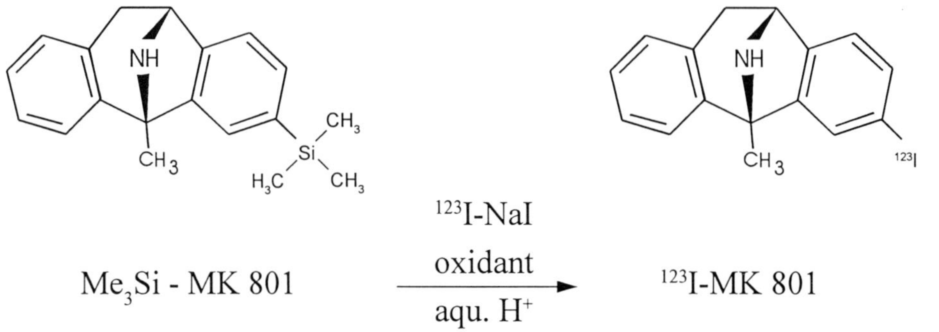

Me$_3$Si - MK 801 $\xrightarrow[\text{aqu. H}^+]{\substack{^{123}\text{I-NaI}\\ \text{oxidant}}}$ ^{123}I-MK 801

Fig. 1: Labeling of ^{123}I-MK 801.

Preparative HPLC isolation of ^{123}I-MK 801 from the reaction mixture was performed with an isocratic reversed-phase system. Column: Nucleosil-100, 5 µm, C18, 4 x 290 mm. Eluent: 60 % (v/v) aqu. ammonium formate, 40 % acetonitrile. Flow: 1.5 ml/min. Detectors: UV 275 nm and Radiometric (scintillation) in series. Calibration: ^{127}I-MK 801. The isolated product peak was vacuum evaporated and the residue taken up in phosphate buffered saline containing 5 % ethanol. For analytical HPLC the same system was used but equipped with a separate analytical column.

TLC was performed on Merck silicagel plates developed in ether: acetonitrile: ammoniumhydroxide (70:30:0.5). Radioactivity distribution was measured with a Berthold Linear Analyzer.

Tissue distribution was measured 4 hours after tail vein injection of 50 µCi, 0.09 nmol, ^{131}I-MK 801 in rats (~ 200 g, n = 7) by dissection (5). Samples were weighed and counted in a NaI (Tl) detector in comparison to injection standards resulting in [% injected dose/g] values.

RESULTS AND DISCUSSION

^{123}I labeling

For introduction of ^{123}I into a predetermined position on a phenyl-ring a preferred method is to use a precursor with a bulky tri-butyl-tin group, a good leaving group, at this same position.

Since TMS-MK 801 was available, we used it as precursor for electrophilic iodo-desilylation in analogy to iodo-destannylation (4) (Fig. 1).

When electrophilic iodo-desilylation was performed using Chloramine-T as oxidant and aqueous dilute hydrochloric acid as solvent, radiochemical yield (Y) was extremely low, ≤ 3 %, and could not be improved by varying other reaction parameters (precursor concentration, reaction temperature and time). Under similar conditions very high and reproducible Y had been obtained in iodo-destannylation with epidepride and β-CIT (4).

The electrophilic cleavage of the TMS-MK 801 precursor is expected to be facilitated by acid (6). Accordingly increasing the acid strength and concentration should promote the reaction. A strong acid with good solvent properties and complete volatility is trifluoroacetic acid (TFA).

When the reaction was performed in concentrated TFA with exclusion of water, ^{123}I-MK 801 was actually obtained in good Y.

Using the optimized reaction parameters shown in table 1, Y of ^{123}I-MK 801 amounted to 60 %.

Table 1: ^{123}I-MK 801 **optimized labeling conditions**

aqu. ^{123}I-NaI evaporated to **dryness**		
Me$_3$Si-MK 801	in **TFA**,	1.0 mM
ClAT	in **TFA**,	1.7 mM
reaction volume	: 20 μl	
reaction temperature	: 25 °C	
reaction time	: 5 min	

Preparative and analytical HPLC

Upon preparative HPLC of the reaction mixture 2 major ^{123}I-peaks were found: inorganic ^{123}I-species, e.g. NaI, eluted at 2.9 min containing about 19 % of the applied ^{123}I and ^{123}I-MK 801 eluted at 15.4 min containing about 60 % and accompanied only by a very small UV-mass-peak (Fig. 2). When this was calibrated with [127]I-MK 801 the specific activity was calculated as ~ 1000 Ci/mmol.

Radiochemical purity, determined by analytical HPLC (Fig. 3) and TLC, was > 97 % and remained stable for > 20 hours.

In vivo tissue distribution

4 hours after injection highest tissue concentration was found in the liver as excretory organ. Blood radioactivity was low at this time. In the central nervous system the concentration was highest in the frontal cortex amounting to 0.1 % dose/g, followed by striatum, thalamus and hippocampus 0.09 % dose/g each, while lowest concentration was in cerebellum 0.06 % dose/g (Fig. 4). This reflects NMDA-receptor distribution and is consistent with previous autoradiographic results (3).

^{123}I-MK 801 may be useful for in-vivo receptor scintigraphy.

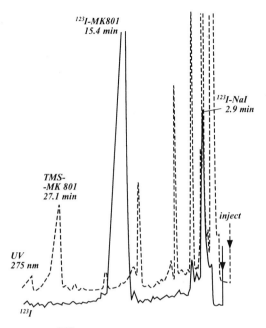

Fig. 2:   Preparative HPLC of ^{123}I-MK 801. For conditions see Material and Methods.
Radioactivity detector in full line, UV detector in dashed line.

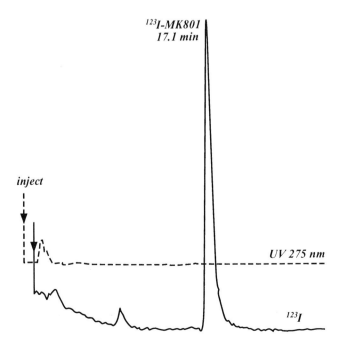

Fig. 3:   Analytical HPLC of ^{123}I-MK 801. For conditions see Material and Methods.
Radioactivity detector in full line, UV detector in dashed line.

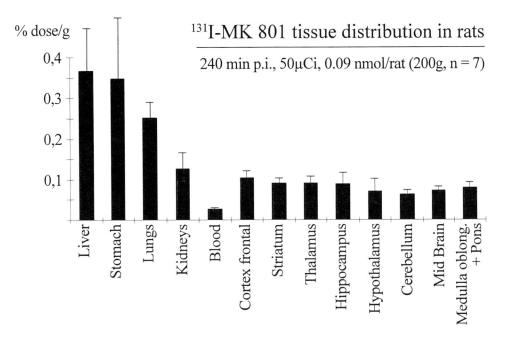

Fig. 4:   Tissue distribution of ^{131}I-MK 801 in rats. For conditions see Material and Methods.

REFERENCES

(1) Woodruff GN, Foster AC, Gill R, Komp IA, Wong EHF, Iversen LL. The interaction between MK-801 and receptors for N-methyl-D-aspartate: functional consequences. Neuropharmacology 1987; 26: 903-909.

(2) Wong EHF, Knight AR, Woodruff GN. (^{3}H) MK-801 labels a site on the N-methyl-D aspartate receptor channel complex in rat brain membranes. J Neurochem 1988; 50: 274-281.

(3) Jacobson W, Cottrell GA. Rapid visualization of NMDA receptors in the brain: characterization of (+)-3-(^{125}I)-iodo-MK 801 binding to thin sections of rat brain. J Neurosci Meth 1993; 46: 17-27.

(4) Angelberger P, Kvaternik H, Portner R, Hammerschmidt F. Optimized preparation of the dopaminergic receptor ligands ^{123}I-epidepride and ^{123}I-CIT. In: Radioactive Isotopes in Clinical Medicine and Research. Bergmann H, Sinzinger H, eds. Birkhäuser, Basel 1995: 281-286.

(5) Glowinski J, Iversen LL. Catecholamine regional metabolism in rat brain. J Neurochem 1966; 13: 655-669.

(6) Wilbur DS, Anderson KW, Stone WK, O'Brien Jr HA. Radiohalogenation of nonactivated aromatic compounds via aryltrimethylsilyl intermediates. J Label Compds Radiopharm 1982, 19: 1171 ff.

Radioactive Isotopes in
Clinical Medicine and Research XXII
ed. by H. Bergmann, A. Kroiss and H. Sinzinger
© 1997 Birkhäuser Verlag Basel/Switzerland

SIMPLE PRODUCTION OF YTTRIUM-90 IN A CHEMICAL FORM SUITABLE TO CLINICAL GRADE RADIOCONJUGATES

M. Chinol, R. Franceschini*, G. Paganelli, A. Pecorale*, A. Paiano*

European Institute of Oncology , Via Ripamonti 435, 20141 Milan, Italy and * Sorin Biomedica Diagnostics, 13040 Saluggia, Vercelli, Italy.

SUMMARY: Although numerous generator systems have been described for the production of yttrium-90 (Y-90), a disadvantage common to all is that the Y-90 is not eluted in a chemical form suitable for direct labeling of chelating agents attached to useful molecules. We have developed a new generator system in which the Sr-90 was bound to a cation exchange resin and the Y-90 was eluted with an acetate buffer solution at pH=5.0-5.5. In the acetate form the activity was used to prepare clinically useful radioconjugates without further manipulations. In addition, the generator was equipped with a safety column connected in series with the first resulting in an eluate free of any Sr-90 breakthrough. The characteristics of this new generator make it suitable for clinical applications.

INTRODUCTION

In a recent evaluation of radionuclides for radioimmunotherapy (1), Y-90 has been selected as one of the four best therapeutic radionuclides for labeling tumor associated antibodies. This selection was based on its suitable half-life (64 hr), absence of gamma-ray emissions, stable daughter, high energy beta emission (E_{max} = 2.3 MeV) and chemical properties suitable for forming stable bindings with various chelating agents. Another important advantage is the fact that it may be obtained by decay of its parent, strontium-90 (Sr-90) ($T_{1/2}$ 28 yr) by means of a radionuclide generator. The nuclear characteristics of the decay system for this pair are shown below :

$$Sr\text{-}90 \xrightarrow{\quad \beta^- (0.54 \text{ MeV}) \quad} Y\text{-}90 \xrightarrow{\quad \beta^- (2.30 \text{ MeV}) \quad} Zr\text{-}90 \text{ (stable)}$$

$$T_{1/2} : 28 \text{ y} \qquad\qquad T_{1/2} : 64.2 \text{ hr}$$

Although solvent extraction methods for the separation of yttrium-90 from strontium-90 have been reported, it is the ion exchange methods that have received the most attention (2). Numerous systems have been described where a cation exchange resin has been used to retain the Sr-90 while the daughter Y-90 activity is eluted with various eluants such as lactate, oxalate, citrate and EDTA. A disadvantage common to all of the above is that the activity is not eluted in a chemical form suitable for direct labeling of chelating agents attached to useful molecules. It is usually necessary to remove these agents prior to protein labeling. One efficient generator system employed 0.003M EDTA as eluant (3) but subsequently this agent has been destroyed prior to the utilization of the Y-90 activity hampering the widespread use of this system. This report describes experiences in the construction, elution and use of a new designed Sr-90/Y-90 generator system.

MATERIALS AND METHODS

Generator Construction

Figure 1 shows the generator system without the lead shielding.

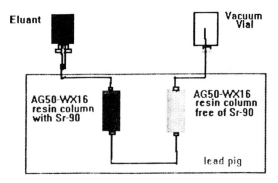

Figure 1. Device for generating Y-90 by radioactive decay of Sr-90 comprising a cation-exchange resin column containing the loading solution and a second column, in series with the first, containing the cation-exchange resin free from Sr-90.

The generator consists of two polycarbonate columns 4.0 cm long and 1.0 cm of diameter with a frit at the bottom and fitted at both ends with plugs. A small diameter tubing is connecting in series the two columns. The inlet and outlet of the generator are fitted with needles where the vial containing the eluting buffer and the evacuated vial are inserted. Both columns were loaded with AG50-WX16 (Bio-Rad) (200-400 mesh, Na^+ form) cation-exchange resin with high degree of cross-linking previously washed with 1M NaOH and water. 185 MBq of Sr-90 in 1M HNO_3 solution were adjusted to pH=4.5 with NaOH and then loaded on one column by means of peristaltic pump. During each elution a sealed glass vial containing 5 mL of 0.6M acetate buffer at pH=5.0-5.5 was inserted in the inlet needle followed by the insertion of a 20 mL evacuated glass vial at the other end.

Strontium-90 breakthrough

A rapid determination of Sr-90 breakthrough may be obtained by paper chromatography and saline eluant where the Sr-90 migrates with the solvent front while the Y-90 acetate remains near the origin (3). A more accurate estimate may be performed subsequently when the Y-90 is partially decayed by liquid scintillation counting as previously described (2).

Preparation of radiopharmaceuticals using generator produced Y-90

The Y-90 in the acetate form was used to obtain two radiopharmaceuticals; particles of $[^{90}Y]$ Ca oxalate to be administered intraarticularly for radiation synovectomy and to label biotin for cancer therapy in a three-step pretargeting approach.

Particle Preparation: 75 MBq of Y-90 acetate were mixed in a test tube to 0.5 mL of 0.1M $CaCl_2$, then the particles were obtained upon addition of 1 mL of 0.1M sodium oxalate as previously described (4).

Biotin Labeling: biotin linked to the macrocyclic chelating agent DOTA was dissolved in 1M ammonium acetate pH=7.0 and then 185 MBq of Y-90 acetate were added without any further manipulation. The labeling efficiency was checked by ITLC (saline as eluant) mixing an aliquot of the reaction mixture with a molar excess of avidin. In this system the labeled biotin bound to avidin remains at the origin while free Y-90 migrates with the solvent front.
The Y-90 labeled biotin was administered to patients with glioma pre-treated with antibody and streptavidin according to a three-step pretargeting protocol (5).

RESULTS

In the five months since its construction, the generator performance remained constant. Elution efficiency was high with more than 90% of Y-90 activity eluted with the 5 mL vial of eluant as shown in figure 2.

Elution yield
(%)

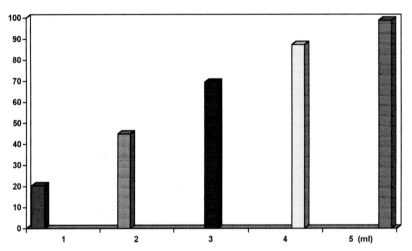

Eluant Volume

Figure 2. Yttrium-90 elution profile.

Also there was no detectable Sr-90 contamination in the eluate. The incorporation of Y-90 into the particles of calcium oxalate ranged from 85 to 95% while the labeling yield of the biotin-DOTA was greater than 95%.

DISCUSSION

There is a large interest in the applications of Y-90 for radiotherapy either associated to inorganic particles for radiation synovectomy (4) or to label molecules such as biotin e/o avidin and monoclonal antibodies for cancer treatment (5-6).

Among the generator systems previously described in literature two appear to be more interesting. One is the generator which employs a solution of 0.5% citric acid as eluant (7) and the second is the one eluted with 0.003M EDTA (3). The main drawbacks of these generators were that the former required large volumes of eluant to achieve good Y-90 yields while the latter required the distruction of EDTA prior of using the Y-90 activity for any application. Both these disadvantages have been overcome with the proposed new generator. In fact, due to an improved cation-exchange resin and to the use of a stronger complexing agent, more than 90% of the activity was eluted in the first 5 mL of acetate buffer. Moreover, the Y-90 in the acetate form, can be transferred to a stronger chelating agent such as DOTA previously attached to clinically useful molecules.

Another important aspect to be considered when the generators are intended for clinical applications is the presence of Sr-90 in the eluate. Due to the extreme toxicity of Sr-90 and its long lifetime, maximum permissible dose fixed in bone has been set at only 2 μCi (8). The above mentioned generators showed a low but detectable Sr-90 breakthrough; 0.1% in the citrate and 0.01% in the EDTA generator. Our system instead, equipped with the second safety column, has produced so far an eluate free of any Sr-90 contamination.

The design of this new generator is also very similar to the commercially available "Moly" generator. Elutions are performed in a similar manner with the vial of buffer and that under vacuum. This offers the advantage that once the buffer solution is checked for sterility and pirogenicity, the eluted activity is also in safe biological conditions for human use.

CONCLUSIONS

This new type of generator offers several advantages reducing the manipulations of the eluate and making easier the labeling with Y-90 of compounds which find their application in cancer therapy and radiation synovectomy.

(ACKNOWLEDGEMENTS)

The authors acknowledge support from the Ministero dell'Università e della Ricerca Scientifica e Tecnologica and from the CNR Fin. Pr. A.C.R.O.

REFERENCES

1. Wessels BW, Rogus RD. Radionuclide selection and model, absorbed dose calculations for radiolabeled tumor associated antibodies. Med Phys 1984; 11: 638-645.

2 . Skraba WJ, Arino H, Kramer HH. A new Sr-90/Y-90 radioisotope generator. Int J Appl Rad Isot 1978; 29: 91-96.

3. Chinol M, Hnatowich DJ. Generator-produced Yttrium-90 for radioimmunotherapy. J Nucl Med 1987; 28: 1465-1470.

4. Davis MA, Chinol M. Radiopharmaceuticals for radiation synovectomy: evaluation of two Yttrium-90 particulate agents. J Nucl Med 1989; 30: 1047-1055.

5. Paganelli G, Chinol M, Grana C, De Cicco C, Cremonesi M, Meares C, Franceschini R, Tarditi L, Siccardi AG. Optimization of the three-step pretargeting approach for diagnosis and therapy in cancer patients. 42nd Annual Meeting, Society of Nuclear Medicine, Minneapolis, MN, June 12-15, 1995. J Nucl Med 1995; 36: Suppl. 5, 225 P.

6. Deshpande SV, De Nardo SJ, Kukis DL, Moi MK, McCall MJ, De Nardo GL, Meares CF. Yttrium-90-labeled monoclonal antibody for therapy: labeling by a new macrocyclic bifunctional chelating agent. J Nucl Med 1990; 31: 473-479.

7. Doering RF, Tucker WD, Stang LJ Jr. A simple device for milking high purity yttrium-90 from strontium-90. J Nucl Md 1963; 4: 54-59.

8. ICRP Publication 30, 1979; Part 1, 2: 77-78.

INVESTIGATIONS INTO BIOKINETICS OF I-123-DIETHYLSTILBESTROL
PHOSPHATE (DSEP) IN TUMOR-BEARING MICE.

K. Schomäcker[1], B. Meller-Rehbein[2], B. Gabruk-Szostak, H. Gerard[1],
K. Scheidhauer[1], A. Scharl[3], M. Bähre[1], E. Richter[3], and H.
Schicha[1].
Departments of [1]Nuclear Medicine and [3]Obstet & Gyn, University of
Cologne, Germany. [2]Clinic of Radiation Therapy and Nuclear Medicine,
University of Lübeck, Germany,

SUMMARY. Diethylstilbestrolphosphate, a nonsteroidal estrogen shows
promising affinity and specificity for estrogen-receptors (ER).
After successful radioiodination of DSEP, our further investigations
focused on biodistribution, in vivo stability and isolation.

100 µl 123I-DSEP solution (3.7 MBq/ml) were injected i.v. into male
mice (6 weeks old DBA mice, 20 g weight) bearing an ER-positive
breast adenocarcinoma of app. 0.5 g in the right upper limb.
Radioactivities accumulated in different organs were measured 10
min, 20 min, 1 h, and 2 h p.i. and calculated as % radioactivity
applied per g organ weight (%/g). The biodistribution of the tracer
was visualized 10 min and 1 h p.i. by a gamma camera. To test
whether the accumulation was mediated by ER, "cold" DSEP was applied
in 100-fold excess prior to the application of 123I-DSEP. The
scintigrams obtained showed the tumor clearly. From 10 min up to 2 h
p.i. high and fairly concentrations of the radioactive compound were
measured in ER-rich tissues of prostate and tumor (app. 50 %/g).
Radioactivities in ER-poor tissues were considerably lower and
decreased with time. This resulted in tumor/background ratios of
app. 50 - 80. The preapplication of "cold" DSEP inhibited the
accumulation of 123I-DSEP in ER-rich tissues like prostate and
tumor.

The results showed that 123I-DSEP is a ER-receptor-specific
radiopharmaceutical which concentrates in ER-rich tissues. This
radiopharmaceutical is promising for ER-imaging.

INTRODUCTION

Three carcinomas which express estrogen receptors account for one
quarter of all tumour-related deaths of women: breast cancer affects
approx. 1 out of 10 women and is the single most frequent cause of
tumour-related lethality accounting for approx. 16 % of tumour-related
deaths in women and for 3% of total female mortality. Endometrial
carcinoma has an incidence of approx. 25 new cases per 10^5 women and
accounts for 1-2% of all tumour-related deaths. The incidence of
ovarian carcinoma is $15/10^5$ women and exceeds that of invasive cervical
cancer. Because of its high lethality it accounts for 5-6% of all
tumour-related deaths (1).

Estrogen receptor status is at present included in the panel of tumour
characteristics which are considered to be relevant for therapy and
prognostic calculations.

A non-invasive technique for identifying receptor status not only in
primary breast tumours but also sites of metastases would be clinically
advantageous. More than 50 % of breast endometrial and ovarian
carcinomas express intracellular proteins, referred to as estrogen
receptors that selectively bind estrogens with high affinity and retain
this steroid in target cells. It has long been appreciated that
radioligand binding to estrogen receptors would be capable of achieving
target/blood ratios suitable for in vivo imaging (2). Most suitable for
this application would be high-affinity, receptor-selective
radioestrogens bearing isotopes decaying with a γ-emission energy
within the optimal sensitivity range of conventional nuclear medicine
scintillation cameras (140 to 280 keV).

The radiosyntheses of γ-emitting estrogens were first reported app. 40
years ago (3-5), whereas labelling using tritium with specific
activities high enough to detect estrogen receptor proteins was
accomplished approximately 10 years later (6-8). Early

radiohalogenations produced products exhibiting low stability that were not characterized biologically or biochemically (3-5). The radiosynthesis of estradiol labelled with iodine 125I at 16alpha in the late 1970s provided a stable radioligand with high specific activity that demonstrated specific and selective receptor-mediated retention in estrogen receptor-containing tissues (9, 10). More recently, additional estrogens radiolabelled with iodine, bromine, and fluorine have been described that demonstrate specific receptor-mediated ligand retention (11-14).

Our own results from a multicenter study using 16alpha-123I-iodoestradiol (123I-E2) showed that the sensitivity of this substance in the detection of primary breast cancer was low, compared to mammography and other methods (15). Therefore a scintigraphic method basing on 123I-E2 cannot be used as screening method. Differentiation of malignant and benign tissue was even more difficult because both may have a positive ER status (mastopathia). However, these data suggest that a scintigraphic method has potential for the non-invasive determination of receptor status in primary and metastatic carcinomas.

Unfortunately, 16alpha-123I-iodoestradiol is not available for sale and it is a patented substance. Furthermore, the tumour/blood ratio of this radioestrogen is too low to achieve bright tumour images in any case.

Searching for another and better tracer with potential affinity to estrogen receptors - especially in cases of breast cancer - a procedure was developed to radioiodinate and to purify diethylstilbestrol (DSEP).
Diethylstilbestrol diphosphate, in Germany known under the trade name Honvan, is a nonsteroidal estrogen analogue (16). Therefore, it is accumulated in estrogen receptor rich tissues. DSEP is dephosphorylated by acid phosphatase, which is especially highly concentrated in the prostate organ , and the resulting DSE (Diethylstilbestrol) exhibits a receptor mediated binding to DNA (17, 18).

Tubis et al. (19) had proposed radiolabelling of DESP for tumor
diagnosis, and prepared and labelled the agent by 131I-Cl addition
to the central double bond of the molecule. First animals
experiments with radioiodinated DSEP produced according this method
were carried out by Mende et al. (20, 21). These preliminary results
were somewhat disappointing, probably due to the insufficient
separation and purification of the radiolabelled DSEP.

Maysinger et al. (22) converted Diethylstilbestrol to their mono-
and polyiodinated derivatives by electrophilic substitution of
positive iodine into the activated aromatic rings using both
chemical and electrochemical procedures. Neither the purity nor the
stability of the final products were sufficient enough to be used as
radioactive diagnostics.

The aim of this study is to present preliminary biokinetic data of
123I-Diethystilbestrolphosphate which was labelled by means of
Chloramine T (21, 22).

MATERIALS AND METHODS

Labelling procedure

50 µl 123I- (37 MBq), 50 µl Chloramine-T-solution and 50 µl DSEP
("Honvan" ASTA Medica AG, 300 mg/5 ml) reacted at pH 2 on a
temperature of 50 °C. The reaction-time was about one hour.

The separation and purification was performed by HPLC, using a RP-
C18-Column:

   Solvents: CH_3OH (A)/H_2O+ 1% C_2H_5COOH (B)
   Gradient: 20% A/ 80 % B - 70 % A/ 30 % B within
        5 min and isocratic with the last
        adjustment until 20 min

```
UV:                    254 nm
Retention time: about 10 min
```

The 123I-DSEP-fraction was evaporated to dryness under N_2

The solution was injected as isotonic solution with a radioactivity concentration of 3.7 MBq/ml

Quality control can be performed using HPLC-method described above. The injected 123I-DSEP had the following properties:

Yield: 70 - 80 %
Stability: 24 h in solution
Radiochemical purity > 97 %

Animal experiments

Estrogen receptor-positive tumours were implanted into one limb of male mice, aged six weeks. After seven days, all animals received 100 µl DSEP labelled with ^{123}I via the tail vein. Groups of animals were sacrificed at different times between 10 min and 48 hours post injection. Radioactivity in selected organs was measured and calculated as "percentage of radioactivity applied per g of organ weight" (%ID/g).

To exclude unspecific binding of the substance in tumour tissue the affinity of 123I-DESP to the receptor had to be investigated. For this purpose, cold DESP (300 mg in 100 µl) were injected 1 h prior to 123I-DESP. 100 µl KI-solution (10 mg/ml) were administered i.v. before the experiments to block the thyroid.

RESULTS AND DISCUSSION

The results of the biopsies within 2 h after injection are demonstrated in fig. 1.

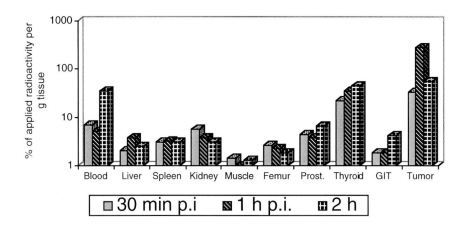

Fig. 1
Results of autopsy 30 min, 1 h, and 2 h p.i.

Already 10 min after injection, nearly 50 %/g of the activity
applied were found in the tumour. High concentrations were also
observed in the prostate. When comparing the tracer accumulation of
certain organs during the 2 hours following the injection, we
observed a maximum radioactivity in the tumour 1 h p.i., a slow
increase in the prostate and a distinct increase of 123I in the
thyroid. This effect could be prevented by thyroid blocking with
"cold" iodine. This demonstrates, that there is an early
deiodination of the tracer in mice.

Long term kinetic data (fig. 2) show the quick renal excretion of
123I-DSEP. Unfortunately, the retention time of the tracer in tumour
tissue is relatively short. According to these findings, imaging
should preferably be performed during the first two hour after
tracer injection.

In contrast, animals in which receptor binding was blocked by cold
estrogen showed a negligible uptake of labelled DSEP in tumour and
prostate, which suggests, that the tracer uptake is receptor-
mediated after preapplication of cold DSEP no increased activity is
present in the tumour in the limb.

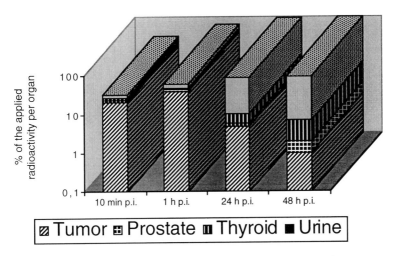

Fig. 2 Long term kinetic data

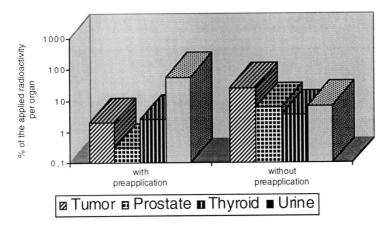

Figure 3
Effect of blockade of estrogen receptors by preapplication of non-radioactive DESP

These results demonstrate an estrogen receptor mediated accumulation
of 123I-DSEP into estrogen-receptor positive tissues including
carcinomas.

References

1. Boring CC, Squires TS, Tong T. Cancer statistics. CA. Cancer J
    Clin. 1992; 42: 19-38.

2. Eckelman WC, Reba RC, Gibson RE, et al. Receptor-binding
    radiotracers: a class of potential radiopharmaceuticals. J Nucl
    Med 1979;20:350-357.

3. Twombly GH, McClintock L, Engleman M. Tissue localization and
    excretion routes of radioactive dibromoestrone. Am J Obstet
    Gynecol 1948;56:260-268.

4. Albert S, Heard RDH, LeBlond CP, Saffran JL. Distribution and
    metabolism of iodo-α-estradiol labeled with radioactive iodine.
J   Biol Chem. 1949;177:247266.

5. Twombly GH, Schoenewaldt EF. The metabolism of radioactive
    dibromoestrone in man. Cancer. 1950;3:601607.

6. Jensen EV. Studies of growth phenomenon using tritium-labelled
    steroids. In: Proceedings of the fourth International Congress
    of Biochemistry. Elmstord, NY: Pergamon Press; 1960;15:119.

7. Glascock RF, Hoekstra WG. Selective accumulation of tritium
    labelled hexoestrol by the reproductive organs of immature
    female goats and sheep. Biochem 1 1959;72:673682.

8. Jensen EV, Jacobson Hl. Fate of steroid estrogens in target
    tissues. In: Pincus G, Vollmer EP, eds. Biological Activities
    of Steroids in Relation to Cancer: Conference on Biological
    Activities of Steroids in Relation to Cancer. Orlando, Fla:
    Academic Press Inc; 1960:161-178.

9. Hochberg RB. Iodine-125-labeled estradiol: a gammaemitting analog of estradiol that binds to the estrogen receptor. Science. 1979;205:1138-1140.

10. Hochberg RB, Rosner W. Interaction of 16α-[^{125}I]iodo-estradiol with estrogen receptor and other steroidbinding proteins. Proc Natl Acad Sci U S A. 1980; 77:328-332.

11. McManaway ME, Jagoda EM, Eckelman WC, et al. Binding charasteristics and biological activity of 17α-[^{125}I]iodovinyl-11ß-methoxyestradiol, an estrogen receptor-binding radiopharmaceutical, in human breast cancer cells (MCF-7). Cancer Res. 1986;46:2386-2389.

12. Zielinski JE, Yabuki H, Pahuja SL, Larner JM, Hochberg RB. 16α-[^{125}I]Iodo-ß-methoxy-17ß-estradiol: a radiochemical probe for estrogen-sensitive tissues. Endocrinology. 1986;119:130-139.

13. Katzenellenbogen JA, McElvany KD, Senderoff SG, Carison KE, Landvatter SW, Welch MJ. 16α-[^{77}Br]bromo-11ß-methoxyestradiol-17ß: a gamma-emitting estrogen imaging agent with high uptake and retention by target organs. J Nucl Med 1982;23:411-419.

14. Kiesewetter DO, Kilbourn MR, Landvatter SW, Heiman DF, Katzenellenbogen JA, Welch MJ. Preparation of four fluorine-18-labeled estrogens and their selective uptakes in target tissues of immature rats. J Nucl Med. 1984;25:1212-1221.

15. Scheidhauer K, Müller S, Smolarz K, Bräutigam P, Briele P. Tumorszintigraphie mit 123I-markiertem Östradiol beim Mammakarzinom-Rezeptorszintigraphie. Nucl Med 1991; 30:84-99

16. Dodds EC, Goldberg L, Lawson W, Robinson R. Estrogenic activity of certain synthetic compounds. Nature 1938; 141: 247-248.

17. Ts'o POP, Lu P. Interaction of nucleic acids. I. Physical
     binding of thymidine, adenine, steroids, and aromatic
     hydrocarbons to nucleic acids. Proc Natl Acad Sci US 1964; 51:
     17-24

18. Blackburn GM, Flavell AJ, Thompson MH. Oxidative and
     photochemical linkage of diethylstilbestrol to DNA in vitro.
     Cancer Res 1974; 34: 2015-2019.

19. Tubis M, Endow JS, Blahd WH. The preparation of 131I labeled
     diethylstilbestrol diphosphate and its potential use in nuclear
     medicine. Nucl Med 1967; 6: 1-15.

20. Mende T, Hennig K, Wollny G, Gens J, Zotter S. Verteilung von
     Jod-markiertem Diäthylstilbestroldiphosphat nach intravenöser
     Injektion. Szintigraphische Darstellung von Mammatumoren im
     Tierexperiment. Gynäk Rdsch 1979; 19: 30-36.

21. Mende T, Hennig K, Wollny G, Gens J. Experimentelle
     Untersuchungen über die Verteilung von intravenös injiziertem,
     jodmarkiertem Cytonal (Diäthylstilbestroldiphosphat. Z Urol u
     Nephrol 1978; 71: 529-534.

22. Maysinger D, Marcus CS, Wolf W, Tarle M, Casanova J.
     Preparation and high-performance liquid chromatography of
     iodinated diethylstilbestrols and some related steroids. J
     Chromatogr 1977; 130: 129-138.

Radioactive Isotopes in
Clinical Medicine and Research XXII
ed. by H. Bergmann, A. Kroiss and H. Sinzinger
© 1997 Birkhäuser Verlag Basel/Switzerland

PREOPERATIVE THORACIC STAGING OF NON-SMALL CELL LUNG CANCER: 18-FDG-PET EVALUATION

C.A. Guhlmann, M. Storck, F. Kocher, J. Kotzerke, L. Sunder-Plassmann, S.N. Reske

Departments of Nuclear Medicine and Thoracic Surgery,

University of Ulm, Germany

SUMMARY: Sixty-one patients with focal pulmonary abnormalities underwent preoperative PET scanning with 2-[F-18]-fluoro-2-deoxy-D-glucose (FDG). Forty-one patients had non-small cell lung cancer (NSCLC), 20 patients had a benign process. The sensitivity, specificity, and accuracy of FDG-PET for characterizing the primary lung lesion as malignant or benign were 97.6%, 80%, and 92%. Overall sensitivity, specificity, and accuracy for thoracic lymph node staging in patients with NSCLC were 84%, 87%, and 85%. FDG-PET identified absence of lymph node tumor involvement in No disease at 100% (13/13). Lymph node metastases in N1 disease were correctly detected at 50% (3/6), in N2 at 81% (13/16), and in N3 at 100% (5/5).

INTRODUCTION

Treatment of bronchogenic carcinoma varies with a number of factors that include cell type and stage at initial diagnosis [1]. Cure of non-small cell lung cancer (NSCLC) is possible if the disease is diagnosed early in its course before mediastinal lymph node or systemic metastases occur. The presence and site of nodal metastatic disease has a significant effect on prognosis and management [1,2]. Metastasis to **contralateral** hilar or madiastinal lymph nodes (N3 disease) indicates unresectable disease.

Current non-invasive methods for staging NSCLC and evaluating the mediastinum include chest radiography, computed tomography (CT) and magnetic resonance imaging (MRI) [3]. In contrast to CT and MRI, which depend primarily on **anatomic** imaging features and are of limited sensitivity and specificity in staging mediastinal nodal metastases [4,5], positron emission tomography (PET) depends primarily on the **metabolic** characteristics of a tissue for the diagnosis of disease.

PET with 2-[F-18]-fluoro-2-deoxy-D-glucose (FDG) has been successfully used to image primary lung cancer [6] and to differentiate with a high degree of accuracy malignant from benign pulmonary nodules [7-13]. In two recent reports, FDG-PET was suggested as a most promising noninvasive technique in detecting mediastinal lymph node involvement of NSCLC [14,15].

PATIENTS AND METHODS

Sixty-one patients (48 male, 13 female) with lung tumors were examined preoperatively by FDG-PET. Of the 61 tumors, 41 were NSCLC (28 squamous cell carcinomas, 9 adenocarcinomas, 4 large cell carcinomas). Additionally, there were 20 benign tumors consisting of 8 pneumonias, 3 florid abscesses, 2 sarcoidoses, 1 aspergilloma, 1 hamartoma, 1 tuberculosis, 1 aneurysm of the subclavian artery, 1 lung fibrosis, 1 echinococcosis, and 1 inflammatory pseudotumor. The final diagnosis and the TN staging in patients with lung cancer were established by means of histopathologic examination based on lobectomy or pneumonectomy including mediastinal lymphadenectomy.

PET was performed with a scanner (Siemens-CTI-ECAT Scanner 931/08/12, Knoxville, Tenn) that produces 15 slices of 6.75-mm thickness. Patients fastet for at least 12 hours before the study. Prior to FDG administration, transmission scans were obtained in at least four bed positions for attenuation correction of emission data. Acquisition time was 10 min per bed position.

^{18}FDG was injected intravenously at a mean dose of 250 MBq (range 200-350 MBq). After a 50-min uptake period, patients were carefully repositioned by using laser guided landmarks to ensure an identical field of view for emission and transmission scanning. Acquisition time for emission scans was 15 min for each bed position. Image reconstruction was performed with an iterative reconstruction algorithm. The resolution was 7 mm for iterative reconstruction for full width at half maximum at the center of the field of view.

Qualitative evaluation of PET scans was performed blinded and independently on transaxial, coronal and sagittal sections by two observers. Areas of FDG uptake in both lung fields were classified according to intensity, size, and shape. A clearly delineated area of intense focal uptake was considered indicative of lung carcinoma. Less intense, diffuse, heterogeneous or multifocal FDG uptake was considered indicative of inflammatory processes.

RESULTS AND DISCUSSION

Based on visual inspection of the images, the PET-FDG scans correctly identified 40 of the 41 malignancies. The false-negative finding was a 1-cm intrapulmonal metastasis of an adenocarcinoma. False-positive results were obtained in one patient with aspergilloma and in three patients with florid abscesses. The sensitivity and specificity of PET-FDG imaging for detecting lung cancer were 97.6% and 80%, respectively. The positive and negative predictive values for detecting malignancy in lung tumors were 91% and 94%, respectively. The accuracy for differentiating benign from malignant primary lung tumors was 92%. Our results with PET-FDG imaging of lung tumors confirm the experience of others [7-13]. Accordingly, false-positive findings were reported in lung diseases such as granulomas and abscesses [7,10,12] that demonstrate acute inflammatory process. It should be noted that semiquantitative evaluation and visual analysis of FDG-PET images have been shown to be equally accurate methods in differentiating malignant from benign focal pulmonary abnormalities [16].

The results of histologic analysis of thoracic lymph nodes (LN) were available from 40 of the 41 patients with NSCLC. Overall sensitivity, specificity, and accuracy for thoracic lymph node staging in patients with NSCLC were 84%, 87%, and 85%, respectively. PET-FDG scans correctly identified the absence of lymph node tumor involvement in all of the patients with histologically negative lymph nodes (13/13). Lymph node metastases in N1 disease were correctly detected at 50% (3/6), in N2 at 81% (13/16), and in N3 at 100% (5/5). In N1 disease we obtained three false-negative findings due to lymph node metastases closely adjacent to the primary tumor. These false-negative readings might have been correctly localized if the spatial resolution of the PET-FDG image had been better. Moreover, anatometabolic fusion images with combined CT anatomic and PET metabolic information may improve the anatomic localization of areas of FDG uptake [14]. With regard to definitive surgical treatment, accuracy of FDG-PET for differentiating patients with N2 disease (ipsilateral mediastinal, carinal or subcarinal LN) from patients with unresectable N3 disease (contralateral hilar or mediastinal LN) was 95%.

CONCLUSIONS

PET-FDG imaging is a very useful noninvasive technique for accurate differentiation of malignant from benign focal pulmonary abnormalities and provides a new and effective method for thoracic lymph node staging in patients with newly diagnosed or suspected NSCLC. In particular, FDG-PET enables with a high degree of accuracy the differentiation of patients with N2 disease from patients with unresectable N3 disease and should be helpful in further treatment selection.

REFERENCES

1.   Bains MS. Surgical treatment of lung cancer. *Chest* 1991; 100:826-837.

2.   Mountain CF. Surgery for stage IIIa-N2 non-small cell lung cancer. *Cancer* 1994; 73:2589-2598.

3.   Armstrong P and Vincent JM. Staging non-small cell lung cancer (review). *Clin Radiol* 1993; 48:1-10.

4.   Webb WR, Gatsonis C, Zerhouni EA, Heelan RT, Glazer GM, Francis IR, et al. CT and MR imaging in staging non-small cell bronchogenic carcinoma: report of the Radiologic Diagnostic Oncology Group. *Radiology* 1991; 178:705-713.

5.   McLoud TC, Bourgouin, PM, Greenberg RW, Kosiuk JP, Templeton PA, Shepard JAO, et al. Bronchogenic carcinoma: analysis of staging in the mediastinum with CT by correlative lymph node mapping and sampling. *Radiology* 1992; 182:319-323.

6.   Nolop KB, Rhodes CG, Brudin LH, Beaney RP, Krausz T, Jones T, et al. Glucose utilization *in vivo* by human pulmonary neoplasms. *Cancer* 1987; 60:2682-2689.

7. Kubota K, Matsuzawa T, Fujiwara T, Ito M, Hatazawa J, Ishiwata K, et al. Differential diagnosis of lung tumor with positron emission tomography: a prospective study. *J Nucl Med* 1990;31:1927-1933.

8. Gupta NC, Frank AR, Dewan NA, Redepenning LS, Rothberg ML, Mailliard JA, et al. Solitary pulmonary nodules: detection of malignancy with PET with 2-[F-18]-fluoro-2-deoxy-D-glucose. *Radiology* 1992; 184:441-444.

9. Hoh CK, Hawkins RA, Glaspy JA, Dahlbom M, Tse NY, Hoffman EJ, et al. Cancer detection with whole-body PET using 2-[18F]fluoro-2-deoxy-D-glucose. *J Comput Assist Tomogr* 1993; 17:582-589.

10. Patz EF, Lowe VJ, Hoffman JM, Paine SS, Burrowes P, Coleman RE, et al. Focal pulmonary abnormalities: evaluation with F-18 fluorodeoxyglucose PET scanning. *Radiology* 1993; 188:487-490.

11. Rege SD, Hoh CK, Glaspy JA, Aberle DR, Dahlbom M, Razavi MK, et al. Imaging of pulmonary mass lesions with whole-body positron emission tomography and fluorodeoxyglucose. *Cancer* 1993; 72:82-90.

12. Dewan NA, Gupta NC, Redepenning LS, Phalen JJ, Frick MP. Diagnostic efficacy of PET-FDG imaging in solitary pulmonary nodules. Potential role in evaluation and management. *Chest* 1993; 104:997-1002.

13. Lewis P, Griffin S, Marsden P, Gee T, Nunan T, Malsey M, et al. Whole-body 18F-fluorodeoxyglucose positron emission tomography in preoperative evaluation of lung cancer. *Lancet* 1994; 344:1265-1266.

14. Wahl RL, Quint LE, Greenough RL, Meyer CR, White RI, Orringer MB. Staging of mediastinal non-small cell lung cancer with FDG PET, CT, and fusion images: preliminary prospective evaluation. *Radiology* 1994; 191:371-377.

15. Scott WJ, Schwabe JL, Gupta NC, Dewan NA, Reeb SD, Sugimoto JT, and the members of the PET-lung tumor study group. Positron emission tomography of lung tumors and mediastinal lymph nodes using [18F]fluorodeoxyglucose. *Ann Thorac Surg* 1994; 58:698-703.

16. Lowe VJ, Hoffman JM, DeLong DM, Patz EF, Coleman RE. Semiquantitative and visual analysis of FDG-PET images in pulmonary abnormalities. *J Nucl Med* 1994; 35:1771-1776.

Radioactive Isotopes in
Clinical Medicine and Research XXII
ed. by H. Bergmann, A. Kroiss and H. Sinzinger
© 1997 Birkhäuser Verlag Basel/Switzerland

ELEVATED EXPRESSION OF GLUCOSE TRANSPORTER GENES AS REASON FOR AN INCREASED F-18 FDG UPTAKE IN HUMAN PANCREATIC ADENOCARCINOMA

K.G. Grillenberger, T. Helfrich, S.N. Reske

Department of Nuclear Medicine, University Hospital, Ulm, Germany

SUMMARY: One of the most common cancer diagnostics in nuclear medicine is based on an increased F-18 FDG uptake observed by PET imaging. We investigated the molecular biological basis for these clinical findings by quantitative determination of glucose transporter (GLUT) expression using polymerase chain reaction (PCR). mRNA of tissue samples from 10 patients with pancreatic adenocarcinoma (APC) served as template for RT-PCR analysis. 10 patients with chronic pancreatitis (CP) served as controls. Quantification of PCR products in relation to an internal standard was performed using HPLC, identity was confirmed by non-radioactive DNA sequence analysis. Average GLUT-1 mRNA concentration was 1.21 nmol/mg tissue for APC and 0.034 nmol/mg for CP. GLUT-4 was detectable in 6/10 patients with CP but only in 1/10 patients with APC.

INTRODUCTION

It is well known that glucose is the main source of energy in cellular metabolism. Accordingly, it is to be expected to find an accelerated glucose uptake in cells with an increased proliferation rate such as cancer cells [1]. Diagnostic nuclear medicine makes use of this fact for identification of various malignant primary or recurrent tumors by the determination of 2-[^{18}F]-fluoro-2-deoxy-D-glucose (FDG) uptake with positron emission tomography (PET) [2,3]. At the cellular level, a family of structurally related proteins has been found to be responsible for transporting glucose across the plasma membrane [4]. Six isotypes of these glucose transporters (GLUT) have been isolated and characterized with distinct tissue distribution [5,6,7]:

GLUT-1 (erythrocyte type), GLUT-2 (liver type), GLUT-3 (brain type), GLUT-4 (muscle/fat type), GLUT-5 (small intestine type), and GLUT-7 (hepatocyte type). GLUT-6 is a pseudogene that is not expressed at the protein level [5]. All known GLUT isotypes have 12 transmembrane segments in common.

Earlier investigations dealed with GLUT expression under physiological and pathophysiologal circumstances such as diabetes mellitus [8], fasting [9], or developmental regulation [10]. Recent studies have shown GLUT-1 and GLUT-3 overexpression in esophagus, stomach, and colon cancer by RNA blotting analysis [11].

We used PCR amplification after reverse transcription of mRNA isolated from tissue material to examine and quantify the expression of GLUT-1 and GLUT-4 in pancreatic adenocarcinoma (APC) and chronic pancreatitis (CP) in order to check if there is any correlation between increased FDG uptake in patients with pancreatic cancer (determined with PET), and expression of glucose transporters. Quantification of PCR products was performed by high performance liquid chromatography (HPLC) related to a with the same primers co-amplified neutral DNA fragment as internal standard.

MATERIALS AND METHODS

Positron-emission-tomography. FDG-PET was performed using an ECAT 931-08-12 scanner (Siemens-CTI-Inc., Knoxville, TN) which produces 15 contiguous slices per bed position (10.1 cm). Slice Thickness was 6.75 mm for primary and secondary slices. Patients were fasted for at least 12 h prior to the study. Transmission scanning for positron attenuation correction was performed prior to emissions scans with a Ge-68/Ga-68 ring source in at least three bed positions starting at the liver dome. Acqisition time was 10 min per bed position. 250-350 (mean 270) MBq FDG were injected into an antecubital vein. 20 mg of furosemide were injected intravenously to reduce artifacts due to high radioactivity in the renal collecting system. After repositioning of the patient with laser-guided landmarks emission scans were recorded 45 min after FDG administration. FDG accumulation was calculated using standardized uptake values (SUV: activity concentration divided by injected dose/body weight).

Tissues and mRNA extraction. The pancreatic tissues were snap-frozen in liquid nitrogen immediately after excision and stored at -196 °C until used. All tissues were histologically classified as pancreatic cancer or chronic panceatitis. Extraction and purification of mRNA was performed on samples of about 30-50 mg (splitted in liquid nitrogen) using guanidinium thiocyanate/oligo(dT)-cellulose chromatography (QuickPrep Micro; Pharmacia No. 27-9255-01). The isolated mRNA was precipitated with ethanol (95%) and redissolved in 20 μl of DEPC-treated water. Concentration of RNA was determined spectrophometrically at 260 nm, purity was calculated by the OD_{260}/OD_{280} quotient. Pure preparations of DNA and RNA have OD_{260}/OD_{280} values of 1.8 and 2.0 respectively. If there is contamination with protein the OD_{260}/OD_{280} will be significantly less than the values given above.

Oligonucleotides. As primers for amplification of GLUT-1, GLUT-4, and the neutral DNA fragment (internal standard IST) the following oligonucleotides were used (table 1):

Table 1: Description of the applied primers.

primer	nucleotide sequence of primer	size of primer	binding site (amino acid sequ.)	size of PCR product
primer1 (GLUT-1)	5'-CAT-CCT-GGA-GCT-GTT-CCG-CT-3'	20-mer	258-265	614 bp
primer2 (GLUT-1)	5'-CTC-ATC-GAA-GGT-CCG-GCC-TT-3'	20-mer	456-462	614 bp
primer1 (GLUT-4)	5'-AGC-CAG-CAG-CTC-TCT-GGC-AT-3'	20-mer	297-303	602 bp
primer2 (GLUT-4)	5'-CTG-GGT-TTC-ACC-TCC-TGC-TC-3'	20-mer	491-497	602 bp
primer1 (IST-1/4)	5'-TTT-GTC-GAC--AGC-CAG-CAG-CTC-TCT--GGC-ATC-ATC-CTG-GAG-CTG-TTC-CGC--TTT-GGA-GAA-GGG-AGA-GCG-TTT-3'	69-mer	------	404 bp
primer2 (IST-1/4)	5'-TTT-CCT-AGG-CTC-ATC-GAA-GGT-CCG--GCC-TTC-TGG-GTT-TCA-CCT-CCT-GCT--CAG-GGC-ATG-TTG-AAA-AAG-CCC-3'	69-mer	------	404 bp

RNA reverse transcription. Reverse transcription of mRNA into cDNA was performed with Moloney Murine Leukemia Virus (M-MuLV) reverse transcriptase using the First-Strand cDNA Synthesis Kit (Pharmacia No. 27-9261-01). The reaction mix was incubated for 60 min at 37 °C, heated to 95 °C for 5 min, and then chilled on ice.

PCR amplification. Polymerase chain reaction was performed at a final concentration of 1x PCR buffer (50 mM KCl and 20 mM Tris-HCl, pH 8.4), 0.75 mM MgCl$_2$, 0.01 μM each dNTPs, 0.5 μM each 5'- and 3'-primers, and 1.25 U Taq DNA polymerase (Gibco BRL No. 18038-018) in a final volume of 50 μl. Simultaneously with the specific cDNA of glucose transporters from tissues a neutral DNA fragment with binding sites for the specific GLUT-1 and GLUT-4 primers was coamplified as internal standard (IST) in a defined concentration. This neutral DNA fragment (442 bp) was synthesized using the PCR MIMIC™ Construction Kit (Clontech No. K1700-1) and the above mentioned 69-mer primers for IST-1/4.

The PCR mixture was overlaid with 50 μl mineral oil and then amplified using a Hybaid OmniGene thermal cycler (30 cycles; denaturation at 95 °C for 30 sec; annealing at 55 °C for 1.5 min; extension at 72 °C for 2 min). After 30 cycles the tubes were kept at 72 °C for 10 min and afterwards stored on ice.

First we determined a calibration by co-amplifying a constant amount of the neutral DNA fragment with various well known concentrations of positive controls for GLUT-1 (a 2.47 kb fragment from the internal BamHI site of Escherichia coli HB 101 containing plasmid [ATCC No. 59630]) and GLUT-4(a 2.0 kb fragment from SalI site of E. coli DH5 alpha containing plasmid [ATCC No. 61616]). By HPLC measuring the area of the different GLUT peaks compared with the IST peaks we were able to establish a standard calibration curve showing the relation between the initial GLUT concentration and the HPLC ratio GLUT : IST. The same amount of neutral DNA fragment (1 pg) was added to every PCR reaction of tissue cDNA.

Electrophoresis and qualitative analysis. For qualitative analysis 10-μl samples of each PCR reaction mixture were subjected to electrophoresis on 6% agarose gels (containing 0.001% ethidium bromide) in 1x TAE buffer.The gels were run at 80 V for 3 h with positive controls for GLUT-1 and GLUT-4 (see above).

Quantitative analysis. Quantification of the amplified PCR products was performed by HPLC analysis. We used a TSK-DEAE-NPR ion-exchange column (Tosohaas) and an aqueous gradient mixture of 0.02M Tris-HCl (pH 9.0) [=A] and 0.02M Tris-HCl + 1.0M NaCl [=B] with a linear gradient of 45% to 60% B within 15 min and a flow of 1.5 ml/min. Detection of the nucleotide peaks was achieved photometrically at 260 nm.

Sequence analysis. Evidence of identity of the amplified PCR products was provided by non-radioactive sequence analysis using digoxigenine labeled primers according to the standard procedures (DIG Taq DNA Sequencing Kit, Boehringer Mannheim No. 1449 443). Detection was performed with alkaline phosphatase linked anti-DIG-antibodies.

RESULTS

Tissues and mRNA extraction. Using oligo(dT)-cellulose chromatography for mRNA extraction from specimens of about 30-50 mg chronic pancreatitis tissue or pancreatic adenocarcinoma tissue we attained mRNA amounts of 1.7-2.8 μg as determined by spectrophotometric measurement. The OD$_{260}$/OD$_{280}$ value of the isolated mRNA was in every case >1.7.

RNA reverse transcription. For reverse transcription we applied 1.0 μg mRNA for each sample.

Qualitative analysis. Qualitative evaluation of GLUT-4 PCR products by electrophoresis and UV detection showed in 6/10 APC tissues a distinct expression of GLUT-4 but only in 1/10 CP tissues (table 2).

Quantitative analysis. HPLC analysis of the PCR reactions yielded in a clear separation of internal standard IST (404 bp) and GLUT-1 (614 bp) and GLUT-4 (602 bp) respectively. Under the above mentioned HPLC conditions the shorter IST nucleotide is detected at 10.4 min and the longer GLUT-1 nucleotide at 11.3 min (fig. 1). Absolute quantification of the HPLC peaks led to the following result (table 2):

The average standardized uptake value (SUV) for pancreatic adenocarcinoma was 3.46, for chronic pancreatitis 0.77. Average GLUT-1 mRNA concentration was 0.034 nmol per mg tissue for chronic pancreatitis and 1.21 nmol per mg tissue for pancreatic adenocarcinoma which is equivalent to an 35 fold increase.

Table 2: Results of HPLC quantification

number (n)	histology	SUV (av. +/-s.d.)	mRNA GL-1 (nmol/mg)	GLUT-4
10 (4m+6f)	pancreatic carcinoma	3.46 +/- 0.97	1.21 +/- 0.92	6 pos. / 4 neg.
10 (8m+2f)	chronic pancreatitis	0.77 +/- 0.32	0.03 +/- 0.05	1 pos. / 9 neg.

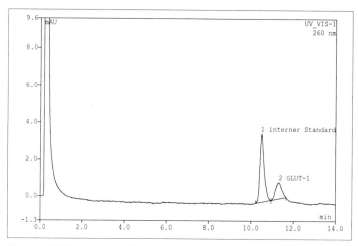

Figure 1: HPLC separation of internal standard and GLUT-1

Sequence analysis. Analysis of the nucleotid sequence of the amplified PCR products for GLUT-1 and GLUT-4 showed complete correspondence with the known sequence of GLUT-1 and GLUT-4 cDNA.

DISCUSSION

The aim of this study was to determine if there is a difference in expression of glucose transporter GLUT-1 and GLUT-4 in malignant diseases such as pancreatic cancer as compared with chronic pancreatitis. GLUT overexpression in various human cancers has already been shown by RNA blotting analysis [11]. We wanted to investigate the use of PCR of cDNA from human tissue samples and HPLC analysis to achieve quantification of GLUT-1 and GLUT-4 expression.

HPLC provides more reliable and reproducable results than radioactive PCR and evades handling of radioactive agents. Using an artificial DNA segment as internal standard is more advantageous than co-amplification of endogenous „house-keeping-genes" like ß-actin. First the initial amount of standard used in the PCR reaction is precisely known. This makes it possible to calculate the absolute level of target mRNA or cDNA present in the native sample. Furthermore the usage of two different primer pairs involves the risk of different amplification rates for standard and target, whereas one primer pair amplifies standard and target with the same efficiacy. Perhaps the greatest advantage of using competitive PCR is that it is not necessary to assay PCR products exclusively during the exponential phase of the amplification because the ratio of target to standard remains constant during amplification [12].

Using this technique we were able to show considerable overexpression of GLUT-1 in malignant pancreatic cells as compared to chronic pancreatitis indicating its important role for the elevated glucose uptake in malignant cells.

REFERENCES

1. Warburg O. On the origin of cancer cells. Science 1956; 123: 309-314.

2. Klever P, Bares R, Fass J, Bull U, Schumpelick V. PET with fluorine-18-deoxyglucose for pancreatic disease. Lancet 1992; 340: 1158-1159.

3. Wahl RL, Cody RL, Hutchins GD, Mudgett EE. Primary and metastatic breast carcinoma: initial clinical evaluation with PET with the radiolabeled glucose analogue 2-(F-18)-fluoro-2-deoxy-D-glucose. Radiology 1991; 179: 765-770.

4. Mueckler M. Facilitative glucose transportes. Eur J Biochem 1994; 219: 713-725.

5. Kayano T, Burant CF, Fukumoto H, Gould GW, Fan Y, Eddy RL, Byers MG, Shows TB, Seino S, Bell GI. Human facilitative glucose transporters. J Biol Chem 1990; 265: 13276-13282.

6. Mueckler M, Caruso C, Baldwin SA, Panico M, Blench I, Morris HR, Allard WJ, Lienhard GE, Lodish HF. Sequence and structure of a human glucose transporter. Science 1985; 229: 941-945.

7. Kayano T, Fukumoto H, Eddy RL, Fan Y, Byers MG, Shows TB, Bell GI. Evidence for a family of human glucose-like proteins. J Biol Chem 1988; 263: 15245-15248.

8. Kahn BB, Charron MJ, Lodish HF, Cushman SW, Fliers HS. Differential regulation of two glucose transporters in adipose cells from diabetic and insulin treated diabetic rats. J Clin Invest 1989; 84: 404-411.

9. Kahn BB, Cushman SW, Fliers JS. Regulation of glucose transporter-specific mRNA levels in rat adipose cells with fasting and refeeding: implications for an in vivo control of glucose transporter number. J Clin Invest 1989; 83: 199-204.

10. Werner H, Adamo M, Lowe WL, Roberts CT, LeRoith D. Developmental regulation of rat brain/Hep G2 glucose transporter gene expression. Mol Endocrinol 1989; 3: 273-279.

11. Yamamoto T, Seino Y, Fukumoto H, Koh G, Yano H, Inagaki N, Yamada Y, Inoue K, Manabe T, Imura H. Over-expression of facilitative glucose transporter genes in human cancer. Biochem Biophys Res Comm 1990; 170: 223-230.

12. Murphy LD, Herzog CE, Rudick JB, Fojo AT, Bates SE. Use of the polymerase chain reaction in the quantification of mdr-1 gene expression. Biochemistry 1990; 29: 10351.

Radioactive Isotopes in
Clinical Medicine and Research XXII
ed. by H. Bergmann, A. Kroiss and H. Sinzinger
© 1997 Birkhäuser Verlag Basel/Switzerland

BIODISTRIBUTION AND KINETICS OF ^{191}Pt IN PATIENTS UNDERGOING THERAPY WITH CISPLATIN

Areberg J, Norrgren K, Björkman S**, Einarsson L***, Lundkvist H***, Mattsson S,
Nordberg B, Scheike O*, Wallin R**,

Dept of Radiation Physics, *Dept of Oncology,** Hospital Pharmacy, Malmö
University Hospital, Malmö,***The Svedberg Laboratory, Uppsala, Sweden.

INTRODUCTION

Cisplatin and carboplatin are two frequently used cytostatic agents. They are often combined with other drugs. Cisplatin is used in therapy of testis, head and neck, ovarian and bladder tumours . Individual variations in the therapeutic results are seen for patients receiving the same cytostatic drug treatment although they have the same histological form of cancer in the same stage.

So far, it has not been possible to optimise clinical treatment schedules for cytostatic drugs, because of the difficulty to determine the drug concentration in tissues. It is therefore urgent to develop quantitative methods to determine the in vivo concentration of the cytostatic agents in the tumour and organs at risk.

In this initial phase of the study we have set up the synthesis of cisplatin and the quality control methods. We have developed methods for gamma camera measurement and phantom calibration to be able to quantify the tissue uptake in patients. So far, 5 patients have been included in the study. In our studies less than 10 % of the ordinary amount of cisplatin was replaced with ^{191}Pt cisplatin, which offers a possibility to determine the individual biokinetics in each patient.

The aim of the study is to characterise the distribution and kinetics of ^{191}Pt cisplatin in humans by in vivo measurements using a gamma camera and to investigate the possibility to correlate the concentration and biokinetics for tumours and normal tissues to the effect of the treatment.

MATERIAL AND METHODS

^{191}Pt production

^{191}Pt is produced at the The Svedberg Laboratory in Uppsala. A gold foil is irradiated with 70 - 75 MeV protons, whereby three main reactions take place.

^{197}Au(p,7n) ^{191}Hg -> ^{191}Au (49min) - > ^{191}Pt

^{197}Au(p,6n)^{191}Au ->^{191}Pt

^{197}Au(p,2p5n) ^{191}Pt

Of these three reactions, the last is dominating. [191]Pt decays by electron capture (EC) to stabile [191]Ir with a halflife of 2.9 days. In the decay X-rays with energies 63-73 keV (131%) are emitted as well as several γ-rays of which the 82 keV (5%), 359 keV (6%), 409 keV (8%), 465 keV (3.4%) and 538 keV (14%) are the most important.

Synthesis of cisplatin

[191]Pt is transported to Malmö University Hospital, where the synthesis is done under sterile conditions. The synthesis takes 12 hours and is carried out in accordance with the method described by Nordberg et al (1), and published by Baer et al (2).
The activity yield of the synthesis is 20- 35 %

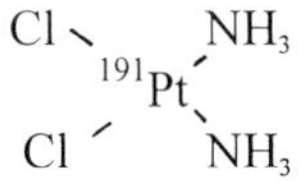

$$Cl \diagdown \underset{Cl}{\overset{NH_3}{\underset{\diagup}{191}Pt}} \diagup NH_3$$

Figure 1. Cisplatin

Quality control

The radionuclide purity was verified by gamma spectrometry (HPGe).
The chemical purity of the [191]Pt -cisplatin was controlled by HPLC and sterility test
    was done.

Gamma camera calibration

To be able to quantify the activity uptake in patients, phantom studies were done. Activity was filled in a MIRD liver phantom and two cylinders simulating kidneys. The liver and kidneys were inserted in an elliptical thorax phantom (adult MIRD) filled with water. The phantom was imaged with the same collimator and collection parameters as in the patient studies.

Patients

Until today 5 patients have been included in the study, 3 male and 2 female. Their age varied between 51 and 72 years. The patients were treated with cisplatin for uroepithelial cancer, cancer of head and neck and lung cancer.
The synthetisized [191]Pt cisplatin was administrated by infusion, mixed with the normal commercially available cisplatin and given after hydration. The synthetisized [191]Pt cisplatin was maximum 10% of the total amount of cisplatin given. The [191]Pt activity was 35-45 MBq.

Biodistribution and kinetics

Directly after end of the infusion, imaging was performed on a gamma camera (Toshiba) equipped with a high energy collimator due to the presence of high energy photons. A 20 percent energy window was centered over the 70 keV X-ray peak.
Imaging was done immediately after end of infusion, then at 24 h and in one case after 7 days. Scanning, anterior and posterior, and static imaging was done over liver and kidney and over areas with known tumours. The collection matrix was 256x256

for static images and imaging time was 10-20 minutes depending on the activity. Scanning was done using a 256x1024 matrix and a scan speed of 10 cm/min.

For quantification, ROI:s were drawn over whole body, kidneys, liver, tumours and other organs. Regions were drawn in anterior and posterior images and the geometric mean was used together with phantom studies to enable quantification of uptake. The halftime for [191]Pt different organs were determined.

RESULTS

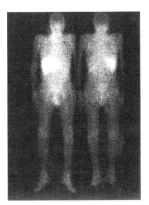 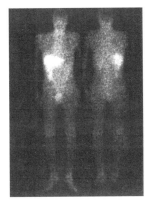 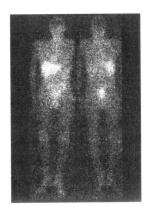

Figure 2. Whole body scintigrams at 2 hours, 24 hours and 7 days after infusion of cisplatin.

The images in figure 2 shows anterior and posterior whole body scans of [191]Pt-cisplatin in a 61 year male patient with a head and neck cancer. The patient received 100 mg cisplatin of which 1.5 mg or 35 MBq was our own syntetisised [191]Pt-cisplatin. The liver is clearly seen in all images. There are also indications of a presence of [191]Pt in the colon. An increased uptake is seen in the neck region, corresponding to the tumour site.

For this patient, the effective halftime for [191]Pt in the whole body was 64 hours. The early phase of the retention curve was not evaluated, since the measurements were started after the infusion was completed. The halftime for [191]Pt in the liver and kidneys was 62 hours.

For all patients in the study, the liver was clearly seen. Presence of [191]Pt in the colon was noted in 2 of the 5 patients and an uptake in the mediastinal region was seen in all patients.

In liver 5 - 12 % of the administered activity was present directly after infusion. The kidney uptake was 0.5 - 1 % of the administered activity.

Dosimetry

Dosimetric calculations were performed based on our own measurements and on literature data (3-5). The absorbed dose to liver was calculated to be 0.4 mGy/MBq. The kidney absorbed dose was 0.6 mGy/MBq and the effective dose was calculated to be 0.15 mSv/MBq

CONCLUSION

We now successfully run the synthesis of [191]Pt cisplatin from [191]Pt. The imaging technique is set up and our five first patient studies have been performed. The liver uptake seen in our images was higher than expected from our earlier XRF measurements (6) but consistent with the data reported by Smith et al. (4). On the other hand the kidney uptake was lower than expected.

Due to the limited number of patients included in the study so far it is not yet possible to draw general conclusions regarding the biokinetics and the tumour uptake.

ACKNOWLEDGEMENT

The authors would like to thank Prof. B Nosslin for analysing of the scintigraphic images.The study was supported by grants from The Swedish Cancer Foundation (grant no 3147-B92-02XBB), The Medical Faculty, Lund University, The University Hospital MAS Cancer Foundation, The Royal Physiographic Society, Lund, The Gunnar Arvid and Elisabeth Nilssons Foundation.

REFERENCES

1. Nordberg B, Björkman S, Mattsson S. Cis- och karboplatins kinetik studerad in vivo med [191]Pt-scintigrafi. Report MA RADFYS 93-01.
2. Baer J, Harrison R, McAucliffe CA, et al. Microscale synthesis of anti-tumour platinum compounds labelled with [191]Pt. Int J Appl Radiat Isot 1985: 36: 181-184.
3. Owens SE, Thatcher H, Sharma N, et al. In vivo distribution studies of radioactively labelled platinum complexes; cis-dichlorodiammine platinum (II), cis-trans-dichlorodihydroxy-bis-(isoproplamine) platinum (IV), dis-dichloro-bis-cyclopropylamine platinum (III), and cis-diammine 1,1-cyclobutanedicarboxylate platinum (II) in patients with malignant disease, using a gamma camera. Cancer Chemother Pharmacol 1985: 14:253-257.
4. Smith PHS, Taylor DM. Distribution and retention of the antitumor agent [195m]Pt-cis-dichlorodiammine platinum (II) in man. J Nucl Med 1973: 15: 349-351.
5. Lange RC, Spencer RP, Harder HC. The antitumor agent cis-Pt(NH$_3$)$_2$Cl$_2$: Distribution studies and dose calculations for [193m]Pt and [195m]Pt. J Nucl Med 1972: 14: 191-195.
6. Jonson R, Börjesson J, Mattsson S, Unsgaard B, Wallgren A. Uptake and retention of platinum in patients undergoing cisplatin therapy. Acta Oncol 1991: 30: 315-319.

Radioactive Isotopes in
Clinical Medicine and Research XXII
ed. by H. Bergmann, A. Kroiss and H. Sinzinger
© 1997 Birkhäuser Verlag Basel/Switzerland

BIODISTRIBUTION PHARMACOKINETICS AND DOSIMETRY OF ^{99m}Tc-D-GLUCARIC ACID IN HUMANS

N.Molea[1], E.Lazzeri[1], L.Bodei[1], L.DiLuca[1], D.Bacciardi[1], B.A.Khaw[2], K.Y.Pak[3], J.Narula[2], H.W.Strauss[4], R.Bianchi[1] and G.Mariani[5]

[1]Regional Center of Nuclear Medicine of the University of Pisa, Pisa (Italy); [2]Northeastern University, Boston, MA 02115; [3]Molecular Targeting Technology Inc., Malvern, PA 19355; [4]Stanford University Medical Center, Stanford, CA 94305 (USA); [5]Nuclear Medicine Service, DIMI, University of Genoa, Genoa (Italy)

SUMMARY: ^{99m}Tc-D-Glucaric acid ([99m]TcGLA) favourably accumulates in animal models of acute ischemia/early myocardial necrosis and in human tumor xenografts. This study evaluated the biodistribution pharmacokinetics and radiation dosimetry (using the MIRD approach) of [99m]TcGLA in 12 cancer patients, based on whole-body scans and blood/urine sampling from 0-46 hours. The pharmacokinetic pattern showed fast removal from the body (about 10% I.D. retained at 46 hr, almost exclusively in the kidneys). The initial and total distribution volumes corresponded to the extracellular and the total body water, respectively. The main radiation dosimetry estimates (mGy/MBq) were: 0.5488 (kidneys), 0.0208 (bladder), 0.051 (liver), 0.0041 (red marrow), 0.0053 (ovaries), 0.0036 (testes) and 0.0041 (whole-body).

INTRODUCTION

Continuing advances of radioisotopic methods has led to better morpho-functional evaluation of various organs and tissues, thus providing complementary information with respect to other imaging techniques such as echocardiography, computerized transmission tomography (CT), and magnetic resonance (MRI).

Early identification of the size, exact location and degree of acute ischemic lesions is crucial for adequate treatment, particularly in the case of heart and brain lesions.On the other hand, CT and MRI evaluation of ischemic brain damages is possible relatively late after the onset of ischemia, while the more recent method for scintigraphic visualization of brain ischemia based on the use of ^{18}F-deoxyglucose (FDG) and Positron Emission Tomography (PET) is not yet widely available because of complexity and high cost of the required equipment.

D-Glucaric Acid [general formula COOH-(HCOH)$_4$-(COOH)] is an endogenous end-product of glycuronic acid conjugation reactions usually found in body fluids and in urines of many mammals, including humans. While it has been used as a chelating agent in [99m]Tc- or ^{111}In-labeling of monoclonal antibodies, experimental studies have shown the favourable targeting potential of ^{99m}Tc-labeled D-glucaric acid ([99m]TcGLA, which behaves *in vitro* and *in vivo* somewhat like fructose) in animal models of severe ischemia or early necrosis of the heart and brain, and in human tumour xenografts. While [99m]TcGLA quickly accumulates in ischemic but still viable tissues, it does not accumulate in normal or transiently ischemic, or in frankly necrotic tissues (1-6).

In this study we evaluated the biodistribution pharmacokinetics and radiation dosimetry of [99m]TcGLA in humans, whist also assessing its tumour imaging potential in cancer patients.

MATERIALS AND METHODS

Twelwe patients (9 women and 3 men, aged 42-78 years) affected by breast cancer (9 cases) or colon cancer (3 cases) were enrolled in this study, after fully informed consent was obtained.

Labeling of [99m]TcGLA was performed by stannous reduction of ^{99m}Tc-pertechnetate (about 1500 MBq, freshly eluted) in an acid medium in presence of sodium glucarate (12.5 mg). The mixture was incubated for 20-30 minutes at room temperature. Radiochemical purity was evaluated by TLC using Watman no. 1 paper, with a mobile phase of acetonitrile:water (60:40). Labeling efficiency was always virtually 100%.

Patients were fasting since at least 12 hours before [99m]TcGLA administration, which was performed as an i.v. bolus (900 MBq). Blood samples were taken at frequent time-intervals from 4-5 minutes until 46-48 hours post-injection, while urines were cumulatively collected at 6-hour intervals. Conjugate-view whole-body scans were recorded at 0.5, 1, 2, 4, 6, 10, 24, 32 and 46 hours post-injection. Planar static images of areas of clinical interest were also recorded at various times after tracer administration.

The MIRD approach was employed to estimate the radiation dosimetry to various organs and tissues, based on radioactivity contents at various sites (corrected for standard attenuation coefficients in biological tissues, but not corrected for the physical decay of ^{99m}Tc) evaluated with the aid of specific regions of interest (ROIs) defined on the conjugate whole-body acquisitions. The MIRDOSE 3 software package kindly provided by the Oak Ridge Institute for Science and Education (Oak Ridge, TN, USA) was employed for the dosimetric estimate analysis, after calculating the transit times of radioactivity for each ROI.

No early or delayed adverse reactions of any type were observed in any of the patients enrolled in the biodistribution study, and no signs of hematologic toxicity or of impairment of liver and/or kidney function were noted, based on the blood chemistry and urinalysis tests performed in all patients.

RESULTS

Evaluation of the serial gamma-camera images showed early visualization of the kidneys (starting few minutes after bolus injection) and prompt urinary excretion of radioactivity; whereas, the liver was clearly outlined in later images (some hours after injection) and some hepato-biliary clearance took place, without however any clear visualization of the gallbladder. Visualization of the kidneys was persistent also in the late scans, about 8-10% of injected activity remaining in these organs, virtually the only site of accumulation by 46-48 hours as shown in Figure 1.

[99m]TcGLA did not appear to cross the intact blood-brain barrier, and no important *in vivo* metabolic degradation of the tracer took place, as no thyroidal uptake of radioactivity was ever detectable also in late scans (46-48 hours).

The plasma clearance curve of TcGLA exhibited in all patients a three-exponential pattern of disappearance, with average half-life values (mean ± SEM) equal to 0.37 ± 0.06 hours (fast distribution component), 1.36 ± 0.24 hours (intermediate distribution component) and 36.82 ± 3.03 hours (terminal clearance component) (see Fig. 2). The mean transit time in plasma was 52.5 ± 3.1 hours, while the overall clearance rate from the body was 1042 ± 105 mL/hour; the initial distribution volume was 11.18 ± 0.72 liters (corresponding to the extracellular volume) and the total distribution volume was 55.47 ± 7.34 liters (corresponding to the total body water volume). Urinary excretion of radioactivity (virtually 100% in the form of intact TcGLA, as shown by chromatographic analysis of urine samples) was 39.32 ± 4.57% of injected activity in the first 6 hours after tracer injection, with a cumulative plateau of 51.49 ± 6.38% of injected dose over the 48 hour experimental interval. By the end of the 46 hour experimental period, about 15-30% of injected activity was removed from the body through an extra-renal route of excretion, by way of hepato-biliary clearance.

Estimation of the radiation dosimetry values based on the biodistribution results obtained demonstrated a very low overall radiation burden both to the whole body and to the target organs, due to the fast clearance of [99m]TcGLA from the body. In fact, the results obtained (normalized to an average reference adult of 70 kg body weight) were very similar to those resulting from a diagnostic test with a high-clearance radiopharmaceutical for kidney function evaluation, such as ^{99m}Tc-MAG3, or a radiopharmaceutical with persistent kidney uptake, such as ^{99m}Tc-DMSA (see Table I).

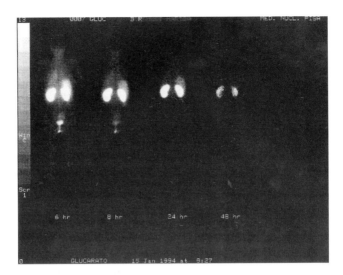

Fig. 1 - Whole-body acquisitions (posterior views) recorded at various times after i.v. injection of ^{99m}Tc-GLA in one of the patients included in the pharmacokinetic biodistribution study. Marked radioactivity accumulation is observed in the kidneys, virtually the only site of uptake at late imaging times.

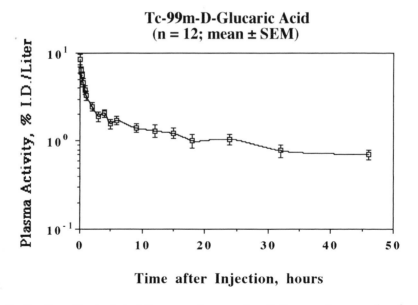

Fig. 2 - Semilogarithmic plot of the mean plasma radioactivity curve (expressed as fraction of injected dose per liter) observed after the bolus i.v. injection of [99m]TcGLA in the patients included in this pharmacokinetic biodistribution study.

TABLE I - Radiation dosimetry estimates (mean ± SEM) derived from the ^{99m}TcGLA biodistribution study in cancer patients, as compared to average values for some of the
radiopharmaceuticals commonly employed for morphofunctional kidney evaluation.

Organ	^{99m}TcGLA	^{99m}Tc-MAG3	^{99m}Tc-DMSA
	mGy/MBq	mGy/MBq	mGy/MBq
Kidneys	0.5488 ± 0.0098	0.017	0.375
Liver	0.0051 ± 0.0007	0.005	0.011
Bladder	0.0208 ± 0.0045	0.127	0.019
Red marrow	0.0041 ± 0.0005	0.003	0.004
Spleen	0.0086 ± 0.0012	n.a.	n.a.
Ovaries	0.0053 ± 0.0007	0.007	0.003
Testes	0.0036 ± 0.0004	0.004	0.001
Whole body	0.0041 ± 0.0005	0.001	0.004

The primary tumours were visualized at early imaging times, with tumour/background ratios
equal to about 2.2 at 0.5-3 hours, and 1.6 at 24 hours (see Fig. 3). In contrast, metastatic
lesions from colorectal adenocarcinoma to the liver did not accumulate ^{99m}TcGLA.

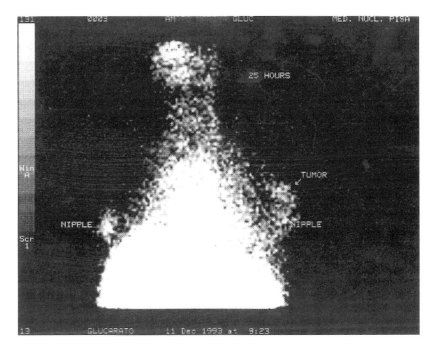

Fig. 3 - Positive tumor imaging observed in one patient with breast cancer after the i.v.
injection of ^{99m}TcGLA (see text).

DISCUSSION

Early diagnosis of myocardial ischemic lesions is of paramount importance for timely therapy. In today's clinical practice, this diagnostic process is based upon clinical criteria, electrocardiographic pattern, and elevated serum levels of specific cardiac enzymes; additional diagnostic criteria can be provided by echocardiographic evaluation which is, however, a highly operator-dependent procedure, while miocardial perfusion studies with thallium-201 or ^{99m}Tc-Sestamibi may also be of some help. As concerns instead direct scintigraphic visualization of the infarcted myocardium, current procedures based on ^{99m}Tc-pyrophosphate or ^{111}In-anti-myosin antibodies are of little help, as they become frankly positive relatively late after the onset of myocardial infarction. A positive scintigraphic indicator of infarcted tissue or tissue severely damaged by ischemia would therefore be highly desirable, particularly if such indicator could provide diagnostic information in the early time-window of infarction. Experimental data cumulated so far in animal models of acute brain or heart ischemia point out the potential of ^{99m}TcGLA for such time-window.

The results obtained in this study point out the overall satisfactory pharmacokinetic and biodistribution properties of ^{99m}TcGLA in humans. In particular, the very low radiation dosimetry estimates demonstrate the safety of this radiopharmaceutical, and open the perspective of further exploring its potential role as a tracer for clinical and pathophysiologic studies, particularly in conditions of severe ischemia or early necrosis of the heart and brain. Our groups are now conducting further investigations to explore the potential role of ^{99m}TcGLA in conditions of severe heart or brain hypoxia.

REFERENCES

1. Khaw BA, Pak KY, Ahmad M, Nossif ND, Strauss HW. Visualization of experimental cerebral infarct: application of a new Tc-99m-labeled compound (abstract). *Circulation* 1988; 78: II-140.
2. Uehara T, Ahmad M, Khaw BA, et al. Tc-99m-glucarate: a marker of acute cerebral damage (abstract). *J Nucl Med* 1989; 30: 901.
3. Yaoita H, Uehara T, Brownell AL, et al. Localization of technetium-99m-glucarate in zones of acute cerebral injury. *J Nucl Med* 1991; 32: 272-278.
4. Yaoita H, Juweid M, Wilkinson R, et al. Detection of myocardial reperfusion injury with Tc-99m-glucarate (abstract). *J Nucl Med* 1990; 31: 795.
5. Orlandi C, Crane PD, Edwards S, et al. Early scintigraphic detection of experimental myocardial infarction in dogs with technetium-99m-glucaric acid. *J Nucl Med* 1991; 32: 263-268.
6. Ohtani H, Callahan RJ, Khaw BA, Fischman AJ, Wilkinson RA, Strauss HW. Comparison of technetium-99m-glucarate and thallium-201 for the identification of acute myocardial infarction in rats. *J Nucl Med* 1992; 33: 1988-1993.

Poster Session I: Dosimetry; Physics

Radioactive Isotopes in
Clinical Medicine and Research XXII
ed. by H. Bergmann, A. Kroiss and H. Sinzinger
© 1997 Birkhäuser Verlag Basel/Switzerland

PROGRESS IN MODELLING OF BIOKINETICS OF ^{131}I

J. Heřmanská, M. Kárný [a], T. Blažek [b], J. Němec

Clinic of Nuclear Medicine, Faculty Hospital Motol, Prague, Czech Republic
[a] Institute of Information Theory and Automation, AV ČR, Prague, Czech Republic
[b] Institute of Medical Biophysics, 2nd Medical Faculty, UK, Prague, Czech Republic

SUMMARY: Kinetics of the cumulated activity in human body determines strongly medical impacts of ionizing radiation. The effective half-life is mostly used as its global descriptor. The effective half-life was found, however, of a limited use as the underlying deterministic relationship time – activity can hardly be taken as (mono)exponential. More complex dependences of activity on time are inspected here. While retaining practical feasibility, a substantial descriptive capability is gained as demonstrated on an extensive set of real data.

INTRODUCTION

The activity administered for diagnostics/therapy has to be large enough to reach the administration aims. Simultaneously, it should not damage healthy tissues. It calls for a reliable estimation of the energy imparted, i.e. of the absorbed dose, to the human body, e.g. (1-2). The Medical Internal Radiation Dose (MIRD) methodology (3) provides the necessary physical and experimental background for it. It needs, however, good estimate of the activity cumulated in considered organs and tissues.

The cumulated activity is the integral under the time trajectory of the instantaneous activity which has to be reconstructed from a few measurements. It is possible only when a curve from a pre-specified class is fitted to noisy measurements. The quality of the resulting estimate is strongly influenced by the class of the fitted curves.

This paper inspects a novel model of the activity evolution for diagnostic/therapeutic applications of ^{131}I. A recently proposed quadratic relationship of ln(*instantaneous activity*) to ln(*time*) (4) and its refinement are evaluated on an extensive set of real data. The quadratic form is much better than the standard model in which ln(*instantaneous activity*) is modelled by a straight line characterized by the effective half-life.

MATERIAL & METHODS

Records used are related to 3000 patients treated for thyroid diseases at the Clinic of Nuclear Medicine, Faculty Hospital Motol, 2nd Medical Faculty, Charles University. The data are stored during routine evaluations by a software system JOD (5). The records containing at least four measurements (greater than the dimension of the estimated parameter) were processed. The selected records contain at most 20 measurements and 1 up to 4 lesions.

In diagnostic phase of treating thyroid diseases by ^{131}I, a diagnostic amount the iodine is administered and accumulation abilities of various lesions are estimated. Assuming invariability of the accumulation ability, the doses absorbed during the therapeutic phase can be predicted and the adequate therapeutic activity administered.

Knowledge of instantaneous and cumulated activities in the therapeutic phase is also useful for controlling the radio-hygienic regime of patients and checking the assumption of accumulation invariability.

The cumulated activity $A_{cum} \equiv \int_0^\infty A(t) \, dt$ where $A(t)$ is instantaneous activity at time $t >$application time=0. The induced counts $a(t)$ corresponding to activity values $A(t)$ are measured in several time instants t_i only $(i = 1, \ldots, m \approx 2\text{-}20)$.

The registered counts a(t) are related to the activity by

$$a(t) = c.A(t).noise$$

where c denotes the calibration factor which can be well estimated (5). The needed estimate of the whole curve can be obtained only when
- the trajectory $A(t)$, $t > 0$, is parametrized by a smooth function containing a few time invariant parameters Θ only;
- the adequate probabilistic noise description is selected.

For computation reasons, the probabilistic modelling is often simplified and logarithmic-normal model is adopted

$$ln(a(t)) = f(t, \Theta) + white\ normal\ noise, \ f(t, \Theta) \approx ln(cA(t)).$$

The usual model is specified by the model M_1

$$f(t, \Theta) = ln(cA(t_1)) - ln(2)t/T_{ef} \ \text{for}\ t > t_1 > 0.$$

The time $t_1 > 0$ separates time interval during which fast and complex transients of the activity distribution occur. T_{ef} denotes the effective half-life. The activity $A(t_1)$ modified by a calibration factor c completes set of unknowns. Thus, the parameters determining this model are $\Theta = (cA(t_1), t_1, T_{ef})$.

By neglecting contribution of the transient phase, the cumulated activity is given by simple formula $A_{cum} = A(t_1)T_{ef}/ln(2)$.

This model was found inadequate in a significant portion of the inspected cases (6,7). For this reason, an alternative solution was searched for.

Available compartmental models suggest $f(t, \Theta)$ as a sum of several exponential functions. Their parameters are, however, individual for each patient and have to be estimated. This is unfeasible task with a few measurements available. Thus, a mild deviation from the standard straight-line form is acceptable only.

The shapes of activity trajectories for the reference man (8) indicated the following model M_2 as a suitable candidate

$$f(t, \Theta) = K_1 + K_2 \ln(t) + K_3 \ln^2(t) - \ln(2)t/T_p$$

where the triple $\Theta = (K_1, K_2, K_3)$ is unknown and T_p is the known physical half-life of ^{131}I.

During experiments reported below, the new model M_3 has been proposed

$$f(t, \Theta) = K_1 + K_2 \ln(t) + K_3 t^{2/3} \ln(t) - \ln(2)t/T_p$$

which replaces the term $\ln^2(t)$ by a faster function of time $t^{2/3} \ln(t)$.

The cumulated activity for the models M_2 and M_3 has to be computed numerically. Both, however, exploit and describe full data set. Similarly as M_1, both have triple of unknown parameters and estimation of all models can be optimally performed by least squares (linear-in-parameters normal model). The procedure can be and should be modified by prior information resulting from Bayesian formulation of finite-sample estimation (7).

The models M_2, M_3 have the following desirable qualitative properties. Trajectories start at zero if $K_1 \geq 0$ (no activity is cumulated at administration time yet). They fall to zero faster than the physical decay if $K_3 < 0$ and are unimodal for $t > 0$. They include explicitly the physical decay so that the individual biological elimination is to be estimated only.

RESULTS

The models are compared according to predictive capabilities for the following reasons:
- Models which are good in the hard extrapolation problem have to grasp substantial invariant features of the reality. Thus they are expected to suit for estimation of the patient's "invariant", his/her ability to accumulate activity.
- The estimated models serve as predictors for radio-hygienic purposes.

Specifically, let us consider any of the tested sets of trajectories $f(t, \Theta)$ parametrized by a multivariate parameter Θ. Let $\hat{\Theta}_m$ be an estimate gained from data recorded *before* time t_m. Then, the relative prediction error of the value $a(t_m)$ is defined

$$\delta(t_m) = \frac{a(t_m) - \exp[f(t_m, \hat{\Theta}_m)]}{a(t_m)} 100 \quad [\%].$$

The entire patient set is judged according to the sample mean μ, standard deviation σ^2 as well as the shortest empirical confidence interval $[\underline{\delta}, \bar{\delta}]$ containing 70% of relative errors. The typical results are summarized in the following Table 1.

Table 1. Comparison of relative prediction errors over the patient set

Model type	t_1 [days]	No. of cases	Mean μ [%]	Dispersion σ^2 [%]	Confidence interval $[\underline{\delta}, \bar{\delta}]$ [%]
M_1	0	2175	95.5	235	$[-16, 112]$
M_1	1	1541	102.5	293	$[-44, 76]$
M_1	2	1177	46.0	183	$[-28, 44]$
M_2	–	2175	30.7	117	$[-32, 44]$
M_3	–	2175	1.2	102	$[-44, 24]$

Note that the selected tests eliminate need for inclusion of calibration task as the estimate of the product cA_1 is needed for predicting the observations $a(t)$.

DISCUSSION

The following phenomena are clearly demonstrated in Table 1:
- Bias μ is substantially decreased for M_2 and it is almost zero for M_3. Just attempts to decrease this bias led to M_3. The model M_3 provided the best results from a wide set of tested models.
- Dispersions σ^2 are lower for these models, too.

– The confidence interval for M_1 is close to those of M_2, M_3 only if almost half of the patient is not evaluated because of lack of data.

– The results presented for the classical model M_1 applied to all data ($t_1=0$) are presented for comparison only. They underline its restricted validity.

The results summarized in Table 1 are typical. Changes in the prior information as well as variations of the significance level led to the same qualitative picture.

Note, that the performed tests are strict as the substantial portion of several-days pre-·dictions is included. It happens always when week end falls into to the measurement period.

Formerly reported improvements for M_1 (7), achieved by considering adequate Poisson noise distribution, support conjecture that the further improvements are achievable for M_2 and M_3. This requires to face a non-trivial problem of multivariate integration (9).

The following methodologically significant conclusion can be drawn from the present-ed study: Improved modelling and estimation of basic quantities met in nuclear medicine may lead to substantial improvement of precision of the obtained results without need for instrumentation improvements.

ACKNOWLEDGEMENT

The research has been partially supported by GA ČR, grant No. 312/94/0679 and by COST OC B2.20 project.

REFERENCES

1. Culver CM, Dworkin HJ. Radiation safety considerations for post-iodine 131 hyperthyroid therapy. J Nucl Med 1991; 32:169–173.
2. Maxon HR, Englaro EE, Thomas SR et al. Radioiodine-131 therapy for well-differentiated thyroid cancer. A quantitative radiation dosimetric approach: outcome and validation in 85 patients. J Nucl Med 1992; 33:1132–1136.
3. Snyder WS, Ford MR, Warner GG, Watson SB. Absorbed dose per unit cumulated activi ty for selected radionuclides and organs. NM/MIRD, Pamphlet No. 11, Oak Ridge National Laboratory, Tenesee, 1975:257 pp.
4. Heřmanská J, Blažek T, Němec J, Kárný M. Beyond effective half-life characterization of radionuclide dynamics. In: Preprints of XVIII. Radiation Hygiene Days, Jáchymov, 1994:78–85.
5. Heřmanská J. Bayesian approach to dosimetric data evaluation for medical use of ^{131}I (in Czech). Docent Thesis. Clinic of Nuclear Medicine, 2nd Medical Faculty, Charles University Prague, 1993:103 pp.
6. Heřmanská J, Němec J, Blažek T, Kárný M. Bayesian prediction of ^{131}I kinetics. J Nucl Med 1994; 21:870–870.
7. Heřmanská J, Kárný M. Effective half-life estimation: Bayesian solution.   Radiation Protection Dosimetry, 1995: in print.
8. Kliment V, Thomas J. Mathematical solution of the iodine retention and excretion mod-el. Jad En 1986; 32:85–88.
9. Guy TV. Multivariate integration problem in Bayesian theory application in nuclear medicine. Technical Report ÚTIA AV ČR. Prague, 1995:12 pp.

Radioactive Isotopes in
Clinical Medicine and Research XXII
ed. by H. Bergmann, A. Kroiss and H. Sinzinger
© 1997 Birkhäuser Verlag Basel/Switzerland

PHARMACOKINETICS AND DOSIMETRY
AFTER COMBINED APPLICATION
OF Sr-89 CHLORIDE AND Re-186-HEDP IN BONE METASTASES

Limouris GS[1], Manetou A[2], Nikoletopoulos S[1], Toubanakis N[1], Stavraka A[1], Vlahos L[1]

[1] Radiology Dept, Nucl Med Div, Areteion Univ Hosp, Athens, Hellas; [2] Nucl Med Dept, NIMTS - Hosp, Athens, Hellas

INTRODUCTION

Sr-89 Chloride[1,2,6,9] and Re-186-HEDP[3,4,6] have been proposed as two very promising radiopharmaceuticals for the palliative treatment of bone metastatic pain. Besides the worldwide efforts to achieve optimal doses for longest possible analgetic duration, the therapeutic results remain still moderate for both radiopharmaceuticals.

PATIENTS AND METHODS

In an attempt to improve the traditional therapeutic schemes in a total of 7 patients with bone metastases due to prostate cancer, 148 ± 15 MBq of Sr-89 Chloride (Amersham Int plc, Backinghamshire) were i.v. administred followed, after a weekly interval, by a second i.v. injection of 1400 ± 100 MBq of Re - 186 - HEDP (Mallinckrodt + Medical BV, Petten). This combined[5] radionuclide application resulted in a marked longer duration of osseous analgesia (x: 4.2 ± 0.9 months) compared to that achieved with Sr - 89 Chloride (x: $1,6 \pm 0.6$ months, 9 cases) or Re-186-HEDP (x: $2,1 \pm 0.7$ months, 11 cases) alone.

Consequently the absorbed doses of the three groups referred, were correlated to the therapeutic effect achieved, using quantitative conjugate-view counting techniques with a gamma-camera in preselected metastatic lesions (Elscint APEX 408, ECT) and the obtained radionuclide to bone retention curves ploted (Figure 1).

Furthermore before any absorbed dose calculation, the following assumptions were taken into consideration:

– both, Sr-89 chloride and Re-186-HEDP,

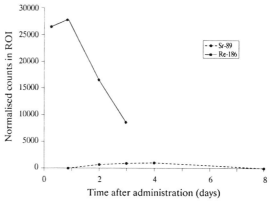

Figure 1. Strontium-89 and Re-186 bone retention at the initiation of the therapy

are **volume seeking** radiopharmaceuticals (they tend to be deposited
uniformly throughout bone tissue),

– on average, **66%** of Sr-89 chloride and
  30% of Re-186-HEDP is retained by the
  skeleton, following i.v. injection,

– on average, activity surrounding metastases is **five** times higher for Sr-89
  chloride and **three** for Re-186-HEDP,

– skeletal mass is **10%** of body mass,

– T1/2 Sr-89 eff = T1/2 Sr-89 phys = 50.5
  days, and

– T1/2 Re-186 eff = T1/2 Re-186 phys =
  3.7 days

Following i.v. injection of 2.2 MBq/kg
body weight (BW) of Sr-89 Chloride and
20 MBq/kg BW of Re-186-HEDP (Figure
1, Figure 2) about 0.72 6 MBq for
radiostrontium (2.2 MBq/kg x 10^{-1} x 0.66 x
5) per kgBW and 1.80 MBq for radio-
rhenium (20 MBq/kg x 10^{-1} x 0.3 x 3) per kg
BW will be found in bone surrounding
skeletal metastases (Figure 3). Using the
formulations:

$$D\beta = 73.8\ E\beta\ TC \quad \text{and}$$

$$d\beta t = D\beta\ (\ 1 - e^{-0.693t/T}\ )$$

for uniformly distubuted radionuclides,
where:

  Dβ: the tumour absorbed dose, up to com-
    plete radionuclide desintegration,

  dβt: the tumour absorbed dose, up to some
    time t (in days) prior to comple-
    te desintegration,

  Eβ: 0.583 MeV for Sr-89 and 0.349 MeV for
    Re-186,

  T: 50.5 days for Sr-89 and 3.7 days for
    Re-186,

  C: 0.726 MBq/kg MW for Sr-89 and 1.8 MBq/kg BW for Re-186

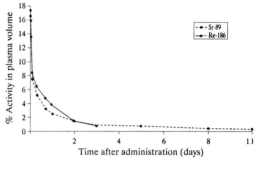

*Figure 1. Strontium-89 and Re-186 plasma activity at the initiation
of the therapy*

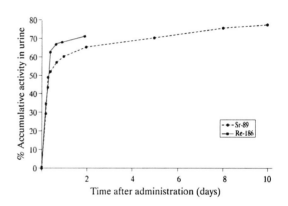

*Figure 2. Strontium-89 and Re-186 urine activity at the initiation
of the therapy*

and according to their disintegration curves **6%** of the activity will have disintegrated 15 days* following Sr-89
and **7%**, 8 days* following Re-186 i.v. injection, depositing about **290 cGy** and **135 cGy** respectively. The tumour
(e.g. bone metastases) absorbed dose up to complete radionuclide desintegration Dβ, was found to be approx **1580
cGy** for Sr-89 and **170 cGy** for Re-186.

In conclusion the sum of the combined radiation delivered is still palliative rather than curative because the
accumulative radiation deposition on the osseous metastases from both radionuclides is approx **1750 cGy**, pretty
below the **4000 cGy**, absorbed from external radiation therapy, considered necessary for healing.

* *initiation time of analgetic effect*

REFERENCES

1. Bos SD. An overview of current clinical experience with strontium-89 (Metastron). Prostate (suppl) 1994; 5: 23-6.

2. Guerrieri P, Madoni S, Parisi S, Fusco V, Oriolo V, Rendina G, Paleani-Vettori PG. Bone formation markers and pain palliation in bone metastases treated with strontium-89. Am J Clin Oncol 1994; 17(1): 77-9.

3. Klerk de JMH, Dijk van A, Schip van het AD, Zonnenberg BA, Rijk van PP. Pharmacokinetics of rhenium-186 after administration of rhenium-186-HEDP to patients with bone metastases. J Nucl Med 1992; 33:646-651.

4. Klerk de JM, Zonnenberg BA, van het Schip AD, van Dijk A, Han SH, Quirijnen JM, Blijham GH, van Rijk PP. Dose escalation study of rhenium 186 hydroxyethylidene diphosphonate in patients with metastatic prostate cancer. Eur J Nucl Med 1994; 21(10): 1114-20.

5. Limouris GS, Manetou A, Shukla SK, Stavraka A, Vlahos L. Combined ^{89} Sr-Chloride / ^{186} Re - HEDP application in bone metastases. Eur J Nucl Med 1995; 22 (8): 808.

6. Porter AT, Ben-Josef E, Davis L. Systemic administration of new therapeutic radioisotopes, including phosphorus, strontium, samarium and rhenium. Curr Opin Oncol 1994; 6(6): 607-10.

7. Samaratunga RC, Thomas SR, Hinnefeld JD, von Kuster LC, Hyams DM, Moulton JS, Sperling MI, Maxon HR. A Monte Carlo simulation model for radiation dose to metastatic skeletal tumor from rhenium-186 (Sn)-HEDP. J Nucl Med 1995; 36(2): 336-50.

8. Serafini AN. Current status of systemic intravenous radiopharmaceuticals for the treatment of painful metastatic bone disease. Int J Radiat Oncol Biol Phys 1994; 30(5): 1187-94.

9. Taylor AJ. Strontium - 89 for the palliation of bone pain due to metastatic disease. J Nucl Med 1994; 35 (12): 2054.

Radioactive Isotopes in
Clinical Medicine and Research XXII
ed. by H. Bergmann, A. Kroiss and H. Sinzinger
© 1997 Birkhäuser Verlag Basel/Switzerland

RHENIUM-186 LABELLED MAb-170: A SUITABLE AGENT FOR RADIOIMMUNOTHERAPY OF OVARIAN CARCINOMA ?

C. Alexander[1], C. E. Villena-Heinsen[2], A. Schaefer[1],
L. Trampert[1], W. Schmidt[2], C.-M. Kirsch[1]

[1]Department of Nuclear Medicine, [2]Department of Obstetrics and
Gynaecology; Saarland University Medical School;
D-66421 Homburg; Germany

SUMMARY: For biokinetic and dosimetry studies the Tc-99m-labelled MAb-170 was administered intraperitoneally in four patients. Assuming equal biodistribution for the Re-186- and Tc-99m-tagged antibody the 48 hours-measurement of whole-body scintigraphy, blood activity concentration and urinary excretion gave a value of 0.35 Gy/370 MBq for bone marrow dose. These results confirm that a RIT with Re-186 MAb-170 might be feasible with activities of up to 3.7 GBq.

INTRODUCTION

The monoclonal antibody (MAb) 170 (Tru-Scint™AD) is a Tc-99m labelled investigational drug for the in vivo diagnosis of adenocarcinomas developed by Biomira Inc., Edmonton, Canada. First clinical results revealed Tc-99m-labelled MAb-170 to be a promising radiopharmaceutical in the diagnosis of adenocarcinoma with emphasis on breast cancer and ovarian carcinoma (1-3). Scintigraphic results showed high tumor-to-background ratios in both primary ovarian carcinomas and peritoneal metastases that seemed to be suitable for intraperitoneal radioimmunotherapy (RIT). This approach might be successful in patients stage FIGO III/IV with minimal residual disease after first-look-surgery. The present study should answer the questions if a Rhenium-186-labelled MAb-170 could be suitable for intraperitoneal RIT.

MATERIALS AND METHODS

Prior to enrollment in this study, all patients had given written informed consent. The population included 4 female patients with ovarian carcinomas and peritoneal metastases aged 50, 57, 65 and 76 years.

In each patient intraperitoneal administration of 972 MBq (mean) of MAb-170 solution, corresponding to 2 mg of MAb-170, was performed.

Scintigraphic imaging was performed by means of a double head gamma camera with a LEHR collimator (MULTISPECT II, SIEMENS, Erlangen, Germany). Ventral and dorsal whole-body scintigraphy was acquired at 5 min, 15 min, 1 h, 4 h and 24 h in three patients and at 48 h after injection in two patients. Additional urine collection and serum sampling were performed for these intervals.

The time-activity-curves of peritoneal cavity, kidneys, liver, spleen, heart lungs and the remainder of the body were evaluated from whole-body-images using the region-of-interest (ROI) technique and calculation the geometric means of opposite ROI's as a percentage of whole-body-activity.

Blood specimen drawn at 5 min, 15 min, 1 h, 4 h, 12 h, 24 h and 48 h p.i. were counted by an automatic gamma sample changer with adaequate standards for technetium activity and the curves of whole blood activity concentration were documented.

The cumulative urinary excretion of Tc-99m MAb-170 was calculated as a percentage of the injected dose (ID).

RESULTS

Assuming identical biodistribution kinetics for the Tc-99m- and the Re-186-labelled MAb-170 we came to the following results:

The urinary excretion gave values of 33.3 % and 57.2 % of ID 24 h and 48 h p.i., respectively. As the hepatobiliary excretion of MAb-170 is neglegible the whole body curve was derived from these values. It showed a monoexponential decay with an effective half-time of 34.5 h (r=0.986).

The ROI-evaluation of scintigrams showed organ activities with am initial accumulation phase that came to a maximum 24 h p.i. and a subsequent exponential elimination curve. Assuming the worst case for dosimetry calculation the period beyond 48 h p.i. was fitted to the physical decay curve of Re-186. The kidneys as the main route of excretion showed the highest accumulation of 5.9 % ID 24 h p.i.. The other maxima of organ activities were 2.40 % ID (liver), 0.93 % ID (spleen), 1.87 % ID (heart), and 1.93 % ID (lung) at 24 h p.i.. The decay of activity in the peritoneal cavity was monoexponential, the effective half-time was 20.6 h (r=0.995).

Mean serum activity concentration gave a maximum of 12.8 kBq/ml 23 h p.i. (370 MBq ID). As the red bone marrow was not visible in planar scintigraphy and as the overlay of blood pool activity in the large vessels avoided an acurate ROI-evaluation, the serum dose was used to guess the red marrow dose.

Table 1. Dosimetry of Re-186 MAb-170 after i.p.-administration of 370 MBq

organ	dose [Gy/370 MBq]
peritoneal cavity	4.09
kidneys	0.37
liver	0.05
spleen	0.19
heart	0.25
lung	0.07
serum	0.35
red bone marrow	< 0.35
remainder of body	0.01
effective whole body dose	0.21

For dose calculations only the main nonpenetrating radiations were considered. Table 1 gives the results of dosimetry calculations.

DISCUSSION

The calculation of Re-186 MAb-170 dosimetry on the basis of Tc-99m MAb-170 biokinetics is a reasonable attempt to achieve dose calculations without exposing study patients to beta irradiation. The chemistries of Tc and Re are similar and the binding mechanism to the antibody is identical. So this approach should be reliable for problem solution. Dosimetry shows the highest organ dose in the kidneys. The limiting factor is the red marrow dose that is guessed to be less than 0.35 Gy/370 MBq. This value includes a large margin of safety because red marrow dose was guessed from serum dose. The latter exceedes whole blood dose by a factor of about two, and in scintigraphy blood pool activity is higher than bone marrow accumulation in the first 48 h p.i.. Another overestimation results from fitting the serum curve to the physical decay of Re-186 for the phase beyond 48 h p.i.. So intraperitoneal RIT should be safe using therapy activities of up to 1.85 GBq Re-186 MAb-170 at least.

REFERENCES

1.   MacLean GD, McEwan AJ, Noujaim AA, et al. Two Novel
      Monoclonal Antibodies Have Potential for Gynecologic
      Cancer Imaging. Antibody, Immunoconjugates, and
      Radiopharmaceuticals 1991; 4:297-308.

2.   McEwan AJB, MacLean GD, Hooper HR, et al. MAb 170H.82: an
      evaluation of a novel panadenocarcinoma monoclonal
      antibody labelled with ^{99}Tc^m and with ^{111}In. Nucl Med
      Commun 1992; 13:11-19.

3.   Alexander C, Villena-Heinsen CE, Trampert L, et al.
      Radioimmunoscintigraphy of ovarian tumours with
      technetium-99m labelled monoclonal antibody-170: first
      clinical experiences. Eur J Nucl Med 1995; 22:645-651.

Radioactive Isotopes in
Clinical Medicine and Research XXII
ed. by H. Bergmann, A. Kroiss and H. Sinzinger
© 1997 Birkhäuser Verlag Basel/Switzerland

BETA-GAMMA DOSIMETRY IN RADIOIMMUNOTHERAPY: EXAMPLES OF MODEL CALCULATION
APPLAYED TO BRAIN GLIOMA AND COMPARISON BETWEEN DIFFERENT NUCLIDES

G. Giorgetti, S. Lazzari and G. Sarti

Health and Medical Physics dpt, Hosp "M. Bufalini" Cesena, I

SUMMARY: The MIRD schema permits the absorbed dose calculation with
convolution integral algorithm. We implemented this kind of algorithm to
take care of non uniform distribution, to improve algorithm convergence
speed and to describe more complex geometry reconducting them to union of
elementary geometrical shapes or even matrix of voxel.
The results obtained in calculations have been verified with the Monte
Carlo results and has revealed to be consistent in the measurement error
range. The time of calculation are increased in typical cases.

INTRODUCTION

As a radioimmunotherapy neediness, when a case of recurrence is
revealed by gamma camera image, the calculation of the dimensions of the
lesion is essential in intralesional therapy because it defines the
concentration of radioisotope (I131 or Y90) to be injected once the
radiologist has determined the activity in the lesion. The size is
established from CT image approximating it to a sphere or an ellipsoid and
then it is elaborated using a Monte Carlo algorithm. With the new
methodology here presented, improvements are detectable in three phases:
VOI detection from CT digital image rather than measuring directly on the
film; data conversion in voxel that can consider each point apart which its
own activity concentration and calculation of energy fraction deposed in
the three regions with convolution integral.

METHODS

The lesion region may be defined in two ways: with the geometrical
parameters of a union of ellipsoids that best describe the region or
directly on the image, using a threshold algorithm or defining the VOI with
the mouse in all the interested slices; the definition of the regions is
always supervisioned so the user can, in every moment, set one image point
or a group as belonging to one or to another region.

The phisical points are converted to voxel according to their dimension and then the algorithm can treat them in the same manner as the geometrical parametrization. The convolution integral algorithm simply sums the contribute of energy deposed in every points of every region from all the source voxels. This contribute only depends on the distance of the two points, if the radioisotope is already been defined, and it is extrapolated from a kernel matrix data. The real difficulty is to treat the zero singularity and we solved this problem running a Monte Carlo for the autoabsorbed energy of the voxel; it depends on the dimension of the voxel and on the isotope considered.

$$\dot{D}(r) = \Delta \int_{\substack{source \\ volume}} C(r_s)\phi(|r - r_s|)d^3r_s$$

Convolutive expression of the dose rate distribution D(r) produced by a nonuniform activity concentration C(r$_s$) in a homogeneous target volume.

$$\phi(r) = \frac{\mu_{en}}{\rho} \cdot \frac{1}{4\pi r^2} \cdot e^{-\mu r} \cdot B_{en}(\mu r)$$

Point isotropic specific absorbed fraction in an unbounded homogeneous medium for photons; for beta particles, this formula is much more complicated and it is not generally integrable, so we used the value from the kernel matrix.

RESULTS

The validity of this algorithm has been verified comparing the results obtained on spherical shells of increasing radius (see the table below) and on complex geometrical structures (simple ellipsoid, ellipsoid perturbed with a small sphere, two and three intersercting ellipsoids) with those obtained by Monte Carlo simulation. As it can be seen clearly, the energy fraction deposed in the regions is the same in the two cases considering the measure errors and, as predicted, the calculation speed is higher for convolutive algorithm in lesion of reasonable dimension.

radius	dose CI	dose MC	speed CI	speed MC
5 mm	94.3%	93.8%	480 s	1 s
10 mm	97.1%	97.2%	480 s	11 s
15 mm	98.0%	98.3%	480 s	111 s
20 mm	98.5%	98.5%	480 s	470 s
30 mm	99.2%	99.1%	480 s	6480 s

The error extimated on the dose calculation is ±0.5% in all the measurements, speeds are calculated with an error of ±0.5s. Monte Carlo simulations are done with 20.000 stories. All the values are calculated on the same 100 Mhz Pentium PC.

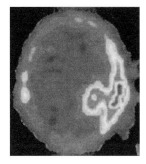

SPECT image of the intralesional therapy which follow the surgical removal of a brain tumor; the red zone show the skull and a possible recurrence.

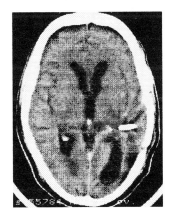

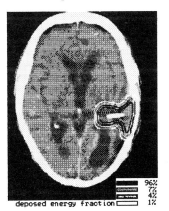

Correspondent CT slice on which the dosimetric calculation are done: extimation of the shape and dimension of the lesion directly on the digitized CT image.

Example of how a isodose curve will appear: it makes easy and immediate to see how the dose fraction is distributed.

DISCUSSION

The success in radioimmunotherapy depends critically on the development of appropriate antibodies which are specific to a given tumor cell antigen for selectively irradiate the tumor cells while sparing the normal tissue and on adequate radioisotope and quantity choice. The methodologies we use to calculate the energy deposition from a non uniform source distribution are already operative. One central problem in radioimmunotherapy is to obtain accurate information on the activity distribution of the radiolabels. Thus the treatment planning procedures should focus on the development of procedures to acquire a more accurate knowledge of the activity distribution in time and the shape and size of target: advances in physic and dosimetric fields are possible with the three dimensional correlations of patient data with other imaging modality such as CT, MR, etc.

Furthermore, the possibility of define the volumes of interest directly on the digitalized images makes the physician able to draw the VOIs with more precision even if they have a very complex shape; as the program itself perform all needed data elaborations, the dose calculation results are obtained by the physician with a sequence of easy mouse operation, no informatic or particle physic knowledges are required. Calculation and printing of isodose curve are a work current in progress and appears to be as a natural development of the present one.

REFERENCES

1. KWOK C.S., PRESTWICH W.V., WILSON B.C. In: Calculation of radiation doses for nonuniformly distributed beta and gamma radionuclides in soft tissue. 04/18/1985.

2. SIMPKIN D.J., MACKIE T.R. In: EGS4 Monte Carlo determination of the beta dose kernel in water, Med. Phys. 17(2) Mar/Apr 1990 pagg. 179-186.

Radioactive Isotopes in
Clinical Medicine and Research XXII
ed. by H. Bergmann, A. Kroiss and H. Sinzinger
© 1997 Birkhäuser Verlag Basel/Switzerland

ABSORBED DOSE ESTIMATION BY COMBINED USE OF CT INFORMATION AND WHOLE BODY SCANNING WITH A DUAL HEAD GAMMA CAMERA IN PATIENTS WITH OSTEOSARCOMA TREATED WITH [153]Sm-EDTMP

A. Skretting, Ø.Bruland ,M. Aas

Departments of Medical Physics and Technology, Oncology and Nuclear Medicine, The Norwegian Radium Hospital, Oslo, Norway

SUMMARY: We have implemented the conjugated view activity quantitation technique on an ADAC dual head whole body scanning system, using a collimated ^{99m}Tc line source to obtain a transmission scan. The aim was to quantitate the uptake of [153]Sm-EDTMP in metastases from osteogenous sarcoma in conjunction with radiotargeting therapy. The posterior-anterior attenuation derived from this scan was modified to take into account the difference in photon energies between ^{99m}Tc and [153]Sm. The validity of this method was checked by experiments. The attenuation was also calculated from series of CT-slices, and excellent agreement was demonstrated between the two methods.

INTRODUCTION

The conjugated view technique (1,2) is frequently used to quantitate the uptake of radioactivity in organs or lesions in the body. We have adapted this technique to the quantitation of [153]Sm-EDTMP uptake in metastatic lesions from osteosarcoma within the lungs and elsewhere in the body. Since we routinely had to use ^{99m}Tc to measure anterio-posterior attenuation, we developed a method to modify this quantity to reflect the attenuation of the 103 keV photons from [153]Sm. We also wanted to investigate whether the attenuation could as well be calculated from a series of CT-slices.

MATERIALS AND METHODS

Whole body scans were acquired on a dual head gamma camera system (ADAC genesys). Prior to injection of the radiopharmaceutical, a transmission scan was obtained by means of a collimated 800 MBq ^{99m}Tc line source that was fixed to the posterior head and thus moved at scanning speed along the patient. The digital whole body images (512 x 1024 pixels) were transferred to a SUN UNIX work station via the hospital network using the COST B2 INTERFILE standard. The programs that were used for analysis and quantitation were written in IDL (Interactive Data Language, Research Systems Inc, CO,USA).

Neglecting for the time being the scatter contribution, the activity is given by the formula:

$$a = c * (I_a * I_p)^{1/2} *(\exp(\int \mu_{Sm}(z) \, dz))^{1/2} \qquad (1)$$

where c is a calibration constant (MBq/count), I_a and I_p are the anterior and posterior counts, respectively, within a region of interest, and the integral is taken along the posterior - anterior path through the patient. $\mu_{Sm}(z)$ is the linear attenuation coefficient of ^{153}Sm. Assuming that the attenuation is dominated by Compton interactions, the difference between the 103 keV photons from ^{153}Sm and the 140 keV photons from ^{99m}Tc was corrected for according to the formula:

$$\int \mu_{Sm}(z) \, dz = (\mu_{Smw} /\mu_{Tcw}) \int \mu_{Tc}(z)dz =(\mu_{Smw} /\mu_{Tcw}) * \ln(\text{incident/Image}) \qquad (2)$$

where μ_{Smw} and μ_{Tcw} are the linear attenuation coefficients in water for photons from ^{153}Sm and ^{99m}Tc, respectively . «Image» is the intensity in an image point of the transmisssion scan and «incident» is the mean intensity in a reference region of the scan where the line source reached the detector without being attenuated by patient, patient fixation or examination table. We used a 15% window, centered over the photopeak for the measurements with ^{99m}Tc, and a 20% window, centered over the photopeak, for measurements of ^{153}Sm. The corresponding values for the linear attenuation coefficients, measured on the camera, were 0.140 cm^{-1} and 0.155 cm^{-1}, respectively.

In order to confirm that this method worked correctly, the above procedure was performed with an Alderson phantom (Alderson laboratories, U S A). It is divided into 2.54 cm thick slabs that are kept together with tightened wires. In addition, a line source was filled with approximately 600 MBq ^{153}Sm and another transmission scan acquired.

The integrals of eq. (2) were also calculated based on a series of CT-slices of the phantom. These images where obtained on a GE CT/PACE and transferred to the SUN work station where they were decoded and rebinned to a 256 x 256 pixel format. (pixel size 1.46 mm). The calculations were based on the work of Battista et al. (reference) who used a Compton scanner together with CT-images to derive a conversion from Houndsfield units (HU) in the CT-image into electron densities relative to water. In Compton interactions, the attenuation coefficient is proportional to the electron density, thus:

$$\int \mu_{Sm}(z) \, dz = \mu_{Smw} \int \rho_r(z)dz \qquad (3)$$

where $\rho_r(z)$ is the electron density relative to that of water. Before the numerical integration, the region corresponding to the CT-examination table had been drawn into one of the CT-images. For each of the CT-slices, this region was excluded from the integration. Thus for each CT-slice, a line projection of the attenuation coefficients within the phantom onto the image plane was created. By linear interpolation between these lines, an image was built that, exept for the different magnification, corresponded to the ones derived from the transmission scans. In the case of the phantom measurement on the camera, the reference region for calculation of the incident intensity was drawn over a part of the examination table (assuming even thickness) to exclude the attenuation in the examination table from the calculation in eq 2.

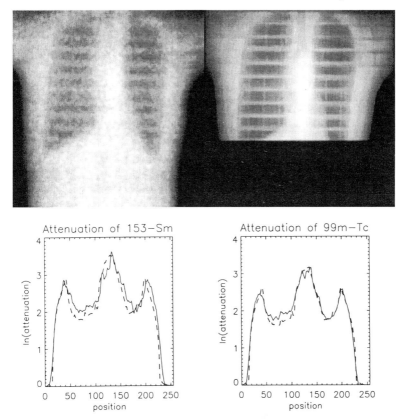

Figure 1.Upper row: the attenuation images for [153]Sm derived from the transmission scan (left) and from the CT images (right) . Lower row: cross section at the level of the lungs through the attenuation images obtained with 153Sm (left) and 99mTc (right). Solid lines denote data derived from line source measurements, and dashed lines have been calculated from the CT-images.

Regions of interest were drawn around the accumulation and a background region, if feasible contralaterally, in the whole body images and copied to the other images. The total net accumulation counts formed the input to eq 1. The tumour contours were drawn in the images where the tumour was visible, and the pixels within all these contours added. Finally the tumour volume was obtained by multiplication with the voxel volume. Since measurements in patients showed that the radiopharmaceutical did not leave the site of uptake, the effective halflife was taken to be equal the physical.

RESULTS

A set of corresponding measured and calculated attenuation images for the case of ^{153}Sm are shown the upper row of figure 1 . These images both show the total anterior - posterior attenuation. The image calculated from the transmission scan has been warped (4) to coincide with the calculated one (right). The agreement between these two images, and between the corresponding two images obtained for ^{153}Sm, were excellent as demonstrated by the cross section through these images, (figure 1, lower row). The dashed curve stems from the CT-images while the solid curve has been calculated from the transmission scan with the ^{153}Sm line source. The difference in attenuation between ^{99m}Tc and ^{153}Sm was significant, indicating that the energy difference must be taken into account.

From the results obtained in the phantom study, it turned out that it would be possible to perform the attenuation correction based on CT-information alone. In this case, the integral of eq 3 was computed along the path from the tumor to the detector.

REFERENCES

1. Myers M J, Lavender J P, de Olivieira JB, Maseri A: A simplified method of quantitating organ uptake using a gamma camera. Brit. J. Radiol. 1981; 54: 1062 -1067

2. Eary J F, Appelbaum F L, Durack L, Brown P Preliminary validation of the opposing view method for quantitative gamma camera imaging. Med. Phys. 1989; 16 :362-387

3. Battista J B, Rider W D, Van Dyk J. Computed tomography for radiotherapy planning . Int. J. Radiation Oncology Biol. Phys. 1980 ; 9: 99-107.

4. Van den Elsen, P A, Pol E.J., Viergever M A, Medical Image Warping - A Review with Classification. IEEE Eng. Med. Biol. 1993; 12: 26 - 39

Radioactive Isotopes in
Clinical Medicine and Research XXII
ed. by H. Bergmann, A. Kroiss and H. Sinzinger
© 1997 Birkhäuser Verlag Basel/Switzerland

NON-IMMUNOGENIC HYPERTHYROIDISM BEFORE AND AFTER RADIOIODINE THERAPY: CELL MASS AND AUTONOMOUS FUNCTION.

Als C, Rösler H, Listewnik M, Lüscher D, Ritter EP.

Department of Nuclear Medicine, University of Berne, Inselspital,
CH-3010 Berne, Switzerland

SUMMARY: A new method, dedicated to the diagnostic quantification of potentially toxic thyroidal areas of non-immunogenic hyperthyroidism is proposed: *the double isotope subtraction scintigraphy*. Regional autonomous function ('toxicity index T') by far exceeds cell density, ('cell density index Q'). T and Q were followed in 53 patients from before radioiodine therapy to 3 and 9 months thereafter. We correlated *1)* T and Q with blood hormone values and *2)* restored euthyroidism with the scintigraphic scarification of the functionally autonomous cell mass.

INTRODUCTION

Non-immunogenic hyperthyroidism (NIH) develops over a latent towards a manifest hyperthyroid stage (1-4). The therapeutic indication is given with scintigraphic decompensation; restored euthyroidism leads to a subjective (5) and objective well-being (6). The presentation of functional autonomy can be unifocal (UFA) or multifocal (MFA) (3,7,8). Echography and fine-needle aspiration cytology are not specific (1,2). A new scintigraphic method investigates as well functional as morphologic regional modifications of the autonomous areas, as compared to the supposed 'healthy' peri-focal thyroid parenchyma (1,2).

MATERIALS AND METHODS

Only patients with NIH entered the protocol. The prerequisites were: the *typical scintigraphic presentation* of 'hot', iodine-avid areas, surrounded by 'cold', functionally suppressed areas and an absence of anti-TSH-receptor antibodies*. *Latent H* was defined as: basal TSH <0.1 mU/l or <0.4 mU/l with blocked TRH-test**, i.e., < 2.5 mU/l increase between the basal and TRH-stimulated values of TSH, both total thyroxine (TT4) and total triiodothyronine (TT3) within normal limits (=mean±2SD). In *manifest H,* TT3 and/or TT4 were above the normal limits.

A multistep processing of sequentially acquired radioiodine and 99mTc-methoxy-isobutilisonitrile (MIBI)***** thyroid scans led to normalized subtraction images of regional function (F) and cell (C) excess (1,2). Two numeric factors were derived from regions of interest (ROI): *T=toxicity index,* indicated the maximal F/C contrast and *Q=cell density index*, compared C in autonomous and suppressed areas. The same ROIs were placed in scans obtained before and after radioiodine therapy (RIT); attention had to be given then to the shrunken pathologic and to the 'apparently enlarged' perinodular area.

The functionally suppressed thyroid is rendered visible with 99mTc-MIBI (1,2). In response to its lipophilicity and a membrane potential, the monovalent cation diffuses passively and non-specifically through cell membranes in the presence of O_2 (9). It is trapped mainly in mitochondria (M). As a high focal accumulation of M has been shown in functionally autonomous thyroid lesions (10), our method rests on the hypothesis that the accumulation of MIBI per volume unit of the thyroid would be a gross measure of the density of M or of viable cells (1,2).

RESULTS

T expanded over a range of 6 – 8735 with UFA (median=165) and with hot areas of MFA (median 15); Q however, never exceeded 61. T was weakly correlated to serum TT3 ($r = 0.41$), but not to autonomous tissue volume, ultrasonographic or cytological criteria. After RIT, the relative excess uptake of radioiodine in hot areas = 'T' decreased from (median) 96 to 1.7 in UFA and from 15 to 1.1 in MFA ($p < 0.001$). In parallel, the autonomous cell mass Q broke down from (median) 4.3 to 1.0 in UFA and from 2 to 1.1 in MFA ($p < 0.0001$). After RIT, 5 functional patterns were observed: euthyroidism (n = 37, 70%), at half with scarred and non-scarred autonomous areas (with low and high T values, respectively), primary hypothyroidism (n=4), residual hyperthyroidism (n=7) and secondary hypothyroidism (n=5). The last two groups had persistent subnormal TSH values, but divergent T values and serum TT3, TT4 levels.

DISCUSSION

Function mirrors the specific metabolic activity of the endocrine cells and is portrayed by radioactive iodine. *Cellularity* (or: *cell density*) reflects the M density, i.e., the mass of viable cells, represented by technetium-MIBI. Both diverge grossly between toxic and perinodular tissue of NIH thyroids. Moreover, a rather small cellular surplus contrasts with a literally exploding function within the suppressive, i.e., toxic area(s) (7). When TSH no longer decreases and TT3 and TT4 only gradually increase, the autonomous function (T) and cell mass (Q) further expand.

Growing autonomous areas have been described to be accompanied by rather slowly increasing toxicity (3,4,7). Our data confirm these observations. But they also trace an initial period of evolution early during adolescence. Thyroid hormone levels rise to overt hyperthyroid stages rather lately (11). A still unpalpable UFA already presents an increased specific function, proven by T ≈ 20. Even an UFA with a Q ≈ 2 but a T of > 40, will be hardly palpable. Only after having reached the stage of Q ≈ 5 (and a T >> 100), the UFA will attract attention by its nodular growth. This knowledge makes understandable why an UFA, arising during adolescence, prevents the growth of a diffuse goiter: the autonomous, i.e., continuous secretion of TT3 (prevalent over TT4) succeeds in adapting the thyroid to iodine deficiency (11).

Double isotope parametric scintigraphy provides the therapist with a quantitative test on the quality of his performance. A significant decrease of Q and T after 131-I therapy was the main study result. A residual T-index > 1 at 3 months must, however, not signify an insufficient treatment result, especially as T did not rise again in any case within another 6 months of observation. Radiation therapy has brought these areas below the "critical" or "relevant" mass of autonomously functioning cells (5).

Admittedly, 131-I treatment 'failed' to exterminate autonomously functioning tissue up to the very last cell in 23/53 patients (43%) with 'warm' residues of their hot nodules or areas. Their collapsed T nevertheless signalized a sufficient therapeutic success, as long-term results have proven further stability (5). Radiation therapy is successful when succeeding in clonogenic death (12); functional death – absent iodine uptake – will follow spontaneously, even if rather late.

CONCLUSION

The standardized *double isotope subtraction scintigraphy* consolidates experiences from visual analysis; the huge T range mirrors the natural evolution over time from euthyroid, scintigraphically compensated over latent hyperthyroid towards manifest hyperthyroid, scintigraphically decompensated autonomous stages of toxicity. T is ruled by inherent features of the autonomous tissue and the response of the imbedding thyroid to TSH stimulation. The increase of Q accords with a general rule that overfunction of an endocrine gland parallels with hypertrophy. Our new technique facilitates individual pre-therapeutic evaluations and post-treatment quality controls.

REFERENCES

* = Trag®, Cis-bio international, Gif-sur-Yvette, France.
** = Relefact® nasal spray, Hoechst AG, Frankfurt, Germany.
*** = Cardiolite®, DuPont, Bad Homburg, Germany.

1. Als C, Listevnik M, Rösler H, Ritter EP. "Separation of Autonomous Function from Cell Density in Non-Immunogenic Hyperthyroidism: (I) Quantification with the Double-Isotope Parametric Scintigraphy." Nuclear Medicine 1995;34:135-140.
2. Als C, Rösler H, Listewnik M. "Separation of Autonomous Function from Cell Density in Non-Immunogenic Hyperthyroidism: (II) Compared quantification before and after radioiodine therapy.'' Nuclear Medicine 1996;35: in press.
3. Hamburger JI. Evolution of toxicity in solitary nontoxic autonomously functioning thyroid nodules. J Clin Endocrinol Metab 1980; 50(6): 1089-1093.
4. Sandrock D., Olbricht T., Emrich D., Benker G., Reinwein D. Long-term follow-up in patients with autonomous thyroid adenoma. Acta Endocrinol 1993; 128: 51-55.
5. Kinser JA, Rösler H, Furrer T, Grütter D, Zimmermann H. Nonimmunogenic hyperthyroidism: cumulative hypothyroidism incidence after radioiodine and surgical treatment. J Nucl Med 1989;30:1960-1965.
6. Theissen P, Kaldeway S, Moka D, Bunke J, Voth E, Schicha H. 31P-Magnetic Resonance spectroscopy: impaired energy metabolism in latent hyperthyroidism. Nucl. Med. 1993;32:134-9.
7. Horst W., Rösler H., Schneider C., Labhart A. 306 cases of toxic adenoma: clinical aspects, findings in radioiodine diagnostics, radiochromato-graphy and histology; results of I-131 and surgical treatment. J Nucl Med 1967; 8: 515-528.
8. Wiener JD. Plummer's disease: localized thyroid autonomy. J Endocrinol Invest 1987; 10: 207-224.
9. Savi A., Gerundini P., Zoli P., Maffioli L., Compierchio A., Colombo F., Matarrese M., Deutsch E. Biodistribution of Tc-99m methoxy-isobutyl-isonitrile (MIBI). Eur J Nucl Med 1989; 15: 597-600.
10. Panke TW, Croxson MS, Parker JW, Carriere DP, Rosoff L, Warner NE. Triiodothyronine-secreting (toxic) adenoma of the thyroid gland. Light and electron microscopic characteristics. Cancer 1978;41:528-537.
11. Als C., Listewnik M., Rösler H., Bartkowiak E. Immunogenic and non-immunogenic hyperthyroidism: recent trends in prealpine Switzerland and in coastal poland. Nucl. Med. 1995;34:92-99.
12. Bloomer WD, Adelstein SJ. The mammalian radiation survival curve. J Nucl Med 1982;23:259-265.

Radioactive Isotopes in
Clinical Medicine and Research XXII
ed. by H. Bergmann, A. Kroiss and H. Sinzinger
© 1997 Birkhäuser Verlag Basel/Switzerland

ARTIFACTS IN RECONSTRUCTED PET-IMAGES DUE TO VARIATION IN DETECTOR SENSITIVITY

R. Weller,J. Ruckgaber,G. Glatting,S.N. Reske
University of Ulm. Department of Nuclearmedicine

SUMMARY: Aim of this study is the quantification of regional insensitivities in reconstructed transversal slices due to detector inhomogeneities of a PET-Scanner. We summarize, that studies measured with a total break down of a block detector or with a 50 % break down of a bucket can be evaluated visually. The regional sensitivity variations of up two 20 % prevent quantitative evaluation of studies.

INTRODUCTION

Quality control gained a growing importance in nuclear medicine. In Germany control procedures for scintillation camera, curimeter etc are regulated under legislative control. Although there are no special regulations for PET, procedures for daily quality assurance are available from any manufacturer. The main observation parameter is the homogeneous sensitivity of the various detectors. The situation is described as standard deviation of the mean sensitivity, or the number of blocks outside a certain level, or by visual presentation of the sinograms. Aim of this study is the quantification and the description of detector problems induced artifacts in reconstructed slices.

MATERIALS AND METHODS

Data acquisition was performed with a ECAT-Siemens 931 PET-Scanner with two detector rings. The rings consist of 64 detector blocks, each block consisting of 32 crystals and 4 photo multipliers. Four blocks are joint together and controlled by a bucket controller. The format of the sinograms is 192 x 256 pixels corresponding to a projection resolution of 192 and 256 angles through 180 degrees. Transversal slices are presented in 128 x 128 matrices. Slices are reconstructed by use of an iterative reconstruction algorithm described by Schmidlin et al.. To maintain quality of the scanner, each month or so or following to any maintenance procedure, a standardization of the scanner has to take place. For this purpose the amplification factors of the detectors are calibrated to its correct energy discrimination levels. In a second step the sensitivity of the single detectors is evaluated and stored to a normalization file as scaling factors. This procedure is done by help of a plane source; it takes about six hours. The stability of the normalization is controlled by a so called "daily check procedure". The plane source is measured, resulting sinograms are visually checked; mean and standard deviation are calculated. With a standard deviation of more than 3 % a renormalisation of the scanner is recommended; with a standard deviation of more than 6 % a renormalisation is required. The connection of these values with the quality of the reconstructed images however remains unclear.

We acquired data from a cylindrical phantom filled with solid Ge-68. Calculated absorption correction was performed. In a second step a mathematical model was calculated. Defects were simulated in the sinograms, by decreasing block or bucket counts in 10 % steps. These modified sinograms were reconstructed and the inhomogeneity and resolution of the transversal slices were quantitatively analyzed and the images were visually inspected for systematic artifacts.

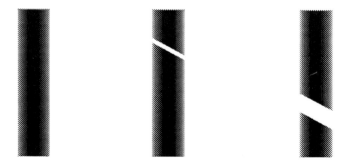

Fig. 1. Normal sinogram and a simulated 100 % depression of a bucket and of a block.

RESULTS

A decreasing sensitivity of a block or bucket shows an increasing inhomogeneity in transversal slices. This growing inhomogeneity is observed with bucket or blocks defects of greater than 50 %. A complete break down of a block increases inhomogeneity from 2 % to 6.5 %. A complete break down of a bucket increases inhomogeneity to 13 %. All values are calculated on simulated data.

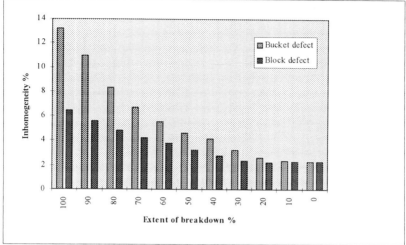

Fig. 2. Partial decrease of sensitivity as consequence of variable size of defect in sinogram, expressed as inhomogeneity.

Increased inhomogeneity is not a consequence of increased noise in transversal slices, but of a regional loss of sensitivity inclining in direction to the defect. An influence on geometric resolution measured in different activity hot spots was not seen. Although on visual inspection of the transversal slice a ray artifact became visible.

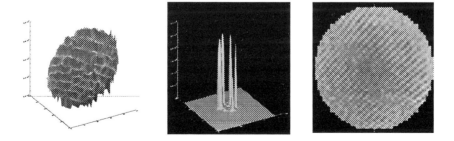

Fig. 3. Left: regional insensitivities in direction to defect ; middle: hot spot phantom with no resolution loss, right: ray artifact in direction to the defect.

CONCLUSION

The increased inhomogeneity is not a consequence of increasing statistical influence but of an inclining regional sensitivity loss up to 20 % in direction to the place of the defect block. A variation of geometrical resolution could not be measured. The visual inspection of reconstructed slices shows ray artifacts originating from the place of defect. In conclusion, PET-Scans acquired with one or more weak detectors, especially in quantitative studies, should be treated very carefully.

REFERENCES

1.   Reist HW,Stadelmann O, Kleeb W. Study on the stability of the calibration and normalization in PET and the influence of drifts on the accuracy of quantification. EurJNuclMed.1989;15(11):732-5

2. Kearfott KJ,Rucker RH. Median polish for quality assurance of a PET scanner. JComputAssistTomogr. 1989 Sep-Oct;13(5):932-9

3. Kearfott KJ. Long-term performance of a multiplanar positron emission tomograph. JNuclMed. 1989 Aug;30(8): 1378-85

4. Doll J, Ostertag HJ, Bellemann ME,Schmidlin P,Kübler WK, Strauss LG, Lorenz WJ. In: Radioactive Isotopes in Cinical Medicine and Research. Bermann H,Sinzinger H, editors. Basel: Birkhäuser Verlag, 1995: 85-90

Radioactive Isotopes in
Clinical Medicine and Research XXII
ed. by H. Bergmann, A. Kroiss and H. Sinzinger
© 1997 Birkhäuser Verlag Basel/Switzerland

Bremsstrahlung Planar and SPECT Imaging: Resolution and Contrast Analysis and Activity Quantitation

Busca F, Lazzari S, Sarti G

"Bufalini" Hospital Cesena, Health Physics Department
Viale Ghirotti 286, I-47023 Cesena, Italy

SUMMARY: Recently Y90, a pure beta emitter, has been raising a great interest in radioimmunotherapy; infact the beta radiation fits very well the problem of cancer penetration without transferring too much energy outside its boundaries. Anyway it's necessary to develope a specific acquisition method in order to acquire Bremsstrahlung images. We used the method suggested by De Nardo and Others about the choice of the energy window and of the collimator, to make contrast and spatial resolution measures. Bremsstrahlung Images have a lower resolution and activity than images obtained using a gamma emmitter; then we used the Chang algorithm to compensate the photon attenuation in SPECT : in fact that algorithm enhances the image strongerly and more precisely than traditional ones, so that it's very suitable to correct the blurred Bremsstrahlung images.

INTRODUCTION

As the Bremsstrahlung spectrum is continuous and the emission is concentrated at low-medium energies and not much abundant, it's necessary to acquire using a large energy window. The aim of this work is to show the results of a large energy window and ME collimator application, and last of an attenuation correction method in quantitative imaging.

METHOD AND MATERIALS

We used a 55-285keV energy window and a ME collimator (when requested). Because of the lower photon emission than for gamma emitters, we made a uniformity test using a 180MBq point source at 2.5m far from the crystal, without collimator (FOV=500mm).

We used the same geometry for acquisition with the bar phantom, in order to measure the intrinsec spatial resolution (without collimator).

About the system spatial resolution, we put the point source about 6cm far from the ME collimator and acquired 4 images: 2 in air and 2 using plexiglass as scatter material; both the former and the latter 2 images were acquired one using energy correction maps and one not. Then we measured the FWHM and MTF, calculated on LSF; MTF (which represents the system frequency response) is a more precise tool than FWHM.

On the same images we calculated the S/B=(Cs-Cb)/Cb, with Cs= source counts and Cb= background counts, and the %FOV= source counts/total counts. The former parameter measures the contrast, the latter one evaluates the scatter effect.

In order to calculate the effective linear attenuation coefficient μ, we used a 10ml spherical Y90 source: fixed the depth (x in cm) we acquired one image in air (No) and one in water (N). Than we made a best fit using the exponential decay law: $N=NoEXP[-\mu x]$. At last, in order to calculate the beta activity of an image, we calculated a proportional coefficient between the real activity (Ci or Bq) and the calculated counts (cps) of a apherical Y90 source. To make that we acquired some SPECTs, then corrected once by the Chang and once by the Hyperbolic Sine one. We made a best fit using a linear relationship, and compared the two techniques. The ROIs were selected using an hystogram method for the threshold evaluation.

RESULTS.

We obtained an integral nonuniformity equal to 4% and a differential nonuniformity equal to 2%, on CFOV, which are two good results for a pure Beta source.

The intrinsec resolution was about 3mm. We could distinguish well the lines uptp 3.2mm distance, and 2,8mm bars too, even if not perfectly.

In system resolution we realized using energy maps was useless. The FWHM was the same also with or without scatter material: 15mm. That means resolution is good in clinical conditions too. MTF which is a more precise tool for resolution measurement, falls zero before 0.5cycles/cm: very quickly. That's a physical limit of Bremsstrahlung images.

S/B was about 30 without plexiglass and 60 with it, near the source. It's a reasonable value, even if not excellent: that is, source and background are well separated. The %FOV was 12% without plexiglass and 18% with it: those results show that scatter effect isn't much interesting for Bremsstrahlung images, in fact the 2 values are very similar.

It was calculated an effective linear attenuation coefficient $\mu=0.14$ cm^{-1} that is a value compatible with literature. We used it in Chang algorithm.

In quantitative analysis we calculated a proportional coefficient equal to 1.02 μCi/cps, using Chang method, and equal to 28.8 μCi/cps using Hyperbolic Sine method. Even if the correlation was very good in both cases, the Chang correction is more suitable than traditional algorithm because it enhances the image activity much more. So that it's better not to trust on Hyperbolic Sine correction for low activity measurements.

CONCLUSION.

Unfortunately Bremsstrahlung images haven't the high resolution of gamma ones, because of the large spectrum. That is shown also by the low frequency response (MTF) and by the contrast (S/B) not so high near the source. Anyway the spatial resolution is reasonable, in clinical conditions too. The FWHM=15mm means that the cancer is recognizable but it will always appear 15mm sized at least, and it will be difficult to distinguish 2 near cancers.

It's possible to make quantitation on image too, but it's necessary to use the Chang correction to compensate photon attenuation, because the traditional methods are not suitable for low activity measures.

REFERENCE.

Shen S, DeNardo GL, Yuan A, DeNardo D, DeNardo SJ.Planar Gamma Camera Imaging and Quantitation of Yttrium-90 Bremsstrahlung.J Nucl Med 1994;35:1381-1389

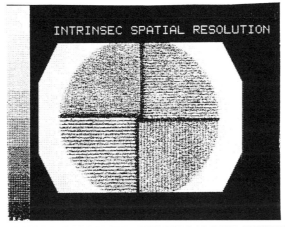

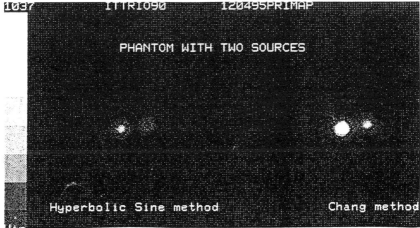

LSF with and without
energy correction maps

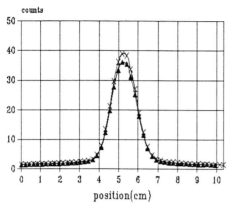

✳ without energy maps ★ with energy maps

MTF

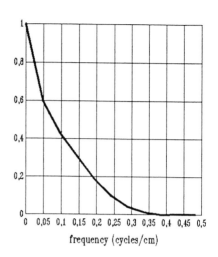

Linear Attenuation Coefficient μ

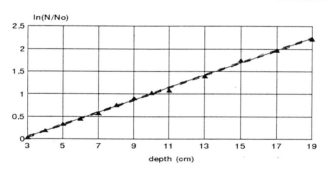

proportional coefficient for Y90
Hyperbolic Sine correction

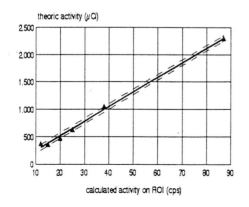

proportional coefficient for Y90
Chang correction

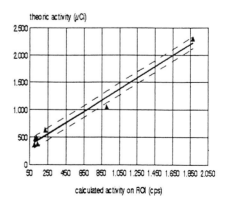

Poster Session II: Radiopharmacology

Radioactive Isotopes in
Clinical Medicine and Research XXII
ed. by H. Bergmann, A. Kroiss and H. Sinzinger
© 1997 Birkhäuser Verlag Basel/Switzerland

STANNOUS ION DETERMINATION: IMPORTANCE AND RELEVANCE FOR RADIOPHARMACEUTICAL KITS

F. Rakias and I. Zolle[*]

National Institute of Pharmacy, Budapest, Hungary
[*]Univ. Klinik für Nuklearmedizin, Radiopharmakologie, AKH Wien, Austria

SUMMARY

A new polarographic method was developed for the determination of tin in the +2- and +4-oxidation state using a square wave polarographic technique. Tin(II) may be determined in 1N sulphuric acid or, using 1N hydrochloric acid and ammoniumchloride buffer as electrolyte solution, both tin(IV) and tin(II) may be quantified in one run. The validation of the method was demonstrated with two HM-PAO kits, namely TromboScint and LeucoScint.

INTRODUCTION

Radiopharmaceutical kits for labelling with ^{99m}Tc-eluate contain tin(II)-ion for the reduction of sodium pertechnetate to lower valency states, which are chemically reactive. It is known that tin(II) salts are easily oxydized, even by the oxygen in air (1). Certain chemicals are also assumed to enhance the oxidation of tin(II) to tin(IV). Therefore, the determination of "active" tin(II) in radiopharmaceutical kits is an important aspect of quality assurance.

We had developed a sensitive method for the spectrophotometric analysis of tin(II) and tin(IV) in radiopharmaceutical kits (unpublished results), however the disadvantages of sample preparation and the slow formation of the coloured complex for absorption measurements have lead us to investigate pulse polarography because of its speed and high selectivity (2). Thus, square wave voltametry has been extended to the measurement of microgram amounts of tin(II) in radiopharmaceutical kits.

The two kits, TromboScint and LeucoScint differ simply by the fact that LeucoScint contains twice the amount of active ingredients, i.e., 0.18 mg HM-PAO and 2.28 µg stannous chloride-dihydrate. LeucoScint is used for labelling leucocytes, and TromboScint is suitable for labelling platelets.

MATERIALS AND METHODS

Apparatus:

- EG & G polarographic analyser (model 384) with a static mercury drop electrode (model 303), and a calomel reference electrode, made in USA. Model 384 is a microprocessor-based polarographic analyser with built-in floppy disc memory to store and recall analytical curves. By controlling each step of the analysis, the microprocessor automates polarographic and voltametric measurements. All experimental parameters may be chosen by the operator. Concentrations are computed automatically and recorded in the range from 0.001 ppb to 9999 ppm.

Chemicals:

- Solvents and reagents were obtained from commercial sources and were analytical grade.
- All solvents were deoxygenated by passing-through nitrogen gas for a minimum of 10 minutes.
- Oxygen-free water was obtained by passing nitrogen gas through 300 mL water for injection for about 30 minutes.

Square wave voltametry of tin(II) and tin(IV)

5 mL of deoxygenated 1N hydrochloric acid + 4N ammoniumchloride buffer (1:1, v/v) was transferred to the dry cell. Sample solutions were prepared by dissolving one kit in 5 mL of 1N hydrochloric acid + 4N ammoniumchloride buffer. This amount was added to the electrolyte solution and recording was started from 0.0 to 0.6 V with the following measuring conditions: scan increment 2 mV, frequency 100 Hz, 10 cycles. The tin(IV)-maximum appeared at -0.25 V and the tin(II) maximum at -0.45 V, as the second peak. If only 1N sulfuric acid is used as an electrolyte, tin(II) may be detected selectively at -0.45 V.

Validation of method

Determination of instrument linearity:

A standard dilution of tin(II) of 1 - 5 mg/mL was used for calibration of the instrument. Linearity was expressed by the correlation coefficient.

Precision of method: A statistically adequate number of samples were measured. From the results we have calculated the mean value, the standard deviation and the coefficient of variation as percent. Since measurements are also affected by the added sample volume, 10 aliquots of a homogenous solution of tin(II) chloride containing 1.14 µg and 2.28 µg of tin(II), respectively, were added to the matrix samples.

Accuracy: Known concentrations of tin(II) (1.14 and 2.28 µg) together with the matrix samples were analyzed twice. Accuracy is expressed by dividing the recovered amount of tin(II) by the added amount of tin(II). A recovery between 97.5 to 102.5% was accepted.

Selectivity: The selectivity of the method was investigated by adding 2 µg of tin(IV) to the test solution. Two sets of samples were analyzed 4-times, with/without addition of 2 µg tin(IV). Data of both determinations were subjected to the Student's 't' test (3).

RESULTS AND DISCUSSION

Classical methods for the determination of tin(II) include the titration with an iodate standard solution, or absorption measurements by spectrophotometric analysis. Both methods have considerable disadvantages for the determination of tin(II) in radiopharmaceutical kits.

Pulse polarography has offered considerable advantages for the determination of the tin(II) content in a number of radiopharmaceutical kits (2). Square wave voltametry shows a considerable increase in sensitivity, suitable for the measurement of very small amounts of tin(II), as used for the reduction of ^{99m}Tc-Na-pertechnetate when labelling radiopharmaceuticals.

Instrument linearity: To identify the highest amount of tin(II) that can be measured with a linear response we have analyzed increasing concentrations of tin(II) up to 5 mg/mL.
A typical calibration curve is shown in Fig. 1. Linear regression analysis of the data showed a correlation coefficient >0.999, indicating linearity of measurements over a wide range of concentrations.

Precision of the method: Measurements were performed with 10 samples of each kit. In the case of TromboScint, the average value of Sn(II) was determined as 1.138 µg/kit (theoretically 1.14 µg Sn(II)/vial) with a standard deviation of 0.050 µg and a coefficient of variation of 4.39%.

In the case of LeucoScint, the average value of Sn(II) was calculated as 2.263 µg/kit (theoretically 2.28 µg Sn(II)/vial), with a standard deviation of 0.089 µg and a coefficient of variation of 3.93% (Table 1).

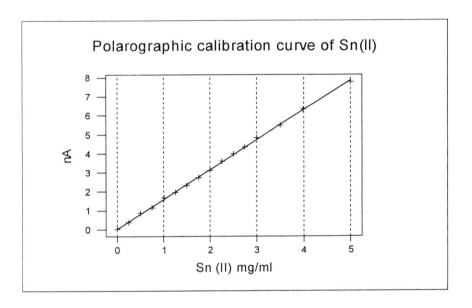

Figure 1.   Calibration curve using increasing amounts of Sn(II) up to 5 mg/mL

Effect of sample volume: Since the vials were filled with 1.0 mL of the dissolved kit content in the production department, there might have been a variation in the amount of tin(II) actually added in this volume. Therefore we have also investigated the precision of the method by analyzing 10 matrix samples to which a homogenous solution of tin(II) chloride containing 1.14 µg and 2.28 µg of tin(II), respectively, had been added. When these known concentrations of tin(II) were analyzed together with the matrix samples, the results were identical with the data shown in Table 1, excluding a volume effect. A recovery between 92.10 and 106.14% was observed (Table 2). The average value of Sn(II) in case of TromboScint was 1.139 µg/kit, with a standard deviation of 0.048 and a coefficient of variation of 4.21%. In case of LeucoScint the average value of Sn(II) was 2.266 µg/kit, with a standard deviation of 0.062 and a coefficient of variation of 2.73% (Table 2).

Table 1.   **Determination of active tin(II)-ion by square wave voltametry**
Precision of method

	TROMBOSCINT 1.14 µg Sn(II)/vial	LEUCOSCINT 2.28 µg Sn(II)/vial
	1.11	2.44
	1.24	2.31
	1.19	2.21
	1.16	2.24
	1.08	2.22
	1.07	2.15
	1.12	2.18
	1.13	2.21
	1.13	2.34
	1.15	2.33
Mean	1.138 ± 0.050	2.263 ± 0.089
Coefficient of Variation	± 4.39%	± 3.93%

Table 2.   **Determination of active tin(II)-ion using square wave voltametry**
Accuracy of method

	TROMBOSCINT µg Sn(II)/vial	Accuracy (%)	LEUCOSCINT µg Sn(II)/vial	Accuracy (%)
	1.13	99.12	2.34	102.63
	1.21	106.14	2.24	98.24
	1.21	106.14	2.25	98.68
	1.17	102.63	2.22	97.37
	1.11	97.36	2.21	96.93
	1.05	92.10	2.21	96.93
	1.13	99.12	2.19	96.05
	1.12	98.24	2.34	102.63
	1.12	98.24	2.35	103.07
	1.14	99.99	2.31	101.31
Mean	1.139 ± 0.048	99.91	2.266 ± 0.062	99.38
Coefficient of Variation	± 4.21%		± 2.73%	

Selectivity: Although it is stated in the literature that Sn(IV) does not interfere with the measurement of Sn(II), we have obtained experimental proof adding 2 µg of tin(IV) to the test solution. When no tin(IV) was added to TromboScint, the average value of Sn(II) was determined as 1.141 µg/kit, with a standard deviation of 0.068 µg and a coefficient of variation of 5.96%. With tin(IV) added to TromboScint, the average value of Sn(II) was determined as 1.126 µg/kit, with a standard deviation of 0.055 µg and a coefficient of variation of 4.88%. Values demonstrating no interference by Sn(IV) are also shown for LeucoScint (Table 3).

Table 3.   **Determination of tin(II)-ion in the presence of Sn(IV)-ion using square wave voltametry**

	TROMBOSCINT		LEUCOSCINT	
	µg Sn(II)/vial without Sn(IV)	µg Sn(II)/vial with 2 µg Sn(IV)	µg Sn(II)/vial without Sn(IV)	µg Sn(II)/vial with 2 µg Sn(IV)
	1.02	1.12	2.41	2.24
	1.09	1.21	2.14	2.47
	1.18	1.08	2.21	2.19
	1.22	1.06	2.24	2.23
	1.21	1.09	2.46	2.41
	1.12	1.20	2.33	2.18
	1.18	1.10	2.22	2.17
	1.11	1.15	2.12	2.22
Mean	1.141 ± 0.068	1.126 ± 0.055	2.266 ± 0.122	2.263 ± 0.112
Coefficient of Variation	± 5.96%	± 4.88%	± 5.38%	± 4.95%

The Student 't' test indicated in case of TromboScint a probability of $t = 0.5150$, and $t_{(0.05, 8)} = 1.761$. In case of LeucoScint $t = 0.5322$, and $t_{(0.05, 8)} = 1.761$. Since $t < t_{(0.05, 8)}$, the 2 populations are similar or in other words, Sn(IV) has no significant effect on the determination of Sn(II).

CONCLUSION

Square wave voltametry has been adapted for the measurement of microgram amounts of tin(II) in radiopharmaceutical kits with high accuracy (>99%). Impurities causing oxidation to tin(IV) have been shown to have no effect on the recovery. Based on the obtained data, square wave voltametry has been shown as a reliable and highly sensitive method for the determination of tin(II) in radiopharmaceutical kits.

REFERENCES

1. Eckelman W, Meinken G, Richards P. Chemical state of Tc-99m in biomedical products. J Nucl Med 1971; 12: 596-600.

2. Rakias F, Kelemen-Küttel I, Tömpe P, Nemeth P, Paal TL. Correlation between the Sn(II)-content of phosphon, fyton, and glucon kits and the quality of the obtained images. In: Radioaktive Isotope in Klinik und Forschung, Band 18, Herausgeber R. Höfer und H. Bergmann, Schattauer Stuttgart, 1988: 417-419.

3. Booster P. In: Statistische Methoden im Laboratorium. Agon Elsevier, 1982: 118-124.

Radioactive Isotopes in
Clinical Medicine and Research XXII
ed. by H. Bergmann, A. Kroiss and H. Sinzinger
© 1997 Birkhäuser Verlag Basel/Switzerland

FEASIBILITY OF THE NONINVASIVE EVALUATION OF GLUCOSE UPTAKE IN SKELETAL MUSCLE USING ^{18}F-FLUORODEOXYGLUCOSE AND A PROBE.

P.G.H.M. Raijmakers, J.J. Bax, F.C. Visser, A. van Lingen,
R. Lengauer, G.J.J Teule.

Free University Hospital Amsterdam, The Netherlands.

SUMMARY: We investigated the feasibility of assessing glucose uptake in skeletal muscle with ^{18}F-fluorodeoxyglucose (FDG) and a probe placed over the upper leg. We studied 6 individuals without diabetes on 2 separate occasions: 1. during hyperinsulinemic glucose clamping and 2. after an overnight fast. Clamping resulted in a significant rise of plasma insulin and a lowering of free fatty acids. Glucose uptake was significantly increased after clamping compared to overnight fasting. This technique represents a simple, noninvasive tool to study glucose uptake in skeletal muscle.

INTRODUCTION

Skeletal muscle plays an important role in glucose homeostasis. Several conditions are characterized by abnormalities in glucose metabolism in skeletal muscle. For example, in patients with type 2 diabetes skeletal muscle glucose disposal is reduced. The tracer ^{18}F-fluorodeoxyglucose (FDG) in combination with positron emission tomography (PET) can be used to study glucose uptake in skeletal muscle (1). Recently, we studied tracer kinetics in the lung using a mobile probe system (2). External detection of radiation with a mobile detection unit allows bedside studies of tracer kinetics in different clinical conditions (2). The aim of the present study was to assess the feasibility of assessing glucose uptake in skeletal muscle using FDG and a mobile probe system. Using this technique we evaluated the influence of hyperinsulinemic euglycemic clamping and overnight fasting on glucose uptake in skeletal muscle in nondiabetic individuals.

MATERIALS AND METHODS

Patients & Study Protocol. Six individuals without diabetes mellitus were studied; 5 men and 1 woman with a mean age of 58±4 years. They had a mean body mass index of 23.4-±3.0 kg.m^{-2} and a fasting plasma glucose level of 5.2±0.4 mmol.l^{-1}. All individuals underwent 2 FDG studies within 1 week in random order. One study was performed after an overnight fast (protocol 1) and the other study was performed during hyperinsulinemic glucose clamping (protocol 2) (3). In protocol 1, 185 MBq FDG was injected intravenously after a 60 min waiting period. In protocol 2, 185 MBq FDG was administered after 60 min clamping. In both protocols, FDG uptake in skeletal muscle was evaluated during 30 min after tracer injection (see below).

Metabolic substrates. In both protocols, venous blood samples were drawn at the time of FDG injection (=at the start of probe measurement) and 30 min later (=at the end of probe measurement) to assess plasma levels of free fatty acids (FFA) and insulin. Glucose was determined every 10 min during the probe measurement.

Probe measurement. Patients were in the supine position and a scintillation detection probe, consisting of a sodium-iodine crystal (1.5·1.5 in., Canberra Packard, Ill.) fitted with a 2.025 cm thick lead collimator (inner diameter 4.45 cm), extending 7.5 cm in front of the crystal, was positioned over the leg, 15 cm cranial of the patella. The probe was connected with a Accuspec/NaI Plus Board (840651A, Canberra Packard, Ill.), installed in a personal computer (M300, Olivetti, Milan, Italy) (2). Starting at the time of injection of FDG, radioactivity was detected in 10 sec frames for the first 2.5 min and in 30 sec frames for the remaining 27.5 min. The 511 keV peak of FDG was used, with a window of 20%. Count rates were corrected for background radioactivity and physical half-live. At 2,3,4,5,7,10,15,20,25 and 30 min after FDG injection, a total of 10 blood samples (2 ml) were drawn from an indwelling i.v. cannula. Each blood sample was weighed and radioactivity of one ml blood was measured by a sodium-iodine well-counter (Berthold, Betron Scientific, Rotterdam, The Netherlands). Also a window of ±20% at the 511 keV peak was used and results were expressed as CPM.g^{-1}.

We used the graphical analysis by Patlak et al (4) to quantify the rate of tracer phosphorylation and therefore trapping of the tracer in the leg (4). Briefly, the X-axis represents the ratio of the intregal of plasma FDG activity divided by the serial FDG plasma activity.

The Y-axis represents the ratio of the leg FDG activity and the time-matched plasma FDG activity. Lineair regression yields a slope constant wich represents the rate constant of FDG uptake in the leg: the K_{FDG}.

Statistical analysis. Data are presented as mean $\pm$ 1 SD. Comparison of the means were made with the (un-) paired Student t test. A P-value $\leq$ 0.05 was considered significant.

RESULTS

Table 1. Metabolic substrates during probe measurement in both protocols.

	Protocol 1	Protocol 2	P-value
Glucose (mmol.l^{-1})	5.2±1.1	4.8±0.6	NS
FFA (mmol.l^{-1})	0.05±0.06	0.36±0.21	<0.01
Insulin (mU.l^{-1})	109.1±24.7	7.3±1.7	<0.01

Protocol 1: overnight fast; protocol 2: hyperinsulinemic euglycemic clamp; FFA: free fatty acids.

During both protocols, plasma levels of glucose, insulin and FFA were constant. The differences between both protocols in metabolic conditions are presented in Table 1. Glucose levels were not significantly different between both protocols. FFA levels were higher in protocol 1, whereas insulin levels were significantly higher in protocol 2.

The K_{FDG} values were significantly lower during protocol 1 as compared to protocol 2: 0.072±0.052 versus 0.026±0.012 (P<0.05). Figure 1 demonstrates the individual K_{FDG} values in both protocols.

DISCUSSION

This study demonstrated the feasibility of assessing FDG (as an indicator of glucose uptake) in skeletal muscle using a mobile probe system. It is well-known that glucose uptake in skeletal muscle is dependent on levels of various substrates, including FFA and insulin (5). While high FFA levels inhibit glucose uptake, high levels of insulin increase glucose uptake (5). In this study we compared FDG uptake after overnight fasting (with high FFA and low insulin levels) with FDG uptake after hyperinsulinemic clamping (with low FFA and high insulin levels). The K_{FDG} values were higher after clamping, indicating increased FDG (and glucose) uptake under these conditions.

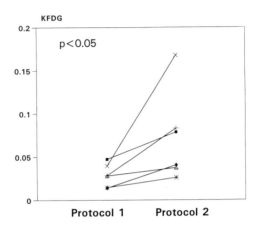

Figure 1. Individual K_{FDG} values obtained after overnight fasting (protocol 1) versus after hyperinsulinemic clamping (protocol 2). Significantly higher K_{FDG} values were obtained after clamping.

This new approach allows a simple, noninvasive assessment of glucose uptake in skeletal muscle and may be useful in patients with diabetes mellitus or altered insulin sensitivity. Further studies in these patients are warranted.

REFERENCES

1. Voipo-Pulkki L, Nuutila P, Knuuti MJ et al. Heart and skeletal muscle glucose disposal in type 2 diabetic patients as determined by positron emission tomography. J Nucl Med 1993;34:2064-2067.

2. Raijmakers PGHM, Groeneveld ABJ, Schneider AJ et al. Transvascular transport of ^{67}Ga in the lungs after cardiopulmonary bypass surgery. Chest 1993;104:1825-1832.

3. DeFronzo RA, Tobin JD, Andres R. Glucose clamp technique: A method for quantifying insulin secretion and resistance. Am J Physiol 1979;237:E214-E223.

4. Patlak CS, Blasberg RG. Graphical evaluation of blood-to-brain transfer constants from multiple-time uptake data. J Cereb Blood Flow Metabol 1985;5:584-589.

5. Nuutila P, Koivisto VA, Knuuti MJ et al. Glucose-free fatty acid cycle operates in human heart and skeletal muscle in vivo. J Clin Invest 1992;89:1767-1774.

Radioactive Isotopes in
Clinical Medicine and Research XXII
ed. by H. Bergmann, A. Kroiss and H. Sinzinger
© 1997 Birkhäuser Verlag Basel/Switzerland

PHARMACOKINETIC EVALUATION OF TWO MONOCLONAL ANTIBODIES AS POSSIBLE IMMUNOSCINTIGRAPHY AGENTS FOR PANCREATIC CANCER IN HUMANS

N. Molea[1], L. Bodei[1], E. Lazzeri[1], D. Bacciardi[1], P.C. Giulianotti[2], D. Balestracci[2],

P. Viacava[4], D. Campani[4], L. Di Luca[3], P.A. Salvadori[3], C. Bonino[5], D.V. Gold[6],

R.M. Sharkey[6], D.M. Goldenberg[6], F. Mosca[2] and G. Mariani[7]

[1]Regional Center of Nuclear Medicine, [2]Institute of General and Vascular Surgery, and
[3]Institute of Morbid Anatomy of the University of Pisa, [4]CNR Institute of Clinical Physiology,
Pisa, [5]SORIN Biomedica, Saluggia (Italy); [6]Center for Molecular Medicine and Immunology,
Newark, NJ 07103 (USA); and [7]Nuclear Medicine Service, DIMI, University of Genoa,
Genoa (Italy).

SUMMARY: In this study we evaluated the biodistribution and potential usefulness for tumor immunoscintigraphy of two recently developed monoclonal antibodies (MoAbs), termed AR-3 and PAM4, in patients with pancreatic cancer. The two MoAbs were labeled with ^{131}I, and their biodistribution and pharmacokinetics were assessed in 5 patients each. The plasma clearance curves of both MoAbs exhibited a biexponential pattern of decay, with average $T_{1/2}$ values equal to 4-6 hours and 40-60 hours, respectively for the fast and the slow components. While imaging with ^{131}I-AR-3 was dubious or weakly positive, immunoscintigraphy with ^{131}I-PAM4 more clearly outlined tumor lesions, both the primary site and locoregional recurrences, particularly at late times after injection (starting usually at about 72-96 hours).

INTRODUCTION

The mucin-like tumour-associated antigen CAR-3, expressed at immunohistochemistry by over 85% of human pancreatic adeno-carcinomas, is defined by the murine IgG_1 monoclonal antibody (MoAb) AR-3 (1,2), which shows favourable tumour-targeting properties in the experimental animal model (3). PAM4 (originally raised against mucin purified from xeno-grafted RIP1 human pancreatic carcinoma) is another MoAb that shows a higher than 85% reactivity with pancreatic adenocarcinomas (4). The high specificity of both MoAbs and their immunoreactivity with pancreatic carcinoma antigens with a secretory-like distribution pattern, particularly intense in the case of PAM4, suggested their potential usefulness as radiolabeled agents for *in vivo* imaging. The aim of the study was to evaluate the tissue biodistribution pharmacokinetics of ^{131}I-AR-3 and ^{131}I-PAM4 in humans, in order to assess their possible clinical use for immunoscintigraphy in patients with pancreatic cancer.

MATERIALS AND METHODS

After labeling the MoAbs with ^{131}I by the iodogen technique and pretreating the patients with potassium iodide, the two tracers (spec. act. 185 MBq/mg) were each administered to five patients (37 MBq as an i.v. bolus) scheduled for surgery because of high-degree suspicion of pancreatic cancer; after the immunoscintigraphic study, pancreatic cancer was confirmed at surgery in eight out of the ten patients. Whole-body scans and spot-views at selected sites were recorded from 0-144 hours by a computerized gamma-camera. Blood samples were also taken at frequent intervals to determine the radioactivity plasma clearance curves, and cumulative urine collection was performed at daily intervals to determine radioactivity removal through the renal route. Scintigraphic images were first interpreted in a totally blind fashion, then reviewed with full knowledge of the surgical results.

RESULTS

No severe adverse clinical reactions of any type were observed in the patients during the study, nor were any abnormal results found in the routine blood chemistry tests performed at the end of the study. However, in one patient injected with ^{131}I-PAM4 an important uptake of activity in the lungs was observed immediately after injection. This was not linked to protein macro-aggregates present in the injectate, although the possibility still exists that particulates were formed due to the presence of, *e.g.*, cold agglutinins circulating in the patient.

Both ^{131}I-MoAbs exhibited similar biodistribution pharmacokinetics, with a biexponential plasma disappearance curve characterized by an initial distribution component with $T_{1/2}$ values ranging from 4 to 6 hours, followed by a slow, terminal component ($T_{1/2}$ 40 to 60 hours).

Nonspecific uptake in the liver, spleen and bone marrow was very low for both tracers, virtually due to the radioactive contents of circulating blood only. When evaluated in a totally blind fashion, ^{131}I-AR-3 immunoscintigraphy did not show clear-cut uptake in tumors; in fact, dubious or weakly positive results were observed in four patients with pancreatic cancer (at 24-48 hours p.i.), while the fifth patient of this group was a true-negative case.

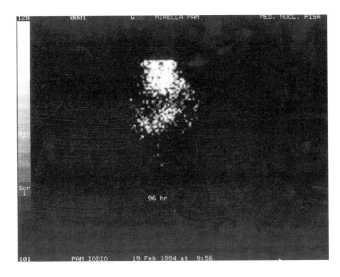

Fig. 1 - Spot view of the abdomen recorded in patient GM01 96 hours after injection of MoAb ^{131}I-PAM4-IgG$_1$. The bulky pancreatic cancer of this patient is clearly outlined (indicated by the arrows), while there is still obvious radioactivity circulating in the cardiac blood pool at this relatively late time after injection.

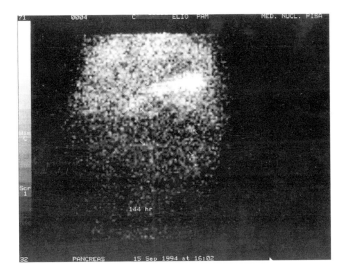

Fig. 2 - Spot view of the abdomen recorded in patient CE04 144 hours after injection of MoAb ^{131}I-PAM4-IgG$_1$. The arrows point to the primary pancreatic cancer, as well as to some of the peritoneal metastatic implants present in this patient (visualization of the gastric area, on the left, is due to free radioiodide). Fast accumulation of the radiolabeled MoAb at these sites of diffuse tumour spreading caused the early, important drop in circulating radioactivity observed in this patient soon after tracer injection (reducing circulating activity to about 30% the levels observed in the other patients at the same time-points).

Immunoscintigraphy with ^{131}I-PAM4 showed, instead, clear radioactivity accumulation in both the primary and recurrent or metastatic tumour lesions, especially at late times post-injection (72-96 hours): four of these patients were true-positive (see Fig. 1) and one was a true-negative case. However, while liver metastases appeared as cold areas during the initial distribution phase of the tracer and gradually accumulated radioactivity in the later scans (until 120-144 hours p.i.), in one patient with massive intraperitoneal metastases (see Fig. 2) the tumour lesions were detectable also in the earlier images (24-48 hours p.i.).

DISCUSSION

Pancreatic cancer is almost invariably fatal, both because it is one of the most aggressive malignant tumors and because its location and silent growth make it difficult to diagnose early by traditional imaging methodologies. Thus, any new diagnostic procedure possibly leading to the earlier detection of primary/recurrent lesions may have value in the management of patients with pancreatic cancer. Based on the favourable tumour-targeting results observed at immuno-histochemistry, we undertook this pilot study, as immunoscintigraphy with radiolabeled MoAbs has shown a considerable clinical usefulness in the non-invasive localization of tumour lesions.

The results obtained point in particular at ^{131}I-PAM4 as a potential tracer for immunoscintigraphy in patients with primary or recurrent pancreatic cancer, but also suggest the possible advantage of using the faster clearance F(ab')$_2$ fragments of both MoAbs, in order to increase the target/background ratios at earlier imaging times and to improve the overall image quality.

REFERENCES

1. Prat M, Morra I, Bussolati G, Comoglio PM. CAR-3, a monoclonal antibody-defined antigen expressed on human adenocarcinomas. *Cancer Res* 1985; 45: 5799-807.

2. Prat M, Medico E, Rossino P, Garrino C, Comoglio PM. Biochemical and immunological properties of the human carcinoma-associated CAR-3 epitope defined by the monoclonal antibody AR-3. *Cancer Res* 1989; 49: 1415-21.

3. Brusa P, Pietribiasi F, Bussolati G *et al.* Blocked and not blocked whole-ricin antibody immunotoxins: intraperitoneal therapy of human cancer xenografted in nude mice. *Cancer Immunol Immunother* 1989; 29: 185-92.

4. Gold DV, Lew K, Maliniak R, Hernandez M, Cardillo T. Characterization of monoclonal antibody PAM4 reactive with a pancreatic cancer mucin. *Int J Cancer* 1994; 57: 204-10.

Radioactive Isotopes in
Clinical Medicine and Research XXII
ed. by H. Bergmann, A. Kroiss and H. Sinzinger
© 1997 Birkhäuser Verlag Basel/Switzerland

PRELIMINARY STUDIES OF SOME ^{99m}Tc LABELED POTENTIAL MYOCARDIAL METABOLIC AGENTS IN RABBITS

J. Környei, M. Antalffy, I. Földes*, I. Szilvási**

Institute of Isotopes Co. Ltd. H-1121 Budapest, Konkoly Thege 29-33,
*Korvin Hospital, **Postgraduate Medical School Budapest, Hungary

SUMMARY: Four groups of new ligands have been designed, synthetized and labeled with [99m]Tc. Each compound possesses either "active" carboxyl groups for interaction with coenzym-A, or are conjugate of glucose, aspartic acid or cystein. Gamma camera imaging in rabbits were carried out and the heart was chosen as target organ. Two compounds, "ASPEC" and "CEPHACYS" were taken up by the myocardium up to 1.1 and 1.63 % of i.d., respectively.

INTRODUCTION

Designed molecules labeled with radionuclides (first of all with ^{99m}Tc) possess an increasing role in radiopharmaceutical chemistry.   In a previous work it was shown that beside the well known N_3S and N_2S_2 cores some surprising structures with proper geometrical arrangement of N, O, S atoms, such as thiazine and thiazolidine rings, can easily form stable complexes with [99m]Tc (1).   On the other hand new ^{99m}Tc-compounds would come into focus of interest if they could enter the myocardial metabolism as till now none of this kind of agents are used in nuclear cardiology.   In the recent work we present our efforts concerning design, labeling and biodistribution studies of new potential myocardial agents.

MATERIALS AND METHODS

Compounds have been designed in four groups according to the type of the complexing core and are shown in Fig. 1.

Group (I)

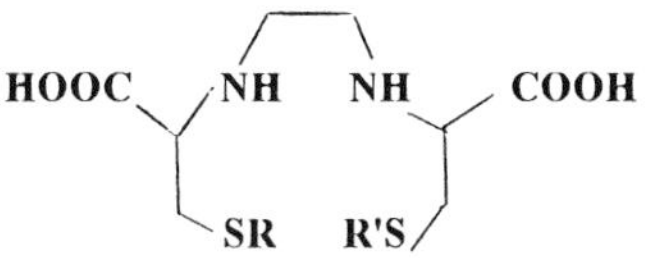

ECACA: R=R'= - CH₂ - COOH
FAEC: R=R'= -CH₂CONHCH₂CHCH₂COOH
                                            CH₃
ASPEC: R= -CH₂-CO-NH-CH-COOH
                                   CH₂COOH , R'=H

Group (II)

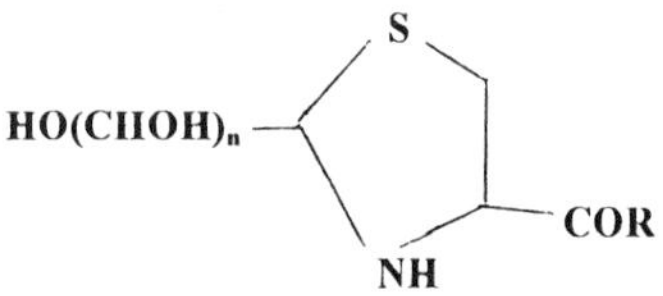

GLTIFA: R= -NH-CH₂-CH-CH₂-COOH
                                      CH₃
GLTI-ASPA-AC: R= -NH-CH-COOH
                                    CH₂-COOH

Group (III)

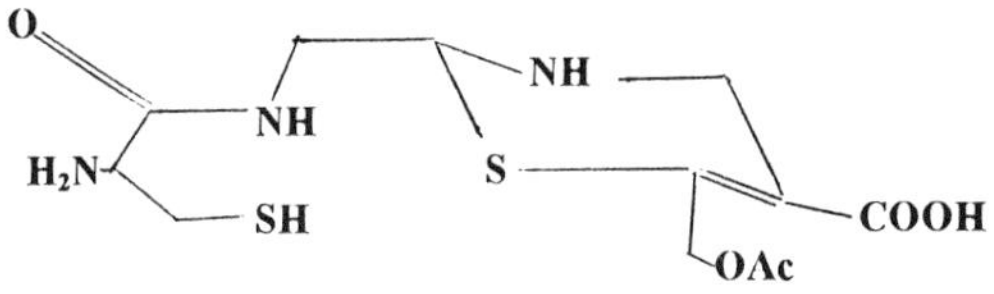

CEPHACYS

Group (IV)

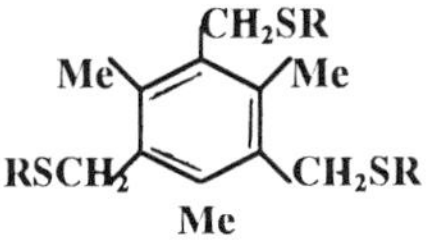

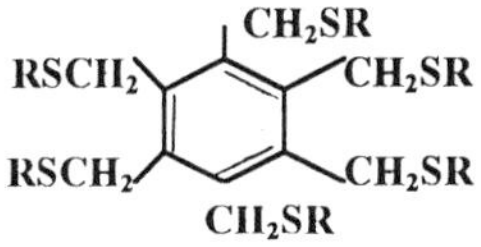

R= -CH₂COOH
        TRIAC   HEXAC

SR= thioglucosyl group
        TRIPS   HEXAPS

Fig. 1.

The new ligands designed, synthetized
and labeled with ^{99m}Tc.

- Derivatives of N,N'-ethylene-L,L-dicystein-(EC).
The EC was built further on its S-terminal with groups containing carboxymethyl groups targeting the interaction with Coenzym-A.
Three derivatives of EC were prepared: ECACA, FAEC and ASPEC, chemical formules are given in Fig. 1.- Group (I).
- Derivatives containing thiazolidine ring. Chemical formules of thiazolidin-4-carboxylic acid are shown in Fig. 1. - Group (II).
- Cystein-conjugate of the 7-amino-cephalosporanic acid can be considered as a new type of N_2S_2 ligands and is presented in Fig. 1.- Group (III).
- Glucose and carboxymethyl derivatives of mercaptomethylene benzene can be seen in Fig.1-Group (IV).

Labeling. All compounds were labeled with ^{99m}Tc in 0.15 phosphate buffer of pH=12 followed by neutralization. Radiochemical purity was determined by TLC method using ITLC SG and Kieselgel 60 layers developed in 5 % glycine and 95 % ethanol, respectively.
Gamma camera imaging was carried out by acquisition of 1 min. frames up to 40 min after i.v. injection. Pharmacokinetic data were obtained using ROI method concerning the heart, liver and kidneys. Maximal heart uptake as % of i.d. was determined by sacrificing the rabbits.

RESULTS

Labeling effficiency data as well as maximal myocardial uptake are listed in Table 1.

Table 1.

Compound	Labeling efficiency, %	Max. myocardial uptake, % of i.d.
ECACA	98.2	0.93
FAEC	90.9	1.04
ASPEC	95.6	1.10
GLTIFA	94.1	1.10
GLTI-ASPA-AC	93.7	0.90
CEPHACYS	96.5	1.63
TRIAC	92.1	0.60
HEXAC	97.3	0.90
TRIPS	94.2	0.55
HEXAPS	98.5	0.76

Pharmacokinetic data are presented in Table 2.

Table 2.
Heart/liver ratios, calculated from the ROI-s, as a function of time

Time, Compound	8 min.	12min.	20 min.	30 min.	40 min.
ECACA	1.40	1.32	1.24	1.00	0.90
FAEC	1.06	0.97	0.87	0.60	0.52
ASPEC	1.48	1.42	1.42	1.36	1.30
GLTIFA	1.22	1.06	0.96	0.90	0.78
GLTI-ASPA-AC	1.42	1.26	1.00	0.90	0.84
CEPHACYS	4.83	4.32	4.10	2.69	1.40
TRIAC	0.63	0.56	0.50	0.40	0.35
HEXAC	1.38	1.25	0.90	0.67	0.55
TRIPS	0.60	0.50	0.80	0.61	0.40
HEXAPS	1.03	0.83	0.80	0.61	0.57

DISCUSSION

It was observed that all the compounds investigated can be labeled with ^{99m}Tc. The new molecules containing new cores and/or designed groups can be taken up by the myocardium in different extent. It should be emphasized that the starting molecules, cores without being conjugated with carboxymethyl groups or glucose, aspartic acid, cystein, can be mainly considered as renal agents (2,3). On the other hand, the designed derivatives provide a relatively clear heart visualization due to the new functional groups conjugated. In case of "ASPEC" and "CEPHACYS" the strong myocardial bound was proved by comparing the myocardial activity before and after washing the heart in "ex-vivo" experiments. The activity decrease was not higher than 10 % in case of the two above mentioned compounds.

It can be established that the myocardial washing out is relatively fast in each case, represented by the decreasing heart/liver ratio as a function of the time. The major route of elimination is the urinary tract accompanied with some hepatobiliary excretion. The carboxymethyl derivatives might be considered as ^{99m}Tc analogs of ^{11}C acetate.

CONCLUSION

Two of the new compounds containing "active" carboxyl group
("ASPEC" and "CEPHACYS") showed myocardial uptake higher than
1 % up to 40-60 min p. i. . The role of the active carboxyl groups of
the new ^{99m}Tc compounds should be clarified in detailed investigations
in the near future.

REFERENCES

(1.) J. Környei, I. Szilvási, Z. Nagy, I. Földes.
      ^{99m}Tc labeling and biodistribution studies of designed molecules.
      in "Radioactive Isotopes In Clinical Medicine and Research,
      Birkhauser Verlag, Basel 1995, pp. 287-292.

(2.) A.M. Verbruggen, D.L. Nosco, Ch.G. Van Nerom, G.M. Bormans,
      P.J. Adriaens, M.J. De Roo.
      ^{99m}Tc-L,L-Ethylenedicysteine, a renal imaging agent
      J. Nucl. Med. 1992, 33, 551-557.

(3.) J. Környei, F. Sztaricskai, Z. Györgydeák, J. Pitlik:
      ^{99m}Tc labeling and biodistribution studies of some dihydro-1,4-
      thiazine and 1,4-thiazolidine carboxylic acid derivatives.
      J. Radioanal. Nucl. Chem. Letters 186 (1) 75-87 (1994).

Radioactive Isotopes in
Clinical Medicine and Research XXII
ed. by H. Bergmann, A. Kroiss and H. Sinzinger
© 1997 Birkhäuser Verlag Basel/Switzerland

EVALUATION OF TUMOUR RESISTANCE USING IODINE-123 LABELLED ANTHRACYCLINES IN CELL CULTURES

H. Wolf, W. Brenner, K.H. Bohuslavizki, C. Stauch, M. Clausen, St. Tinnemeyer, E. Henze

Clinic of Nuclear Medicine, Christian-Albrechts-University, Kiel, Germany

SUMMARY: The aim of this study was to label various anthracyclines (doxorubicin, iododo-xorubicin, daunorubicin) with I-123, and to determine their uptake both in sensitive and anthracycline-resistant tumour cell cultures compared to the standard [C-14]DOX. Three of the four anthracyclines showed different uptake in both cell lines. The uptake in resistant cells seems to be independent of the chemical structure of the anthracyclines, whereas the uptake in sensitive cells was affected by iodination.

INTRODUCTION

One limitation of cancer chemotherapy is the emergence of chemoresistant cell populations in malignant tumours. A well-known and extensively studied mechanism of resistance to cyto-toxics is the p-170 glycoprotein-associated multidrug resistance. P-170 decreases the intracellular concentration of several antineoplastic drugs by enhancing the efflux of the substance out of the cells [1]. Drug resistance to the widely used anthracyclines like doxorubicin (DOX), daunorubicin (DNR) and iododoxorubicin (IDOX) is known [2, 3]. Therefore, the aim of this study was to label DOX, IDOX and DNR with iodine-123 and to estimate the uptake kinetics of these radioiodinated anthracyclines in experimental cell cultures as a function of sensitive versus resistant tumour cells and to compare their uptake with $[^{14}C]$DOX.

MATERIALS AND METHODS

Radioiodination: DOX, IDOX (both from Farmitalia Carlo Erba, Milan, Italy) and DNR (Sigma Chemie, Deisenhofen, Germany) were radioiodinated by the Iodogen method [4]: 10 µg Iodogen (1,3,4,6-Tetrachloro-3α-6α-diphenylglycoluril, Pierce, Oud-Beijerland,

Netherlands) was plated onto the bottom of a test tube and 1 µg of the anthracycline, mixed with 100 µl phosphate buffer (pH 6.8) and I-123-iodide-solution (Amersham Buchler, Braunschweig, Germany), was added. After a reaction time of 60 min the radioiodinated tracer was separated by Sep-pak C-18 reversed-phase extraction cartridge (Millipore, Eschborn, Germany) in the ethanolic extraction solution. The ethanol was evaporated with a speedvac and the radioiodinated anthracyclines were taken up in isotonic solution. Radiochemical purity was higher than 98 % in all cases, and stability at room temperature was observed during 6 hours.

The resulting radiochemical yields (mean ± s.d., n = 10) for I-123–DOX, I-123–IDOX and I-123–DNR were 69,7% ± 8,3%, 58,2% ± 9,5% and 63,1% ± 7,9%, respectively.

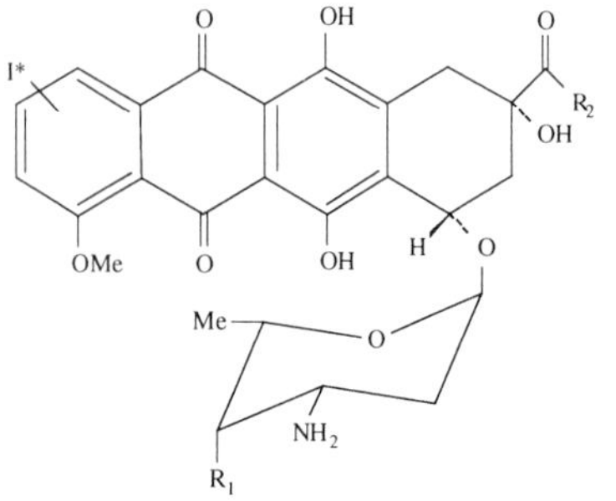

R1	R2	
H	OH	I-daunorubicin
OH	OH	I-doxorubicin
OH	I	I-iododoxorubicin

Fig. 1: Chemical structure of radioiodinated anthracyclines

Cell lines: The sensitive human gastric carcinoma cell line (EPG 85-257 P) and the daunoblastin resistant variant (EPG 85-257 DB) were maintained in L-15 medium (Boehringer Mannheim, Germany) supplemented with 50 ml fetal calf serum (Biochrom, Berlin, Germany), 2.5 ml L-glutamin (200 mmol/l, Biochrom, Berlin, Germany) and 1 ml gentamycin (0.05 mg/ml) per 500 ml. The resistant cell line shows the classical multidrug resistance phenotype in which anthracyclines are actively extruded from the resistent tumour cell via a P-glycoprotein-mediated process [5].

The cell lines grew well in vitro as a monolayer and had doubling times of approximately 35 h. A Fuchs-Rosenthal counting chamber was used for cell counting and the trypan blue exclusion method for viability determination was conducted using an inverted Leitz microscope. The total number of cells ranged from 2.1 to 3.5 million cells per tube with a median of 2.7 million. Cell viability was higher than 90 %.

Uptake measurements: The exponentially growing tumour cells were incubated with I-123-labelled anthracycline in a quantity of 3 kBq/ml medium for each test at 37 °C. Uptake was stopped at different incubation times (10 min to 4 h) by removing the medium. Subsequently, cells were cooled down to 4° C by washing 3 times with 10 ml cold saline solution, and cells were harvested with trypsin-EDTA (Biochrom, Berlin, Germany). The radioactivity was measured with a gamma well counter at constant geometry. Total activity per culture tube was obtained before removing the medium. The cellular uptake was determined after the washing phase.

The commercially available standard [C-14]DOX (Amersham, Braunschweig, Germany) was used in a quantity of 0.3 kBq/ml medium. The incubation and washing procedure was similar, only the measurements were done with a scintillation counter (Canberra Packard, Frankfurt/M., Germany).

Cellular uptake of the 4 tracers was determined in the sensitive cells and in the resistant variants in 60 culture tubes, each (n = 480). Cellular accumulation was normalized both to the activity added to the medium and to one million cells. After correction for physical decay, the results were expressed as a percentage of added activity.

RESULTS:

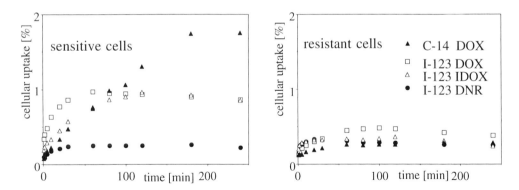

Fig. 2: Cellular uptake as percent of radioiodinated DOX, IDOX and DNR in comparison to [^{14}C]DOX in sensitive and resistant gastric carcinoma cells over time. Results are given as median (n = 5).

Seen in figure 2, the uptake of iodinated daunorubicin was low and very similar in both cell lines. Radioiodinated IDOX and DOX and [^{14}C]DOX showed approximately 2 to 5 times higher uptake in sensitive than in resistant cells. However, the kinetics of [^{14}C]DOX in the sensitive cells differed from the iodinated compounds.

The sensitive cells accumulated [^{14}C]DOX continuously up to a maximal uptake of 1.82 ± 0.23 %, whereas the highest uptake of I-123 DOX and I-123 IDOX was seen after 60 resp. 120 min. In the resistant cells a roughly time-independent uptake of approximately $0.25 \pm 0.1\%$ was observed for the tracers.

DISCUSSION

Cellular resistance to DOX in solid tumours is usually associated with cross-resistance to other anthracyclines [2, 5, 6]. In fact, in sensitive and in resistant gastric carcinoma cells used, differences in uptake of 3 of the 4 tracers were found. Up to 60 min of incubation time the uptake kinetics of [^{14}C]DOX, I-123-DOX and I-123-DOX were very similar. After an incubation time of 60 to 90 min the uptake was affected by iodination, seen in the sensitive cells. In contrast, in the used anthracycline-resistant cells all four tracers showed similar results, an only insignificant uptake of 0.25 %. The resistant cells did not differentiate between iodinated anthracyclines and the original molecule [^{14}C]DOX.

In conclusion, the uptake in sensitive cells was affected by iodination. In resistant cells, however the efflux mechanism seems to be independent of the chemical structure of the anthracyclines. Therefore, certain radioiodinated anthracyclines might be useful for prospective evaluation of tumour drug resistance in patients.

REFERENCES

1. Pastan I, Gottesman M. Multiple drug resistance in human cancer. N Engl J Med 1987; 316: 1388-1393.
2. Davis HL, Davis TE: Daunorubicin and adriamycin in cancer treatment: an analysis of their roles and limitations. Cancer Treat Rep 1979; 63: 809.
3. Mross KB, Mayer U, Hamm K, Burk K, Hossfeld KD. Pharmacokinetics and metabolism of iodo-doxorubicin and doxorubicin in humans. J Clin Pharmacol 1990; 39: 507-513.
4. Fraker PJ, Speck JC. Protein and cell membrane iodination with a sparingly soluble chloramide, 1,3,4,6-tetrachloro-5,6-diphenylglycouril. Biochem Biophys Res Commun 1978; 80: 849-857.
5. Seidel A, Hasmann M, Löser R, Bunge A, Schäfer B, Herzig I, Steidtmann K, Dietel M: Intracellular localization, vesicular accumulation and kinetics of daunorubicin in sensitive and multidrug-resistant gastric carcinoma EPG 85-257 cells. Virchows Archiv 1995; 426: 249-256.
6. Kaye S, Merry S: Tumor cell resistance to anthracyclines. A review. Cancer Chemother Pharmacol 1985; 14: 96.

Radioactive Isotopes in
Clinical Medicine and Research XXII
ed. by H. Bergmann, A. Kroiss and H. Sinzinger
© 1997 Birkhäuser Verlag Basel/Switzerland

PLATELET LABELING WITH ^{67}Ga (^{67}Ga-OXINE, -TROPOLONE, -MPO)

Karanikas G., Rodrigues Margarida*, Granegger Susanne, Havlik E., Sinzinger H.
Department of Nuclear Medicine, University of Vienna, Austria.

SUMMARY: ^{68}Ga-labeled platelets could be useful for positron emission tomographic studies (PET) of thrombosis and / or atherosclerosis. In order to identify the best chelate for radiolabeling of platelets with ^{68}Ga, we investigated the platelet uptake of ^{67}Ga (^{67}Ga-oxine, -tropolone, and -MPO). The influence of platelet-density (1.10^7-1.10^9), temperature ($4°$, $22°$ and $37°C$) and time (1, 5, 10, 20, 30 minutes) of incubation and the amount of radioactivity (0.01-$1\mu Ci/ml$), were analysed. The platelet uptake of ^{67}Ga-oxine and -tropolone is very low (5%). The platelet uptake of ^{67}Ga-MPO on the other hand increases with density of platelets (highest at 10^9 platelets/ml). The labeling efficiency is also dependent on both temperature ($37°C>22°C>4°C$) and time of incubation (highest at 30 minutes), but independent on the amount of radioactivity. Our data provide information about the ^{67}Ga (^{67}Ga-oxine, -tropolone, and -MPO) uptake and mechanism and may have some relevance for the clinical use of ^{68}Ga-labeled platelets for PET studies.

INTRODUCTION

Positron emission tomography (PET) is a new noninvasive diagnostic technique that permits reconstruction of cross-sectional images of the human body which depict the biodistribution of PET tracers. A large variety of physiological PET tracers is available and allows the in vivo investigation of organ perfusion, metabolism and biomolecular processes in normal and diseased states (1). Platelets labeled with generator produced ^{68}Ga could be useful for PET-studies of platelet behaviour in thrombosis and / or atherosclerosis (2). Preliminary reports of ^{68}Ga thrombus imaging in rabbits and dogs suggested that the method might be successfully applied to humans (4). In-vivo results indicate a good viability of ^{68}Ga-MPO-labeled autologous human platelets, but poor visualization of clots by PET imaging, due to the high blood background (5). Systematic in-vitro labeling data, however, are lacking so far. In order to identify the best chelate for radiolabeling of platelets with ^{68}Ga, we investigated the platelet labeling characteristics of ^{67}Ga (^{67}Ga-oxine, -tropolone, and -MPO).

---

*Dr. Margarida Rodrigues is on leave from the Oncology Hospital, Lisbon, Portugal.

MATERIAL AND METHODS

In-vitro studies

Platelet separation and labeling was performed using the technique described by Sinzinger (6).

Blood (7ml) was drawn from the cubital vein without occlusion into a Monovette vial using 2ml ACD as anticoagulant. After removing the handle, the Monovette vial was closed with a plug. Ten minutes were allowed for sedimentation of the red blood cells at room temperature. The vial was centrifuged at 150 g for 5 minutes. The supernatant platelet rich plasma (PRP) was transferred into a 10ml vial using a butterfly needle. The PRP-containing vial was centrifuged at 500 g for 10 min. The platelets were sedimented in a pellet at the bottom of the vial. The supernatant platelet poor plasma (PPP) was withdrawn, carefully preserving the pellet. The pellet in the vial was gently resuspended in 1ml tyrode buffer by shaking the tube gently; then the tracer was added (final concentration about 10 μg/ml). The vial was closed with the plug and incubated in a water bath at the respective temperature. The incubation mixture containing the labeled platelets was resuspended with the platelet-poor plasma preserved for this purpose. The solution-containing vial (pellet, tyrode buffer, tracer, PPP) was centrifuged at 4° C, at 500 g for 10 min. The platelets were sedimented again in a pellet at the bottom of the vial. The supernatant platelet poor plasma (PPP) was withdrawn, carefully preserving the pellet, and aspirated in another vial. The two vials (the first vial containing ^{67}Ga labelled platelets and the second one the supernatant) were counted in a gamma counter. The last step was to calculate the percent of radioactivity uptake by the platelets.

The influence of the following conditions in the above steps was examined: platelet-density (1.10^7, 1.10^8, 1.10^9 platelets / ml), amounted radioactivity (0.01, 0.1 and 1μCi ^{67}Ga-oxine, -tropolone, and -MPO), temperature (4°C, 22°C and 37°C) and time of incubation (1, 5, 10, 20, 30 minutes). Six probes of each combination of the following conditions were studied.

^{67}Ga-oxine, -tropolone and -MPO was obtained from the Department of Chemistry, Research Center, Seibersdorf, Austria.

Results are presented as mean values ± standard deviation; calculation for significance was carried out by Stambolidis Nikolaos. A *p<0.01 was considered as being significant.

RESULTS

The platelet uptake of ^{67}Ga-oxine and -tropolone is very low (5%). The platelet uptake of ^{67}Ga-MPO on the other hand increases with density of platelets (highest at 10^9 platelets/ml). The labeling efficiency is also dependent on both temperature (37°C, 22°C, 4°C) and time of incubation (highest at 30 minutes) (Figures 1, 2 and 3), but independent on the amount of radioactivity.

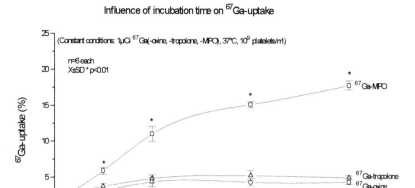

Figure 1.

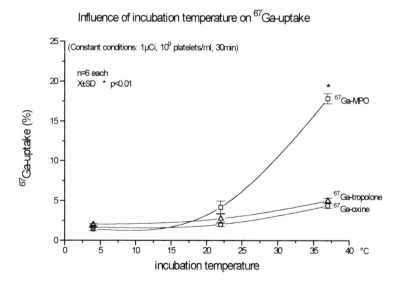

Figure 2.

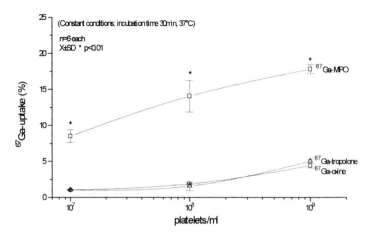

Figure 3.

DISCUSSION

Platelet scintigraphy not only reveals the location of the thrombus but also gives a nonivasive functional assessment of the thrombotic activity of the suspected structures. Since ^{111}In itself does not cross cell membranes, chelating agents have to be used in order to form a lipid-soluble complex for the labeling of platelets. Various chelators such as oxine, oxine-sulphate, tropolone, MPO, acetylacetone and chlorotetraphenylporphyrin have been studied in an attempt to achieve a high labeling efficiency without losing platelet viability (3). Results from in-vivo studies indicate good viability of ^{68}Ga-MPO-labeled autologous human platelets, while there was poor visualization only of clots by PET imaging, due to the high blood background at early times (5). Our in-vitro findings indicate a process being dependent on the cellular density, incubation temperature and time, independent on the amount of radioactivity and provide a minimal affinity of ^{67}Ga-oxine, -tropolone and a low affinity of ^{67}Ga-MPO as compared with those of ^{111}In-chelates.

References:

1. Huang SC , Hoffmann EJ , Phelps ME and Kuhl DE. Quantitation in positron emission tomography: 2.Effects of inaccurate attenuation correction. J Comput Assist Tomogr 3:804-814, 1979.

2. Yano Y. , Budinger T.F. , Ebbe S.N. , Mathis C.A. , Singh M. , Brennan K.M. and Moyer B.R. Gallium-68 lipophilic complexes for labeling platelets. J Nucl Med 26:1429-1437, 1985.

3. Rodrigues M. and Sinzinger H. Platelet labeling and clinical applications. Thromb Res 76: 399-432, 1994.

4. Welch M. J. , Thakur M. L. and Coleman R. E. Gallium-68 labeled red cells and platelets: new agents for positron tomography. J Nucl Med 18: 558-562, 1977.

5. Goodwin D.A. , Lang E. V , Atwood J.E. , Dalman R.L. , Ransone C.McK. , Diamanti C.I. and McTigue M. Viability and biodistribution of ^{68}Ga MPO labeled human platelets. Nucl Med Comm 14: 1023-1029, 1993.

6. Sinzinger H. , Kolbe H. , Strobl-Jäger E. and Höfer R.: A simple and safe technique for sterile autologous platelet labelling using "Monovette" vials. Eur J Nucl Med 9:320-322, 1984.

Radioactive Isotopes in
Clinical Medicine and Research XXII
ed. by H. Bergmann, A. Kroiss and H. Sinzinger
© 1997 Birkhäuser Verlag Basel/Switzerland

IMPROVED SYNTHESIS AND IN VITRO STABILITY TEST OF RHENIUM-188 LABELED RADIOPHARMACEUTICALS FOR POTENTIAL USE IN RADIATION SYNOVECTOMY

K.G. Grillenberger, S.N. Reske

Department of Nuclear Medicine, University Hospital, Ulm, Germany

SUMMARY: One therapeutic approach to rheumatoid arthritis and other inflammatory arthropathies besides surgical or chemical removal of inflamed synovium is radiation synovectomy using beta-emitting radionuclides to destroy the affected synovial tissue. In this study we compared ^{188}Re labeled hydroxyapatite particles and ^{188}Re rhenium sulfur colloid for their potential use in radiation synovectomy. After optimizing labeling conditions we achieved a labeling yield of more than 80 % for ^{188}Re hydroxyapatite and more than 90 % for the rhenium sulfur colloid. In vitro stability studies showed that ^{188}Re labeled hydroxyapatite particles lost about 80 % of their activity within 5 d in synovial fluid. Rhenium sulfur colloid on the other hand proved to be very stable with a remaining activity of more than 93 % after 5 d in diluted synovial fluid.

INTRODUCTION

Rheumatoid arthritis is a widespread disease causing pain and physical disability for the patients, as well as considerable economic disadvantages for general public. One therapeutic approach to this disease involves the use of radiopharmaceuticals for ablation of inflamed synovium [1]. Radiation synovectomy is an alternative to surgical or chemical synovectomy. It is based on intra-articular injection of a beta-emitting radionuclide in colloidal or particulate form. The most important disadvantages of existing procedures are the high radiation doses delivered to non target organ systems like liver, spleen and lymph nodes due to considerable leakage of radioactivity from the injected joint, unfavorable biodistribution of the leaked material and difficulties in accurately calculating patient dosimetry.

The most widely used isotopes today are ^{32}P and ^{90}Y because of the high energies of their beta emission [2,3]. However, these isotopes do not emit imageable gamma rays, so it is impossible to obtain quantitative dosimetric informations and none of the administered substances fulfills all criteria for a optimal radiopharmaceutical.

We used ^{188}Re for labeling of hydroxyapatite particles and for preparation of a rhenium sulfur colloid.

Hydroxyapatite, a physiological substance of skeletal bone matrix, has already been labeled with ^{186}Re and ^{153}Sm with promising results [4]. Rhenium sulfur colloid labeled with ^{186}Re is commercially available and has been used in radiation synovectomy for years [5].

Rhenium-188 (^{188}Re) with a 17 h half-life and an intensive high energy beta-emission (E_{max} = 2.12 MeV) is an attractive isotope for radiation synovectomy. The average tissue penetration is 3.8 mm [6]. With emission of a gamma photon (155 keV, 15 %) it permits the imaging of radiopharmaceutical biodistribution by routinely available gamma camera systems. Carrier-free ^{188}Re can be obtained from a ^{188}W/^{188}Re generator which makes it suitable for clinical use.

In this study we labeled hydroxyapatite particles and sulfur colloid with [188]Re, optimized the labeling procedure, and analyzed the in vitro stability of both agents in various challenge solutions to compare their possible applicability for radiation synovectomy in clinical practice.

MATERIALS AND METHODS

[188]Re production. Carrier-free [188]Re was obtained as [188]Re perrhenate (ReO$_4^-$) from an alumina-based [188]W/[188]Re generator (Oak Ridge National Laboratory, Tenn., USA) by elution with normal saline purged with nitrogen for two hours prior to use [7]. High performance liquid chromatography (HPLC) analysis of the eluent showed a radiochemical purity of >99% perrhenate.

Preparation of [188]Re hydroxyapatite. Commercially available hydroxyapatite (Fluka, Neu Ulm, Germany) was labeled with [188]Re according the method of Chinol et al. [4]. Preparation of [188]Re-hydroxyethylidene-diphosphonate (HEDP) was followed by incubation of [188]Re-HEDP with hydroxyapatite particles. Chinol et al. used 10.0 mg Na$_2$HEDP, 3.5 mg tin(II)chloride SnCl$_2$·2H$_2$O, 3.0 mg gentisic acid and 1.0 ml Na[[186]Re]ReO$_4$ solution. We used for our first experimental phase 10.0 mg HEDP (free acid) instead of Na$_2$HEDP, 3.5 mg SnCl$_2$·2H$_2$O, 3.0 mg gentisic acid and 1.0 ml of the eluent from the above described [188]W/[188]Re generator. The resultant solution was heated in a constant water bath for 20 min at 100 °C. After that radiochemical purity was determined using silica gel ITLC (Gelman). To determine the amount of free [188]Re perrhenate we used methyl ethyl ketone (MEK) as mobile phase which leaves [188]Re-HEDP at the origin and takes free [188]Re-ReO$_4^-$ to the solvent front. A system of ITLC/saline was used to separate [188]Re-ReO$_4^-$ and [188]Re-HEDP (both at the front) from reduced hydrolyzed [188]Re species (ReO$_2$) (at the origin). Quantitative analysis of ITLC plates was performed by a Linear-Analyzer Trace 96 (Berthold GmbH, Munich, Germany).

The radiolabeling of hydroxyapatite with [188]Re-HEDP was carried out by addition of 40.0 mg hydroxyapatite, 100 μl of a 4.0 mg/ml solution SnCl$_2$·2H$_2$O in nitrogen-purged water, 50 μl of a 20 % Triton-X 100 solution in water, 100 μl of [188]Re-HEDP solution and 750 μl nitrogen-purged normal saline. The mixture was incubated for 1 h at room temperature and subsequently analyzed for labeling efficiency via centrifugation (see below).

These standard labeling conditions were modified by variing the concentration of SnCl$_2$·2H$_2$O (2 mg, 5 mg) and of gentisic acid (1 mg, 5 mg), by variing the pH value (addition of different amounts of sodium bicarbonate NaHCO$_3$: 4 mg, 6 mg, 7 mg, 8 mg, 9 mg, 10 mg, 12 mg), by changing the water bath for an autoclav, and by using sealed reaction vials instead of open glass tubes.

Preparation of [188]Re sulfur colloid. [188]Re sulfur colloid was prepared using the method by Venkatesan et al. [5] modified by Wang et al. [6]. In a glass reaction vial is added 40.0 mg sodium thiosulfate, 4.8 mg EDTA disodium salt, and 0.8 mg sodium perrhenate. To the vial is then added 1-2 ml eluent from the [188]W/[188]Re generator followed by 3.0 ml 1 N hydrochloric acid. After adjusting the solution to pH 1 the colloid immediately begins to precipitate. The vial is sealed and heated at 100 °C for 30 min in a water bath or an autoclav (sterile conditions). Upon cooling the solution is centrifuged to determine the labeling yield of the reaction (see below).

Determination of labeling yield. Analysis of the labeling yield of [188]Re labeled hydroxyapatite and sulfur colloid was performed by counting the whole reaction vial in a gamma counter. After centrifugation (2000 rpm, 10 min) the clear supernatant was removed and the pellet was slurried again in saline. Additional centrifugation and removal of the supernatant was repeated until the radioactivity of the supernatant was <0.5 % of the radioactivity measured in the pellet. Labeling yield was defined as the percentage of radioactivity in the pellet after washing (n_x) compared with total radioactivity measured before centrifugation (n_0).

$$\text{Labeling yield} = 100\ n_x / n_0.$$

In vitro stability test. For analysis of in vitro stability of the radiolabeled particles we incubated an aliquot of the centrifuged pellet with an excess (3.0 ml) of various challenge solutions (water, normal saline, 1:4 diluted synovial fluid) at 37 °C. At various times (0 h, 2 h, 24 h, 48 h, 115 h) radiolabeled particles in the incubating fluid were centrifuged at 2000 rpm for 10 min and activity in the pellet and supernatant was measured in a gamma counter.

RESULTS

^{188}Re-hydroxyapatite preparation. In a first labeling reaction following the procedure described in the literature [4] and using HEDP (free acid) instead of Na_2HEDP we achieved a radiolabeling yield of 72.4 % after 30 min and 73.3 % after 80 min incubation time. By addition of various amounts of $NaHCO_3$ the labeling yield increased to 81.2 % after 20 min incubation time (the optimum was 9 mg $NaHCO_3$). Using 12 mg $NaHCO_3$ the labeling yield decreased to 42.0 % after 20 min. This indicates the appreciable pH lability of the reaction. ITLC analysis of the different HEDP reactions showed in every case 0 % free ^{188}Re-ReO$_4^-$ and 0.5 - 7 % ^{188}Re-ReO$_2$ depending on the $NaHCO_3$ concentration. The lowest amount of ReO$_2$ was determined with 9 mg $NaHCO_3$ therefore all following reactions were performed using 9 mg $NaHCO_3$.

Reducing the concentration of $SnCl_2 \cdot 2H_2O$ from 3.5 mg to 2.0 mg resulted in no remarkable change of labeling yield whereas the addition of 5 mg $SnCl_2 \cdot 2H_2O$ decreased the yield to less than 60 %. Variation of the amount of gentisic acid had no effect on the labeling yield. ITLC analysis showed in every case (except the reaction with 5 mg $SnCl_2 \cdot 2H_2O$) no free ^{188}Re-ReO$_4^-$ but the amount of ^{188}Re-ReO$_2$ varied markedly. Especially changes in gentisic acid concentrations led to higher levels of this by-product. Therefore in the following reactions we only reduced $SnCl_2 \cdot 2H_2O$ to 2.0 mg.

Using an autoclav (20 min/121 °C/2 10^5 Pa) instead of a water bath led to a decreased yield of 70 %.

In vitro stability of ^{188}Re hydroxyapatite. In vitro stability of ^{188}Re labeled hydroxyapatite particles in water and normal saline was very similar and dropped to 61.7 % and 66.0 % after 115 h incubation time. In diluted synovial fluid the labeled particles lost much more of their activity and after 115 h only 19.3 % of the ^{188}Re was still bound to hydroxyapatite.

^{188}Re sulfur colloid preparation. Preparing ^{188}Re sulfur colloid in a closed glass tube by using a water bath for heating we achieved a labeling yield of 83.6 %. By replacing the water bath with an autoclav the labeling yield increased to 88.8 %. In one reaction we performed the labeling with 80 mCi ^{188}Re-ReO$_4^-$ and yielded (after decay correction) in 73.7 mCi ^{188}Re sulfur colloid which is equivalent to 92.1 % labeling yield.

In vitro stability of ^{188}Re sulfur colloid. In vitro stability of synthesized ^{188}Re sulfur colloid was very high in water, normal saline and diluted synovial fluid. Even after an incubation time of 115 h more than 93 % of the radioactivity was bound to the pellet.

DISCUSSION

The aim of this study was to compare the suitability of ^{188}Re labeled hydroxyapatite and rhenium sulfur colloid for use in radiation synovectomy. Carrierfree ^{188}Re can be obtained from an inhouse ^{188}W/^{188}Re generator system which makes it easily available for clinical use. Its physical half-life (17 h versus 3.7 d with [186]Re), its beta energy (E_{max} = 2.12 MeV versus 1.07 MeV with [186]Re) and its tissue penetration (max. 11.0 mm versus 3.6 mm with [186]Re) makes [188]Re an attractive isotope for radiolabeling of pharmaceuticals for therapeutic use. We optimized the known labeling procedures and achieved more than 80 % labeling yield for hydroxyapatite and more than 90 % for rhenium sulfur colloid. Both procedures are easy to handle, not labour intensive and can be performed under sterile conditions using an autoclav. Incubation tests in various challenge solutions showed high in vitro stability for rhenium sulfur colloid (> 93 % after 115 h) but instability of the hydroxyapatite - rhenium binding (< 20 % after 115 h).

These in vitro results give evidence for the unsuitability of rhenium labeled hydroxyapatite for therapeutic use. By contrast the present data for [188]Re rhenium sulfur colloid are promising enough to continue the investigation of this new radiopharmaceutical. Additional experiments will be necessary to investigate biodistribution and in vivo stability.

CONCLUSION

In conclusion [188]Re rhenium sulfur colloid is a new potential radiopharmaceutical for radiation synovectomy based on the already available [186]Re colloid. Due to more favourable physical properties the use of this new isotope would result in several advantages (higher therapeutic efficiency, lower radiation doses). Based on the reported in vitro results and outstanding in vivo data [188]Re rhenium sulfur colloid promises to become an additional approach for radiation synovectomy in the treatment of arthritic diseases.

REFERENCES

1. Deutsch E, Brodack JW, Deutsch KF. Radiation synovectomy revisited. Eur J Nucl Med 1993; 20: 1112-1127.

2. Onetti CM, Gutierrez E, Hliba E, Aguirre CR. Synoviorthesis with ^{32}P-colloidal chromic phosphate in rheumatoid arthritis - clinical, histopathological and arthrographic changes. J Rheumatol 1982; 9: 229-238.

3. Stucki G, Bozonne P, Treuer E, Wassmer P, Felder M. Efficiacy and safety of radiation synovectomy with Yttrium-90: a retrospective longterm analysis of 164 applications in 82 patients. Br J Rheumatol 1993; 32: 383-387.

4. Chinol M, Vallabhajosula S, Goldsmith SJ, Klein MJ, Deutsch KF, Chinen LK, Brodack JW, Deutsch EA, Watson BA, Tofe AJ. Chemistry and biological behavior of samarium-153 and rhenium-186-labeled hydroxyapatite particles: potential radiopharmaceuticals for radiation synovectomy. J Nucl Med 1993; 34: 1536-1542.

5. Venkatesan P, Shortkroff S, Zalutsky MR, Sledge CB. Rhenium heptasulfide: a potential carrier system for radiation synovectomy. Nucl Med Biol 1990; 4: 357-362.

6. Wang SJ, Lin WY, Hsieh BT, Shen LH, Tsai ZT, Ting G, Knapp FF Jr. Rhenium-188 sulphur colloid as a radiation synovectomy agent. Eur J Nucl Med 1995; 22: 505-507.

7. Ehrhardt G, Ketring AP, Turpin TA, Razavi MS, Vanderheyden JL, Fritzberg AR. An improved tungsten-188/Re-188 generator for therapeutic applications. J Nucl Med 1987; 28: 656-657.

Radioactive Isotopes in
Clinical Medicine and Research XXII
ed. by H. Bergmann, A. Kroiss and H. Sinzinger
© 1997 Birkhäuser Verlag Basel/Switzerland

TRAINING IN RADIOPHARMACEUTICAL QUALITY CONTROL

Decristoforo C, Scherer O*, Schöpf M

Univ Klinik f.Nuklearmedizin, Anichstr.35, 6020innsbruck, *BSM Diagnostika, Alserstr.25, 1080Wien

SUMMARY: 43 persons from Nuclear Medicine departments in Austria particiated in training courses about radiopharmaceutical quality control. Results from practical training showed a low incidence of artefacts and that quality control can be perfomed in any Nuclear Medcine department, if the staff is properly trained.

INTRODUCTION:

Quality Control of radiopharmaceuticals and especially the determination of the radiochemical purity has still found only limited acceptance in the daily Nuclear Medicine routine. The main reasons are: limited time for the analysis, a confusing number of different methods available (mini colums, HPLC, thin layer chromatography, etc., a summary can be found in (1)), limited experience especially in departments without a radiochemist or radiopharmacist. To improve the situation in Austria a radiopharmaceutical training course was started. The aim was to have at least one person trained in this field available in every Nuclear Medicine department in Austria.

MATERIALS AND METHODS:

Until now 43 persons, among them 32 technicians and 11 medical doctors, were trained in 4 courses. To enable a good practical training the courses were performed with a small number of participants (max.12). The course consisted of a theoretical part with an overview on purity parameters, chromatographic methods, radioanalytical methods and possible artifacts followed by a practical training. The practical part (max.6 participants) emphasized chromatographic methods for the determination of the radiochemical purity of ^{99m}Tc-radiopharmaceuticals and included filtration, mini columns, instant thin layer chromatography (ITLC), and conventional thin layer chromatography (TLC) (Tab.1). Routinely used radiopharmaceuticals (e.g.: ^{99m}Tc-MAG3, ^{99m}Tc-MIBI, ^{99m}Tc-DPD, ^{99m}Tc-MAA, and ^{99m}Tc-DTPA) were tested. For the analysis of TLC-plates a chromatographic scanner, electronic autoradiography, a conventional gamma camera, a dose calibrator or a scintillation well counter was used. The participants had also to distinguish between preparations of good quality and preparations of unacceptably low quality.

Tab 1: **Program of the course „radiopharmaceutical quality control"**

Theoretical part: *Duration 4 hours 9-12 participants*	Practical part: *Duration 5 hours, 2 groups of 5-6 participants*
- Quality parameters for radiopharmaceuticals	- Determination of the radiochemical purity with ITLC, 1-strip method (DPD)*
- Quality control performance	
- Methods for the determination of the radionuclidic purity	- Determination of the radiochemical purity with TLC, distinction between good and bad quality (MIBI)*
- Methods for the determination of the radiochemical purity	
- Methods for the determination of other quality parameters: chemical purity, sterility, apyrogenicity, particle size	- Determination of the radiochemical purity with ITLC, 2-strip method, calculation (DTPA or HMPAO)*
- Methods for quantification of chromatograms: Cut and count, radiochromatography scanner, autoradiography, electronic autoradiography, Linear Analyser, gamma camera	- Determination of the radiochemical purity with mini columns (MAG3)
	- Determination of the radiochemical purity: Filtration (MAA)
- Chromatographic artifacts	- 99Molybdenum breakthrough test
- Documentation as part of quality assurance	** Quantification with radiochromatographic scanner, Linear Analyser, Instant Imager, Ionisation chamber or Gamma Camera*
- Quality control of the Ionisation Chamber	

RESULTS AND DISCUSSION:

All participants managed to perform the required radiochemical purity determinations. „Bad" preparations were clearly distinguished from „good" preparations (Fig.1). Only three results (out of more than 200 analyzed preparations) were „ false negative" (i.e.: a good preparation was considered as insufficient) due to artefacts in chromatography. Different analytical methods or a different professional background (academic vs. non-academic) did not have a significant influence on the results. It could be shown that with a good knowledge, including especially a practical training, radiopharmaceutical quality control can be performed successfully in any Nuclear Medicine department. This training course will be continued in Austria and the future will show, whether a successful training will be translated in daily clinical routine.

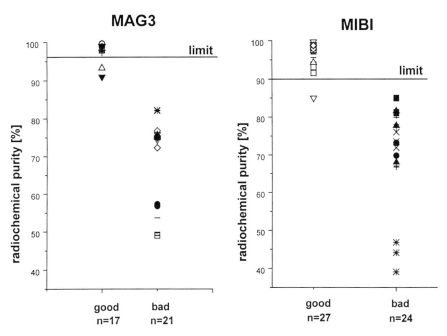

Fig.1.: Results of radiochemical purity determinations. All samples were analysed by people performing the technique for the first time. „Bad" preparations (n=45) could be clearly distinguished from „good" preparations (n=34). Only three good preparations were regarded as insufficient („false negative"). On the left side the results of 99mTc-MAG3 are shown, method: SEPPAK Mini column; eluent1: 0,001N HCl, eluent2: 50% Ethanol/saline. The right side shows results for 99mTc-MIBI, method: TLC, Aluminium oxide / Ethanol.

REFERENCES:

1. Theobald A.E. Quality Control of Radiopharmaceuticals. In: Textbook of Radiopharmacy. Sampson CB, editor. Second Enlarged Edition. Amsterdam: Gordon and Breach Publishers, 1994: 103-123

Radioactive Isotopes in
Clinical Medicine and Research XXII
ed. by H. Bergmann, A. Kroiss and H. Sinzinger
© 1997 Birkhäuser Verlag Basel/Switzerland

STUDIES ON TUMOUR CELL-TARGETING WITH RADIOMETALS

G.Kampf, W.-G.Franke, G.Knop, G.Wunderlich, P.Brust*, B.Johannsen*

Klinik und Poliklinik für Nuklearmedizin, Universitätsklinikum der Technischen Universität Dresden, *Institut für Bioanorganische und Radiopharmazeutische Chemie, Forschungszentrum Rossendorf, Germany

SUMMARY: Radiometal uptake by cultured cells was studied for a better understanding of basic uptake processes using ^{169}Yb and ^{111}In as model nuclides. The results demonstrate the role of protein-binding of different metal-ligand complexes for the cellular uptake, and the principal possibility of loading the cells with metal atoms in order to estimate the potential therapeutic efficacy. In the absence of proteins metal colloids are formed from the citrate complexes which are taken up in high amounts by the cells. Protein-binding prevents colloid formation, and as a sequel cellular metal uptake is decreased. Thus a cell can be loaded in vitro with about 10^{10} metal ions which should be sufficient for a palliative therapeutic effect.

INTRODUCTION

Trivalent radiometals have potencies for vizualizing soft tissue tumours and bone metastases (γ-emitters) as well as for palliation of skeletal pain caused by the secondaries (β^--emitters). In this context the group of the radiolanthanides is especially important as it comprises both kinds of emitters. The principal feasibility has been proved by experimental and clinical approaches; however, uptake in the tumours is not satisfactory. Therefore the challenge for nuclear medicine has been to elucidate the basic uptake processes of radiometals in tumours. In our preceding studies on radiometal uptake by cultured cells different dependences of ^{169}Yb uptake on the metabolic activity of the cells and on the cell type (normal or tumour) were observed (1,2).

Protein-binding of the metals plays an important role for their transport in the blood (3) and possibly for their uptake by the cells. In this study we intended to reveal the influence of the metal and the ligand species on protein-binding and its consequences for cellular uptake with ^{169}Yb and ^{111}In as models for lanthanides and other trivalent metals, respectively. Further, the principal possibilities of targeting tumour cells with radiometals were to be studied. Such knowledge is especially important for evaluation of a potential therapeutic approach.

MATERIALS AND METHODS

The compounds tested were complexes of ^{169}Yb and ^{111}In with the chelators citrate and the aminopolycarbonic acids nitrilotriacetic acid (NTA), ethylenediamine tetraacetic acid (EDTA), and diethylenetriaminepentaacetic acid (DTPA). The sources were ^{169}YbCl$_3$ (Swierk, Poland, spec.act. 15 Gbq/mg Yb) and carrier-free ^{111}InCl$_3$ (Mallinckrodt).

Protein-binding was determined by ultrafiltration through Centricon-30 tubes (Amicon). As proteins those of the fetal calf serum (FCS) used normally for cell growth were added.

For the cell-targeting experiments non-radioactive YbCl$_3$ or InCl$_3$ was added as carrier for achieving defined metal concentrations with the citrate and NTA complexes in the incubation medium. Checking by TLC showed that complex formation was not influenced by the carriers.

Growing and incubation of the cells were performed in RPMI 1640 medium with various portions of FCS. For these studies the malignant cell line KTCTL-2 (human adenocarcinoma of the kidney, from Heidelberg) was used after having seen in previous studies that the normal cell line V79/4 behaves principally in the same way.

After intensive rinsing of the monolayers (12-times phosphate-buffered saline, PBS), trypsinization, and 3-times washing of the cells their radioactivity was measured in a COBRA II Autogamma (Packard).

RESULTS AND DISCUSSION

When the metal complexes are added to the protein-free incubation medium (RPMI 1640), metal colloids are formed from the citrate complexes, with Yb already at very low metal concentrations (3.5×10^{-8} mMol/ml), with In only at higher ones (3.5×10^{-7} mMol/ml). The colloids were detected by prefiltration through a Dynagard (Microgon) sterile filter (0.2 μm) of the solutions intended for ultrafiltration in the protein-binding assay.

Fig.1 demonstrates the relation between protein-binding, colloid formation, and cellular uptake of the metals with the citrate and NTA complexes. The In complexes show greater affinity to the serum proteins than the Yb complexes, and the citrates of both metals are bound to a greater extent than the aminocarbonic acid complexes.. As revealed by TLC, the complexes are bound as a whole to the proteins. The colloids once formed are not bound to the serum proteins.

As shown with the example of Yb citrate, the metal colloids are taken up by the cells in high amounts, however, if protein-binding occurs colloid formation is inhibited. Already a small serum content (3-5%) leads to a drastic drop of the metal uptake.

With Yb and In complexes principally the same dependence of cellular uptake on protein-binding is observed, however, with In citrate, colloid formation occurs only at higher concentrations (3.5×10^{-7} mMol/ml). In Fig.1 the results with 3.5×10^{-8} mMol/ml are depicted. As In citrate shows higher affinity to proteins than Yb citrate, with 3% serum content already 90% of the complex in the low concentration are protein-bound. In protein-free medium the low concentration of ^{111}In is possibly associated to another constituent and cannot lead to colloids.

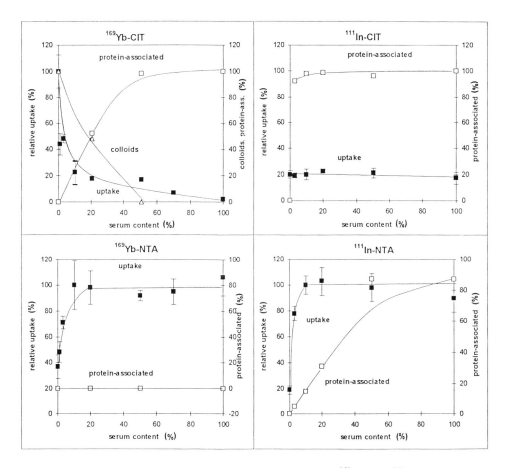

Fig.1. Protein-binding, colloid formation, and cellular uptake of [169]Yb and ^{111}In complexes with citrate (CIT) and NTA in dependence on the serum content of the incubation medium. For the citrate complexes the highest uptake of colloids was taken as 100%.

By contrast, uptake of the aminocarbonic acid complexes of both metals is stimulated by small doses of proteins (simple matrix effect). The complexes of both metals with EDTA and DTPA are not associated to proteins (not depicted).

Protein-binding of the metal complexes is influenced by both the complex ligand and the metal species. By contrast, uptake of the metals by the cells is not influenced by the nuclide except via concentration, but decisively by the ligand coordinated to the metal. With both metals, the normal as well as the tumour cells studied prefer uptake of the colloids rather than the complexes.

The results of the carrier experiments are exhibited in Fig.2. Metal uptake proceeds exactly proportional to the concentration, this is the case with all complexes and colloids studied. The uptake of In and Yb from the citrate complexes is comparable.

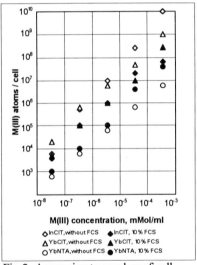

Fig.2. Approximate number of cell-associated metal atoms in dependence on complex concentration. n=6.

With the colloids a cell can be loaded in vitro with about 10^{10} metal atoms per cell, and there is no indication of saturation yet.

Regarding radiation biophysical aspects, about 3×10^4 β^--emitting nuclide particles per cell are necessary for a survival rate of 10^{-12} cells. The metal concentrations reached with the colloids and also with the complexes lie hence far above the level necessary for cell inactivation and should be therapeutically effective also with inhomogeneous distribution in the tumour using the clinically applied nuclides with energies causing crossfire. The problem remains the exploitation of such results for clinical purpose, the selective transport into tumour cells or tumour-accompanying tissue in vivo.

REFERENCES

1. Kampf,G., Knop,G., Matys,S., Kunz,G., Wenzel,U., Bergmann,R., Franke,W.-G. Beziehungen zwischen der [169]Yb-Aufnahme in Normal- und Tumorzellen und deren metabolischer Aktivität in Abhängigkeit von der Ligandspezies. Nucl.-Med. 1994; 33: A 82
2. Kampf,G., Knop,G., Wenzel,U., Wunderlich,G., Bergmann,R., Franke,W.-G. Studies of radiometal uptake by cultured normal and tumour cells. Eur.J.Nucl.Med. 1994; 21: 874
3. Keppler,B., Hartmann,M. Interactions of new tumor-inhibiting metal complexes with biomolecules. GIT Fachz.Lab. 1993: 829-837

This study was partly supported by Mallinckrodt Radiopharma.

Poster Session III: Cardiology; Varia

Radioactive Isotopes in
Clinical Medicine and Research XXII
ed. by H. Bergmann, A. Kroiss and H. Sinzinger
© 1997 Birkhäuser Verlag Basel/Switzerland

REGIONAL PERFUSION AND METABOLISM BEFORE REVASCULARIZATION COMPARED WITH FUNCTIONAL OUTCOME.

J.J. Bax, J.H. Cornel*, F.C. Visser, P.M. Fioretti*,
A. van Lingen, R.A. Lengauer, C.A. Visser.

Free University Hospital Amsterdam, *Academic Hospital Rotterdam, The Netherlands.

SUMMARY: Regional perfusion and metabolism (assessed with FDG SPECT) were compared in 21 patients undergoing revascularization. Segments were classified as 1.normal, 2.viable with FDG-perfusion mismatch, 3.viable without mismatch and 4.scar tissue. Functional outcome was assessed with 2D echo 3 months after revascularization. Wall motion improved in segments with normal perfusion or a mismatch pattern, but not in segments with viable tissue without a mismatch or scar tissue, indicating that in mild perfusion defects a mismatch pattern is needed for functional recovery.

INTRODUCTION

Revascularization may lead to improved left ventricular (LV) function in patients with coronary artery disease if viable myocardium is present (1). Reversibility of regional dyssynergy after revascularization can be predicted with PET or SPECT in combination with ^{18}F-fluorodeoxyglucose (FDG) (2,3). The hallmark of viability is increased FDG uptake in areas of hypoperfusion (FDG-perfusion mismatch). The mismatch pattern is predictive for functional recovery after revascularization, whereas the presence of similarly decreased perfusion and FDG uptake (FDG-perfusion match) is predictive for absence of recovery. In several recent FDG PET studies, a mild reduction in perfusion and/or FDG uptake, without a mismatch pattern, was also considered as viable tissue (4,5). In these studies however, functional outcome after revascularization was not studied. The present study evaluated functional outcome after revascularization in myocardium with these different patterns of viability.

MATERIALS AND METHODS

Patients & Study Protocol. Twenty-one patients with regional dyssynergy on 2D echo, scheduled for revascularization (8 PTCA and 13 CABG) were included (19 men, mean age 63±8 years). Eighteen patients had a previous myocardial infarction. They had a mean number of stenosed vessels of 2.3±0.8 and a mean left ventricular ejection fraction of 46±15%.

Each patient underwent early resting Tl-201 SPECT to evaluate regional perfusion (3), followed by FDG SPECT during hyperinsulinemic glucose clamping (3). The SPECT studies were performed with a dual head rotating gamma camera system (ADAC Laboratories, Milpitas, CA, USA), equipped with 511 keV collimators for the FDG study.

Corresponding series of Tl-201 and FDG images (long- and short-axis) were displayed on a videoscreen. The left ventricule was divided into 9 segments: 1 apical, 4 distal and 4 basal segments (anterior, lateral, inferior and septal). Two experienced observers interpreted segmental Tl-201 and FDG uptake using a semiquantitative scoring scale: 1=normal uptake, 2=mildly reduced, 3=severely reduced, 4= absent uptake, comparable to background activity.

Viability was assessed by comparing perfusion with FDG uptake. Normal myocardium was defined as normal Tl-201 uptake regardless of FDG uptake. Mildly reduced Tl-201 and FDG uptake (score 2) was considered viable myocardium without a mismatch. Mildly/severely reduced or absent Tl-201 uptake (scores 2,3,4) with normal/mildly reduced FDG uptake (scores 1,2) was considered viable myocardium with a mismatch. Severely reduced or absent Tl-201 and FDG uptake (scores 3,4) was considered scar.   Regional wall motion was evaluated with 2D echo before and 3 months after revascularization. The left ventricle was divided into 9 segments, matching the SPECT segments. Each segment was assigned a wall motion score (WMS), ranging from 0: normal to 3: dyskinetic. Recovery was defined as improvement in WMS ≥1 grade after revascularization. The study protocol was approved by the Ethical Committees of both hospitals.

Statistical analysis. Results are expressed as mean±1 SD. Data were compared using the Student's t-test for (un-) paired data. A P-value < 0.05 was significant.

RESULTS

Table 1. Baseline characteristics of 179 segments.

	Perfusion	FDG uptake	WMS
normal (n=97)	1.0±0.0	1.08±0.27	0.16±0.47*
V - mm (n=29)	2.0±0.0	2.0±0.0	0.90±0.88
V + mm (n=31)	2.48±0.50	1.42±0.49	1.06±0.84
scar (n=22)	2.91±0.73	3.27±0.45	1.55±0.72*

FDG: ^{18}F-fluorodeoxyglucose; V - mm: viable without mismatch; V + mm: viable with mismatch; WMS: wall motion score. *:P<0.01 vs all other groups.

Baseline data. Of 189 segments that were analyzed initially, 10 (5%) segments were not revascularized adequately and were excluded from further analysis. The baseline characteristics of the remaining 179 segments are presented in Table 1. Ninety-seven (54%) segments were classified as normal, 60 (34%) as viable (31 with and 29 without a mismatch) and 22 (12%) segments as scar tissue.

SPECT data versus functional outcome. In the segments with normal perfusion, the WMS decreased from 0.16±0.47 to 0.05±0.22 (P<0.01) after revascularization. In the viable segments without a mismatch pattern the WMS did not change significantly: 0.90±0.88 vs 0.79±0.80 (NS), whereas in the viable segments with a mismatch pattern the WMS decreased from 1.06±0.84 to 0.52±0.56 (P<0.01). In the scar segments the WMS remained unchanged: 1.55±0.72 vs 1.64±0.77 (NS).

DISCUSSION

This study evaluated the use of FDG SPECT imaging to predict functional recovery in dyssynergic segments after revascularization using different criteria of viability. The segments with scar tissue on SPECT imaging did not improve in function after revascularization. Conversely, wall motion did improve in viable segments with a mismatch. These findings are in line with previously published data (2,3). Although several studies have used a mild perfusion defect with mildly decreased FDG uptake (viable without mismatch) as a criterium of viability (4,5), these segments did not improve in wall motion after revascularization. Similar results were reported by Vom Dahl et al (6). These segments are likely to represent an area of subendocardial necrosis, that will not improve in wall motion after revascularization.

REFERENCES

1. Dilsizian V, Bonow RO. Current diagnostic techniques of assessing myocardial viability in patients with hibernating and stunned myocardium. Circulation 1993;87:1-20.

2. Tillisch J, Brunken R, Marshall R et al. Reversibility of cardiac wall motion abnormalities predicted by positron tomography. N Engl J Med 1986;314:884-888.

3. Bax JJ, Cornel JH, Visser FC et al. The role of FDG SPECT in predicting reversibility of regional wall motion abnormalities after revascularization. In: Van der Wall EE et al, Eds. Cardiac PET. Viability, perfusion, receptors and cardiomyopathy. Kluwer Academic Press;Dordrecht. 1995;75-85.

4. Bonow RO, Dilsizian V, Cuocolo A, Bacharach SL. Identification of viable myocardium in patients with chronic coronary artery disease and left ventricular dysfunction: comparison with thallium scintigraphy with reinjection and PET imaging with ^{18}F-fluorodeoxyglucose. Circulation 1991;83:26-37.

5. Soufer R, Dey HM, Lawson AJ, Wackers FJT, Zaret BL. Relationship between reverse redistribution on planar thallium scintigraphy and regional myocardial viability: a correlative PET study. J Nucl Med 1995;36:180-187.

6. Vom Dahl J, Eitzman DT, Al-Aouar ZR et al. Relation of regional function, perfusion and metabolism in patients with advanced coronary artery disease undergoing surgical revascularization. Circulation 1994;90:2356-2366.

Radioactive Isotopes in
Clinical Medicine and Research XXII
ed. by H. Bergmann, A. Kroiss and H. Sinzinger
© 1997 Birkhäuser Verlag Basel/Switzerland

CORONARY ARTERY DISEASE (CAD): ROC-ANALYSIS OF Tc-99m-MIBI-SPECT VERSUS Rb-82-PET

G. Glatting, M. Heß, R. Weller, J. Kotzerke, S.N. Reske

Abteilung Nuklearmedizin, Universität Ulm, D-89070 Ulm, Germany

SUMMARY: A quantitative comparison of the assessment of regional perfusion by Tc-99m-sestamibi (MIBI) SPECT and rubidium-82 (Rb) positron emission tomography (PET) is given. A receiver operating characteristc (ROC) analysis is performed for both methods using coronary angiography (stenosis < 70 %) as gold standard. Both methods differ significantly ($p < 0.05$) in the area under the ROC curve. Therefore we conclude that Rb-PET is advantageous to MIBI-SPECT in discriminating patients with coronary artery disease (CAD) from normal.

INTRODUCTION

Although the non-invasive assessment of coronary artery disease (CAD) with rubidium (Rb) and positron emission Tomography (PET) [1,2] is superior to the Tc-99m-MIBI-SPECT technique [3], the origin of the differences is not clear. With the help of receiver operating characteristic (ROC) analysis [4,5], which quantifies the performance of a modality, it may be possible to assign the origin of the differences.

Therefore the purpose of the study was to quantitatively measure the accuracy to detect CAD by Rb-82-PET and Tc-99m-MIBI-SPECT compared to the gold standard of coronary angiography separately for the perfusion territories in order to trace back the cause for the observed differences.

MATERIALS AND METHODS

Patients

55 patients, age (58 ± 10) years, including 11 women were prospectively investigated. 42 of them had a documented infarct and coronary angiography (> 70 % stenosis) revealed 6, 14, 29 patients with 3, 2, 1-vessel disease, respectively.

Radiopharmaceuticals

^{82}Rb, a potassium analog with half-life 76 s, was provided by a ^{82}Sr/^{82}Rb generator (Mallinckrodt) and applicated dose was (1.92 ± 0.46) GBq at rest and stress. Stress and rest dose of ^{99m}Tc Methoxyisobutylisonitrile (Sestamibi) were (326 ± 26) MBq and (902 ± 37) MBq, respectively.

Rb-PET

A Siemens/CTI ECAT 931-08-12 PET was used. After transmission with a ^{68}Ga ring source for attenuation correction a dynamic acquisition after i.v. infusion of ^{82}Rb of in total 7 min (12 x 5 s, 12 x 30 s) was started. Filtered backprojection (Hanning filter, cutoff 0.25) was used for reconstruction.

MIBI-SPECT

A Siemens ZLC-Orbiter 3700 with 180° rotation angle (30° RAO -210° LPO) and 32 projections (30 s per projection was used. Filtered backprojection (Butterworth filter, cutoff 0.5) was used for reconstruction.

Imaging Protocol

Rb-PET and MIBI-SPECT studies were performed on a one-day protocol (Fig. 1). After the Rb rest study 0.7 mg/kg dipyridamole was infused over 4 min to induce coronary vasodilatation. 4 min later MIBI was injected simultaneously with the start of the Rb infusion. The second MIBI study was performed 3-4 hours later. For detailed information see [6].

Image interpretation

The uptake images obtained with both modalities were reoriented according to cardiac axes and shown as a polar map. The left ventricle short axis slices were divided into 13 segments (Fig.

2). The perfusion territories were assumed to consist of the following segments: LAD = 1,6,7,12, LCX = 3,9, RCA = 4,10. The activity values were normalized to the pixel with the higest uptake. The ratio of stress to rest for every perfusion territory was compared to coronary angiography (stenosis > 70 % was assumed as CAD). As result of the ROC analysis the area under the ROC curves were calculated. An area of 0.5 corresponds to a decision by chance and an area of 1.0 is exact.

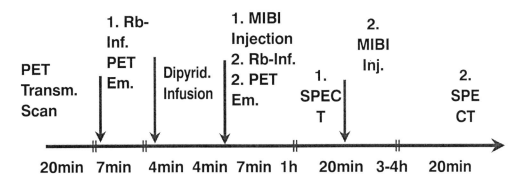

Figure 1. Diagram showing order and time spans of the clinical protocol of Rb-PET and 99mTc-SPECT.

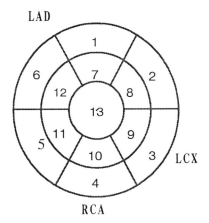

Figure 2. Polar map of the left ventricle from apex (central region) to base (outer circle) with numbered segments.

RESULTS

The results of the ROC analysis are shown in figs. 3 and 4 for [82]Rb-PET and ^{99m}Tc-MIBI-SPECT, respectively. Whereas the ROC curves for the three perfusion territories are have an area A of about 0.8 for SPECT, the curves obtained by Rb-PET range from 0.88 to 0.97.

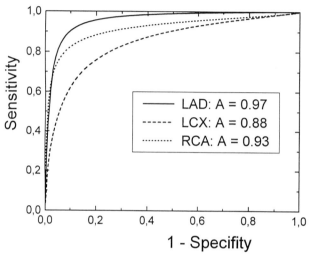

Figure 3. ROC curves for perfusion territories for [82]Rb-PET investigation.

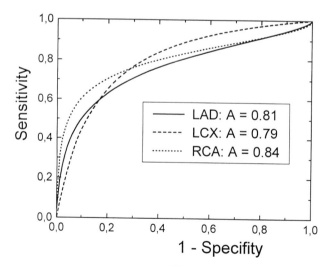

Figure 4. ROC curves for perfusion territories for ^{99m}Tc-MIBI-SPECT investigation.

DISCUSSION

The differences seen between both modalities in this investigation may originate from the different tracer characteristics (lipophilic cationic ^{99m}Tc complex vs. potassium analog), from the improvement due to the correct absorption correction, which is possible for PET, or it may be a consequence of the better resolution of PET. The latter point is at first sight not relevant in our investigation, as we used large segments, but a better resolution may result in better reorientation according to cardiac axes and thus influence the results.

CONCLUSION

[82]Rb-PET is better correlated with coronary angiography for all perfusion territories. The LCX territory shows lowest correlation for both modalities. The differences between perfusion territories are not significant for ^{99m}Tc-MIBI-SPECT, whereas for Rb-PET LAD, RCA and LCX are correlated in descending order.

REFERENCES

1. Stewart RE, Schwaiger M, Molina E, Popma J, Gcioch GM, Kalus M, Squicciarini S, Al-Aouar ZR, Schork A, Kuhl DE. Comparison of rubidium -82 positron emission tomography and thallium-201 SPECT imaging for detection of coronary artery disease. Am J Cardiol 1991; 67: 1030-1310.

2. Grover-McKay M, Ratib O, Schwaiger M, Wohlgelernter D, Araujo L, Nienaber C, Phelps M, Schelbert HR. Detection of coronary artery disease with positron emission tomography and rubidium 82. Am Heart J 1992; 123: 646-652.

3. VanTrain KF, Areeda J, Barcia EV, Cooke CD, Maddahi J, Kiat H, Germano G, Silagan G, Folks R, Berman DS. Quantitative Same-Day Rest-Stress Technetium-99m-Setamibi SPECT: Definition and Validation of Stress Normal Limits and Criteria for Abnormality. J Nucl Med 1993; 34: 1494-1502.

4. Swets JA. Measuring the Accuracy of Diagnostic Systems. Science 1988; 240: 1285-1293.

5. Metz CE. ROC Methodology in Radiologic Imaging. Invest Radiol 1986; 21: 720-733.

6. Grab B, Glatting G, Hess M, Henrich M, Breuer H, Hombach V, Reske SN. A prospective study comparing myocardial perfusion imaging with rubidium-82 PET and Tc-99m MIBI-SPECT. In: Limouris GS, Shukla SK, Biersack HJ, Radionuclides for Cardiology - current status and future aspects, 117-127, Mediterra Publishers, Athens, 1994.

Radioactive Isotopes in
Clinical Medicine and Research XXII
ed. by H. Bergmann, A. Kroiss and H. Sinzinger
© 1997 Birkhäuser Verlag Basel/Switzerland

DETERMINATION OF THE MYOCARDIAL RUBIDIUM EXTRACTION FRACTION: THEORETICAL INVESTIGATION

G. Glatting, R. Weller and S.N. Reske

Abteilung Nuklearmedizin, Universität Ulm, D-89070 Ulm, Germany

SUMMARY: The analytical solution of a two compartment model without backdiffusion is used to rigorously connect the model parameters with experimental results in humans. The resulting extraction fraction depends on flow F and permeability surface product PS according to E=PS/(PS+F), with PS=0.87ml/g/min, a normal value for mammals. This result should replace the earlier result E=0.55 exp(-0.22 F).

INTRODUCTION

Noninvasive assessment of myocardial perfusion is of major importance for the detection of ischemic heart disease and for objective evaluation of the efficiency of treatments designed to augment myocardial blood flow.

A variety of tracers already have been described for quantitative measurement of myocardial blood flow (^{15}O, ^{13}N, ^{11}C, [82]Rb) with positron emission tomography (PET). Among these, the generator-produced nuclide rubidium ([82]Rb) is suitable for carrying out positron emission tomography without the necessity of an on-site cyclotron. Another advantage of [82]Rb is its short halflife of 75s, which facilitates repetitive studies. A potential drawback can be seen in the fact that Rb is only partially extracted by the myocardium after a single capillary passage and that the extraction depends on blood flow F. Therefore, knowledge of the regional extraction fraction E(F) [1-3] depending on the regional blood flow F is essential.

Partially extracted radiotracers have been used for measuring regional blood flow F (ml/g/min) by assuming that flow and extraction E are coupled according to [4]

$$F \bullet E(F) \quad = \quad U(T) / \int_0^T C_a(t)dt \quad . \quad (1)$$

U(T) is the radiotracer uptake at time T in MBq per g tissue and $C_a(t)$ is the arterial blood activity concentration at time t in MBq per ml blood. Note that the extraction fraction E depends on various parameters, especially on blood flow F and on the permeability P and surface area S of the membranes across which the tracer is extracted [3].

In this paper we formulate a rigorous theoretical description for the measurements of Mullani/Goldstein [4,5] in the frame of a two compartment model and show, how this improves their widely used result, which has been under discussion since then [6-8].

MATERIALS AND METHODS

The well established two compartment model [3,4] is used. The two compartments are the cellular and the extracellular, i.e., vascular and interstitial, space (Fig.1). The corresponding differential equations

$$C_1(t) \quad = \quad V_2/V_1 \ \{F \ [C_a(t)-C_v(t)] - PS \ C_1(t)\} \qquad (2)$$

$$C_2(t) \quad = \quad PS \ C_1(t) \qquad (3)$$

can be solved for given input function $C_a(t)$.

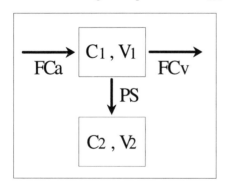

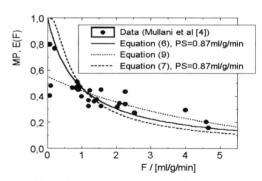

Figure 1. Two compartment model used to describe rate of uptake of Rb from blood to cell. The parameters of the model are: $C_1(t)$, $C_2(t)$ activity concentrations in the compartments; V_1, V_2 volumes; $C_a(t)$, $C_v(t)$ arterial and venous concentration of Rb; F blood flow; PS transfer rate constant from extracellular to cellular compartment.

Figure 2. Experimental data of Mullani et al [4] together with the fitted equations (9) and (7). Note that the error of measurement is extremely large for low blood flows. The Rb extraction fraction (6) is also plotted.

As Mullani et al [4] we assume that the activity concentration of the extracellular compartment $C_1(t)$ has the functional form

$$C_1(t) = B t \exp(-At),\qquad (4)$$

with arbitrary constants A and B. This first assumption is mathematically equivalent to specifying the input function. Secondly the measured parameter MP is [4]

$$MP(t_m) = \frac{V_2\, C_2(t_m)}{V_1\, C_1(t_m) + V_2\, C_2(t_m)}.\qquad (5)$$

In the latter equation, t_m is the time of maximum activity in both compartments.

A straightforward, rigorous derivation of the dependence of equation (5) on the model parameters F and PS for the two compartment model is performed, based only on equations (2)-(4). To determine the parameter PS the resulting expression is fitted to data obtained for dogs by Mullani/Goldstein [4,5]. Then the unidirectional extraction fraction on the basis of the two compartment model [3] reads

$$E(F) = PS / (PS+F).\qquad (6)$$

RESULTS

Under the assumption that equation (4) holds, straightforward calculation of expression (5) for the used two compartment model (Fig.1) yields:

$$MP(t_m) = \{x\, (\exp(1+x) - x - 2)\} / \{x \exp(1+x) + 1\}, \quad x = PS / F.\qquad (7)$$

The fit of equation (7) to the experimental data obtained by Mullani/Goldstein [4,5] yields (Fig.2)

$$PS = (0.87 \pm 0.07)\ \text{ml/g/min}\qquad (8)$$

which is in good agreement with mammalian rate constants (Table 1).

DISCUSSION

The Rb extraction fraction (6) together with equation (8) should be used instead of the result

$$E(F) = a \exp(-bF) \quad , \quad \text{with } a = 0.55 \text{ and } b = 0.22 \text{ g/min/ml } [4,5] \quad , \qquad (9)$$

because the assumption of Mullani et al [4] that $MP(t_m)$ is the extraction fraction is false (compare equations (6) and (7)) and the mathematical derivation of the extraction fraction is inconsistent, as the extraction is not expressed by the model parameters PS and F, but by parameters a and b not connected with the model (equation (9)). Also, extraction fraction for zero flow must be unity (because backward transfer rate was assumed to be zero). This is correctly described by equation (6), but not by (9).

Table 1: Experimentally determined rate constants PS for Rb from literature

authors	model	PS/[ml/g/min]
here*)	dogs	0.87
Budinger et al [9]	dogs/humans	0.90
Huang et al [10]	rabbit	0.99
Reske/Glatting et al [11,12]	humans	0.82

*) this study (correct interpretation of data from [4])

The residuals of the data points in Figure 2 deviate systematically from the fit due to the use of a two compartment model instead of a continuous model, as for example the Renkin-Crone model [1,2], and because of a possible systematic error in the assumption (4). In addition the inherent inaccuracy of the method to measure t_m [4] is extremely large for small flows, because then the noise is of comparable size as the height of the maximum to be determined.

CONCLUSION

The experimental data of Mullani/Goldstein [4,5] can be described by a two compartment model and the functional dependence for the rubidium extraction fraction E on blood flow F from their data is given by equation (6) with PS = 0.87 ml/g/min. This result may form the basis for more accurate quantitation of myocardial blood flow with Rb and positron emission tomography.

REFERENCES

1. Renkin EM. Transport of potassium-42 from blood to tissue in isolated mammalian skeletal muscles. Am J Physiol 1959; 197: 1205-1210.

2. Crone C. The permeability of capillaries in various organs as determined by the use of the "indicator diffusion" method. Acta Physiol Scand 1963; 58: 292-305.

3. Huang SC, Phelps ME. Principles of tracer kinetic modeling in positron emission tomography and autoradiography. In: Phelps ME, Mazziotta JC, Schelbert HR, editors. Positron emission tomography and autoradiography. Principles and applications for the brain and heart. New York: Raven Press, 1986: 287-346.

4. Mullani NA, Goldstein RA, Gould KL, Marani SK, Fisher DJ, Jr. O'Brien HA, Loberg MD. Myocardial perfusion with rubidium-82. I. Measurement of extraction fraction and flow with external detectors. J Nucl Med 1983; 24: 898-906.

5. Goldstein RA, Mullani NA, Marani SK, Fisher DJ, Gould KL, Jr. O'Brien HA. Myocardial perfusion with rubidium-82. II. Effects of metabolic and pharmacologic interventions. J Nucl Med 1983; 24: 907-915.

6. Cherry SR, Carnochan P, Babich JW, Serafini F, Rowell NP, Watson IA. Quantitative in vivo measurements of tumor perfusion using rubidium-81 and positron emission tomography. J Nucl Med 1990; 31: 1307-1315.

7. Yen CK. Re: First-pass measurement of regional blood flow with external detectors [letter]. J Nucl Med 1984; 25: 830.

8. Mullani NA, Gould KL. First-pass measurement of regional blood flow with external detectors (reply) [letter]. J Nucl Med 1984; 25: 831-836.

9. Budinger TF, Yano Y, Moyer B, Twitchell J, Huesman RH. Myocardial extraction of Rb-82 versus flow determined by positron emission tomography [abstract]. Circulation 1983; 68:III-81.

10. Huang SC, Williams BA, Krivokapich J, Araujo L, Phelps ME, Schelbert HR. Rabbit myocardial [82]Rb kinetics and a compartmental model for blood flow estimation. J Physiol 1989; 256: H1156-H1164.

11. Reske SN, Henrich MM, Mate E, Weller R, Glatting G, Grimmel S, Weismüller R, Stollfuß J, Hombach V. Nichtinvasive Bestimmung der myokardialen Ruhedurchblutung mit [82]Rb PET bei Patienten im Vergleich zur Argon-Methode. Nucl-Med 1993; 32: 276-281.

12. Glatting G, Bergmann KP, Stollfuß JC, Weismüller P, Kochs M, Hombach V, Reske SN. Myocardial Rb Extraction Fraction: Determination in Humans [abstract]. JACC 1995; 25[suppl]: 364A.

Radioactive Isotopes in
Clinical Medicine and Research XXII
ed. by H. Bergmann, A. Kroiss and H. Sinzinger
© 1997 Birkhäuser Verlag Basel/Switzerland

COMPARISON OF FILTERED BACK PROJECTION WITH ITERATIVE RECONSTRUCTION IN Tl-201 SCINTIGRAPHY

Maschek W.(1), Pichler R.(1), Huber H.(1), Hatzl M.(1), Leisch F.(2), Kerschner K.(2)

1 Dep. of Nuclear Medicine. 2 Dep. of Cardiology.- General Hospital LINZ, Austria

The purpose of this study was to compare two different image reconstruction modalities in patients who underwent Tl-201 single photon emission computed tomography (SPECT).(1,2,3)

PATIENT POPULATION

31 PATIENTS (pts) 25 m; 6 f;   age 61+/-9 years. CORONARY ANGIOGRAPHY was performed within 14 +/-18 days before or after Tl-201 Sc (Jan.-Dec.1994).

17/31 pts with CORONARY ARTERY STENOSIS > 70%

9 single, 8 two vessel (11 LAD, 5 CX, 9 RCA); 4 pts with history of coronary artery bypass, 3 pts. with akinesia.

EXERCISE PROTOCOL

Ergometer bicycle in upright position; symptom limited; started at 25 W, increased by 25 W every 2 min.

All pts were asked to discontunue anti-ischemic drugs at least 20 hrs before the procedure.

Peak heart rate +/- SD (beats/min) 133 +/-15; Watt 115 +/-32.

In the last minute of peak exercise 70-110 MBq of 201 Tl (depending on the pt`s weight) was injected intravenously. Stress images were obtained 10 min and rest images 3,5-4 hours after the injection.

ACQUISITION

PRISM 1000 (Picker); Motion type:S&S; Collimator: MEGAP parallel; Matrix: 64x64,
Angular step: 3 degree; Number of steps: 60; Magnification 1.6; Acquisition time: 22 min.
Two energy windows (70 and 167 keV, 20 % energy window).

PROCESSING

Filtered back projection and iterative reconstruction was performed with ODYSSEY VP
Computer.

FILTERED BACK PROJECTION (FBP)

Pre-Filtering: Low Pass; Transaxial images were reconstructed using a Ramp Filter.

Transaxial sections were reoriented into vertical long-, horizontal long- and short-axes images.

ITERATIVE RECONSTRUCTION (IR)

Attenuation coefficient: 0.16; Parameter: Iter Nr.1-Iter Nr.5

Transaxial sections were reoriented into vertical long-, horizontal long-and short axes images

IMAGE ANALYSIS

Activity scores from polar map (FBP and IR)

1 = normal, 2 = equivocal, 3 = abnormal, 4 = severly abnormal

were assigned to five myocardial segments: apex- anterior- septal- lateral- inferior.

Three independent observers appraised visually the homogeneity of filtered back and iteratively
reconstructed images separately without knowlege of angiographic results.

STATISTICAL ANALYSIS

SPSS for windows, Version 5.0.1 1992 was used for statistical analysis.

The significance of differences between filtered back and iteratively reconstructed images of
Polar Map was determined by Chi-Square Kendall Coefficient of Concordance and linear
regression correlation. Chi-Square Pearson was used to assess the relationship between filtered
back and iteratively reconstructed images for three independent observers.

RESULTS

Polar Map results: Sensitivity   of 82 %,   Specificity   of 91 % and   Accuracy   of 88 %.
Activity scores of polar map FBP versus IR show a significant difference apical (p <0,05),
but no significant difference anterior, septal, lateral and inferior (p >0,5) (Linear regression
correlation: Fig. 1).

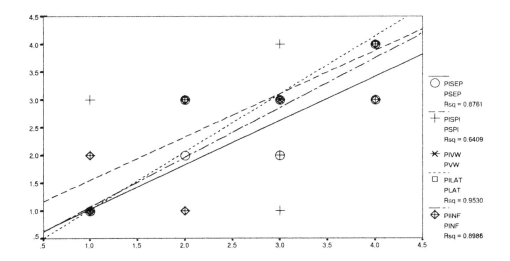

Fig. 1
Linear correlation of Polar Map results between FBP (x axis) and IR`ly (y axis) reconstructed
images: PISEP: IR septum, PSEP: FBP septum; PISPI: IR apical, PSPI: FBP apical; PIVW: IR
anterior, PVW: FBP anterior;PILAT: IR lateral, PLAT: FBP lateral; PIINF: IR inferior, PINF:
FBP inferior. Rsq = Correlation Coefficient.

Visually analysis of three independent observers described more homogeneity for iteratively
reconstrucet images than for filtered back projection (p<0,05).

CONCLUSION

Initial data between differences of filtered back projection and iteratively reconstructed images suggest that:

1. iteratively reconstructed images show more homogeneous tracer distribution than filtered back projection

2. iteratively reconstructed images show a decrease of activity apical- dependent on anatomic wall thinning.

References:
1 LUIG H. Rekonstruktionsverfahren in der Gammaquanten-Tomographie/SPECT. Der Nuklearmediziner 1991; 2:65-73.

2 Patterson RE. Horowitz StF. Eisener RL. Comparison of Modalities to Diagnose Coronaray Artery Disease. Seminars in Nuclear Medicine 1994; VOL XXIV, No 4:286-310.

3 English RJ. Brown SE. In SPECT. Published by the Society of Nuclear Medicine, Inc 1986: 9-23 and 69-90.

Radioactive Isotopes in
Clinical Medicine and Research XXII
ed. by H. Bergmann, A. Kroiss and H. Sinzinger
© 1997 Birkhäuser Verlag Basel/Switzerland

MEASUREMENT OF THE ABDOMINAL RETENTION OF ^{75}Se-HOMOTAUROCHOLIC ACID (SeHCAT) IN PATIENTS WITH DIARRHOEIC SYNDROMES.

J. Martín-Comín, P.A. de Lima, X. Xiol*, M. Roca, M. Castell, X Cervantes*,
R. Puchal, J. Mora, Y. Ricart and M. Ramos.

Serveis de Medicina Nuclear i Gastroenterologia*.
Hospital Universitari Príncep d'Espanya. Barcelona. Spain.

SUMMARY: We investigated the clinical usefulness of SeHCAT test in management of 28 patients with diarrhoeic syndrome using a collimated gammacamera. Abdominal retention of ^{75}Se (AR) lower than 8% suggests ileal disfunction that decreases the absorption of bile acids, as the cause of the diarrhoea. In patients with diarrhoeic syndromes this decrease can be used as criterion to establish specific treatment. In patients with normal AR other causes of diarrhoea must be looked for.

INTRODUCTION

^{75}Se-Selena-Homotaurocholic Acid (SeHCAT) is a synthetic, conjugated bile acid, labelled with ^{75}Se a gamma-ray-emitting isotope, that presents behaviour identical to natural bile acids (1).

The bile acids are reabsorbed by an active transport mechanism in the terminal ileum as part of enterohepatic circulation (2).

Ileal malabsorption can lead to failure of colonic sodium reabsorption, with consequent reduction in water absorption and diarrhoea. In clinical mangement the bile acids agents, Chrolestiramine or Aluminium Hydroxide are usually used (3).

The SeHCAT test consists of measuring the whole body or abdominal retention of ^{75}Se using a whole body counter or an uncollimated gammacamera (2,4-6). In 1990, we validated the method using a collimated gammacamera (7).

The aim of the work was, retrospectively, to investigate the clinical usefulness of ileal function measurement with SeHCAT in the management of diarrhoeic syndromes.

MATERIAL AND METHODS

Twenty-eight patients were studied (13 male and 15 female), mean age was 51.7 ± 15 years (range: 19-79 years). Six patients had undergone ileal resection, 10 unspecific chronic diarrhoeic syndromes, 4 cases of inflammatory bowel disease, 5 diarrhoeic syndromes post-cholecystectomy and 3 malabsorption syndromes.

After overnight fast, the patients received orally a capsule containing 10 μCi of SeHCAT. The anterior (AV) and posterior (PV) abdominal activities as well as the background activity (BA) were measured for 5 minutes at 3 hours, 4 days and 7 days post capsule intake, using a gammacamera fitted with a low-energy parallel-hole high sensitivity collimator. Two energy windows (20%) were centered on the photopics of 136 and 264 KeV of ^{75}Se.

The abdominal activity at 3 hours (AA_0), 4 days (AA_4) and 7 days (AA_7) was calculated as follow:

$$AA = [(AV - BA) + (PV - BA)]/2$$

The abdominal retention of ^{75}Se at 4 days (AR_4) and 7 days (AR_7) was calculated as follow:

$$AR_{4 \text{ or } 7} = (AA_{4 \text{ or } 7}/AA_0) * 100$$

The normal values were considered as $AR_4 > 25\%$ and $AR_7 > 10\%$.

RESULTS

Abdominal Retention

Seventeen patients showed decreased AR of ^{75}SeHCAT at 4 and/or 7 days post-tracer administration: 6 patients with ileal resection ($AR_4=0\%$); Five patients with chronic diarrhoeic syndrome (AR:2.2-8%); 4 out of 5 patients with diarrhoeic syndromes post-cholecystectomy (AR: 0-6.7 %) and 2 patients with ileal Crohn's disease (AR: 0-3 %).

Eleven patients presented normal SeHCAT test. The final diagnosis of these patients was: chronic pancreatitis and hepatic cirrhosis (1 case), diarrhoea secondary to bacterial overgrowth (3 cases) and irritative colon (2 cases), ulcerative colitis (2 cases) and malabsorption syndrome (3 cases). In the last group pancreatic insufficiency, malabsorption syndrome associated with nephrotic syndrome and digestive haemorrhage and anaemia respectively were identified.

Treatment and Evolution

Nine out of 17 patients with positive SeHCAT test received specific treatment for bile acid malabsorption with Cholestiramine (7 cases) or Aluminium Hydroxide (2 cases). The depositional habit normalized in 3 of them and 6 patients improved their clinical status. The frequency of deposition only normalized in 1 out of the 8 patients who did not received specific therapy for BAM (a self-limited diarrhoeic syndrome).

In the 11 remaining cases where the AR was normal, the depositional habit normalized in 8 of them while the other 3 improved with specific treatment for their disease.

DISCUSSION

The utilization of whole body counting limits the use of SeHCAT test in clinical practice because of the limited availability of this equipment. As the activity remains in the enterohepatic circulation, it is possible to change the whole body measurement for the abdominal activity measurement using an uncollimated gammacamera (5) if there are not injected patients, or high activity doses, close to the examination room. To avoid this limitation, we have validated a method using a collimated gammacamera with equivalent results to previous report (7).

In this study, the AR of ^{75}Se was abnormally low in all patients with ileal resection and ileal Crohn disease previously diagnosed, while the patients with ulcerative colitis presented normal abdominal retention of [75]Se. These results agreed with previous reports (8). In patients affected with inflammatory bowel disease, the SeHCAT test was able to identify the Crohn disease cases with ileal affectation. However, the test is not advised for ileal Crohn disease diagnostic because a normal AR does not excluded the disease (9).

Four out of 5 patients with diarrhoea post-cholecystectomy presented abnormal SeHCAT test. These results agreed with a previous publication (10), indicating that bile acid malabsorption is an important etiopathogenic factor to post-cholecystectomy diarrhoea.

Two patients presented $AR_4 > 25\%$ and AR_7 of 6.6% and 8% respectively. According to Merrick et al (3), $AR_7 < 8\%$ is the suitable cutoff value for diagnostic proposals. Using this criterion the second patient did not present BAM. Actually, this patient presented self-limited diarrhoea that resolved spontaneously in a few weeks.

Chronic diarrhoea is a common problem in medical practice and usually these patients require establishing the causal agent, complementary examinations and high cost. The SeHCAT test allows the identification of patients that could profit from specific treatment. However, it is not able to differentiate between the different types of diarrhoea. Therefore, the SeHCAT test is not recommended in the routine investigation of patients with diarrhoea (9).

All patients with positive SeHCAT test that received specific treatment for BAM, presented favourable evolution and clinical improvement, while non-treated patients did not show changes in their depositional habit.

In conclusion, the decrease of the AR of SeHCAT suggests the existence of a disturbance of the ileal absorption, which decreases the absorption of bile acids, as causing the diarrhoea. In patients with diarrhoeic syndromes this decrease can be used as criteria to establish the specific treatment. In patients with normal AR, other causes of diarrhoea must be searched for.

REFERENCES

1. Thaysen EH, Orholm M, Arnfred T, Carl J, Rodbro P. Assessement of ileal function by addominal counting of the retention of a gamma counting bile acid analogue. *Gut* 1982; 23:862-5.

2. Nyhlin H, Merrick MV, Eastwood MA, Brydon WG. Evaluation of ileal function using 23-Selena-25-Homotaurocholate a γ-labelled conjugated bile acid. *Gastroentorology* 1983; 84:63-8.

3. Merrick MV, Eastwood MA, Ford MJ. Is bile acid malabsorption underdiagnosed? An evaluation of accuracy of diagnosis by measurement of SeHCAT retention. *Br M Journal* 1985; 290:665-8.

4. Delhez H, Van der Berg JWO, Van Blankestein MAND, Meerwald JH. New method for the determination of bile acid turnover using ^{75}Se-homocholic acid taurine. *Eur J Nucl Med* 1982; 7:269-71.

5. Hames TK, Condon BR, Fleming JS, Phillips G, Holdstock G, Smith CL, Howllet PJ, Ackery HAD. A comparison between the use of shadowshield whole body counter and an uncollimated gammacamera in the assessment of seven-day retention of SeHCAT. *Br J Radiol* 1984; 57: 581:4.

6. Schroth HJ, Berberich R, Feifel KP, Muller KP, Ecker KW. Tests for the absorption of Se-75-labelled homocholic acid conjugated with taurine (SeHCAT). *Eur J Nucl Med* 1985; 10:455-7.

7. Martín-Comín J, Bonnin D, Baliellas C, Roca M, Xiol X, Ricart Y, Puchal R, Casais L, Ramos M. Medición de la función ileal con ^{75}Se-SeHCAT utilizando una gammacámara colimada en pacientes con enfermedad inflamatoria intestinal. *Rev Esp Med Nucl* 1990; 9:91-5.

8. Holdstock G, Phillips G, Hames TK, Condon BR, Fleming JS, Smith CL, Ackery DM. Potential of SeHCAT retention as an indicator of terminal ileal involvement in inflammatory bowel disease. *Eur J Nucl Med* 1985; 10:528-30.

9. Orholm M, Pedersen JO, Arnfred T, Rodbro P, Thaysen EH. Evaluation of the applicability of the SeHCAT test in the investigation of patients with diarrhoea. *Scan J Gastroenterol* 1988; 23: 113-7.

10. Sciaretta G, Furno A, Mazzoni M, Malaguti P. Post-cholecystectomy diarrhoea: Evidence of bile acid malabsorption assessed by SeHCAT test. *Am J Gastroenterol* 1992; 87: 1852-5.

Radioactive Isotopes in
Clinical Medicine and Research XXII
ed. by H. Bergmann, A. Kroiss and H. Sinzinger
© 1997 Birkhäuser Verlag Basel/Switzerland

FOLLOW-UP OF CARDIAC TOXICITY OF ANTHRACYCLINE CHEMOTHERAPY WITH EQUILIBRIUM RADIONUCLIDE ANGIOGRAPHY

F. PATROIS[1], C. ROUSSEAU[1], F. MONTRAVERS[1], K. KERROU[1]
N. YOUNSI[1], V. IZRAEL[2], J.N. TALBOT[2]

[1] Service de Médecine Nucléaire, Hôpital Tenon, 4, rue de la Chine, 75020
PARIS, France
[2] Service d'Oncologie Médicale, Hôpital Tenon, 4, rue de la Chine, 75020
PARIS, France

SUMMARY : We tested a new schedule for follow up of anthracycline therapy using radionuclide angiography (RNA) in our hospital : just suspend the treatment for one cycle when the absolute LVEF <50 % (or 30 % if the initial LVEF was already abnormal) or if a drop > 10 % occured. Anthracycline treatment could then be restarted if the LVEF was retored, RNA being then performed at the beginning of each cycle. A remission was obtained in 25 cases. A complete remission could even be obtained in a patient whose LVEF was <50 % during treatment.

INTRODUCTION :
The concept of a maximal cumulative dose (550 mg/m^2) limiting the chemotherapy by anthracycline is of little practical value : some patients suffer from congestive heart failure for lower doses and other tolerate higher doses (900 mg/m^2) without cardiac toxicity (1). The follow-up by radionuclide angiography (RNA) with left ventricular ejection fraction (LVEF) measurement has been proposed to detect more accurately this side effect.

MATERIALS AND METHODS
We studied 40 cancer patients with histologic diagnosis of breast carcinoma of sarcoma (mean age 56 yr, range 19-85) eligible for chemotherapy including doxorubicin. 7 of them had previous cardiac disease, 17 had previously received chemotherapy and 19 mediastinal radiotherapy. None of them had evidence of mediastinal or cardiac metastases.
Chemotherapy consisted of cyclophosphamide, doxorubicin and 5-fluorouracil. The doses administered depended of the type of cancer. Chemotherapy cycles were repeated every 3 wk, preceded by a hematologic control.
115 LVEF were measured before and during anthracycline treatment at least 3 wk after the end of a chemotherapy cycle. On average, 3 RNA (range 2-6) were performed in each patient. 20 min after in vivo red blood cell labeling with 950 MBq of technetium-99m, the patient was placed in the supine position ; gated blood-pool scans were acquired with a large field of view camera (General Electric 600XR with a all purpose low energy collimator linked to a General Electric STARCAM 3200

computer) in the LAO 45° projection and no caudal tilt. The cardiac cycle was divided into 24 64x64 frames with a minimum of 4,800,000 counts collected. LVEF was determined using a semiautomatic edge detection processing. Fourier phase and amplitude images were generated to help to trace the region of interest.

RESULTS

In 24 % of RNA, we found a LVEF<50 %. With our proposed schedule, a remission was obtained in 25 cases and the treatment had to be stopped because of cardiac toxicity only in 13 cases ; we observed just one case of clinical failure. Two patients had pretherapeutic LVEF values <50 % but were included after discussion and were followed according to our schedule. A complete remission could even be obtained in a patient whose LVEF was <50 % during treatment which would have lead to a withdrawal of anthracycline with the conventional criteria and would have impaired the favourable therapeutic result.

DISCUSSION

Patients under anthracycline therapy need close cardiac monitoring to identify those at risk of developing heart failure, when the schedule of doses can still be modified, and to reduce mortality or severity of clinical heart failure. Patients at risk can still receive high cumulative doses if the schedule of administration is modified to avoid heart failure (2, 3, 4).

The incidence of congestive heart failure is less than 2 % at total cumulative dose of 400 mg/m^2, 7 % at 550 mg/m^2 and may rise to more than 20 % at cumulative doses above 700 mg/m2. It happens more frequently in patients with previous risk factors, such as mediastinal radiotherapy, hypertension or previous cardiac disease (5). However, there is a considerable individual variability ; with a dose of 500 mg/m^2, some patients can safely receive further treatment, while others present with heart failure at lower doses. It is difficult to fix arbitrarily a ceiling for cumulative dose limit of Doxorubicin (3, 6). The current strategy is to administer Doxorubicin up to a point beyond which further therapy would result in cardiotoxicity. It therefore requires an ability to monitor for cardiotoxicity and safely titrate the cumulative dose of Doxorubicin accordingly (4, 7). A significant reduction in the incidence of severe Doxorubicin cardiotoxicity has been archieved with the use of this approach.

Radionuclide angiocardiography at rest monitors LVEF, an important physiologic index of cardiac function. Overt congestive heart failure is preceded by a progressive fall in left ventricular ejection fraction (LVEF). Serial studies can detect a change in cardiac function over time and Doxorubicin administration can be stopped when a perdetermined reduction in LVEF is observed. Both the level of final LVEF and the magnitude of the fall are important determinants (7). Schwartz et al. have described guidelines for serial radionuclide angiocardiography at rest during the course of Doxorubicin therapy, based upon an experience derived from almost 1,500 patients over a 7-yr period (2, 7). Over four-fold reduction in the incidence of overt cardiac failure was observed when these guidelines were followed. Moreover, if congestive heart failure did develop, it was mild and responsive to routine therapy. True baseline measurements, prior to any chemotherapy, to differentiate between subclinical pre-existent reduction of LVEF and early toxic anthracycline-induced effects are required. To avoid the influence of the transient positive inotropic effect which accompanies and follows acute administration of anthracyclines (10), testing should be performed at least 3 weeks after the last anthracycline dose and just before the next dose. In our past experience, a significant improvement in LVEF was sometimes observed between measurements done less than 3 weeks after the end of a cycle of chemotherapy and measurements done more than 3 weeks after this end. Consequently, we only considered in the present study only the last type of measurements and that gave us the idea to repeat LVEF measurement after a pause corresponding to one cycle (a total of 7 wk without chemotherapy), to look for a possible spontaneous improvement (table 1).

CONCLUSION :

In conclusion, in the serial monitoring of cardiac function during chemotherapy including anthracyclines, LVEF determination to study the systolic function remains at present a widely used parameter to detect cardiotoxicity ; a new schedule is proposed which permitted to obtain remission doses in some patients without rise of toxicity.

Table 1 : Proposed schedule for monitoring Doxorubicin cardiotoxicity by serial radionuclide angiocardiography.

Baseline radionuclide evaluation at rest

I. Patients with normal baseline value :

A. Second study at ½ cheduled dose and then at each cycle.

B. Repeat study after a pause of one cycle if LVEF<50 % then restart if LVEF>50 % or stop if LVEF<50 %.

II. Patients with baseline LVEF<50 %.

A. Study at each cycle.

B. If drop of LVEF>10 % or LVEF<30 %, pause one cycle, then repeat LVEF study : if steady, stop ; if reduction of the drop and LVEF>30 %, study at each cycle.

References

1. Borow KM, Henderson IC, Neuman A. Assessment of left ventricular contractility in patients receiving doxorubicin. *Ann Intern Med.* 1983 ; 99 : 750-756.

2. Schwartz RG, McKenzie MB, Alexander J. Congestive heart failure and left ventricular dysfunction complicating doxorubicin therapy. *Am J. Med.* 1987 ; 82 : 1109-1118.

3. Hortobagyi GN, Frye D, Budzar U. Decreased cardiac toxicity of doxorubicin administered by continuous intravenous infusion in combination chemotherapy for metastatic breast carcinoma. *Cancer* 1989 ; 63 : 37-45.

4. Choi BW, Berger HJ, Schwartz PE. Serial radionuclide assessment of doxorubicin cardiotoxicity in cancer patients with abnormal baseline resting left ventricular performance. *Am Heart* J 1983 ; 106 : 638-643.

5. Legha SS, Benjamine RS, Mackay B. Reduction of doxorubicin cardiotoxicity by prolonged continuous intravenous infusion. *Ann Intern Med* 1982 ; 96 : 133-139.

6. Dardir MH, Ferrans VJ, Mikhael SY. Cardiac morphologic and functional changes induced by epirubicin chemotherapy. *J Clin Oncol* 1989 ; 7 : 947-958.

7. Schwartz RG, Zaret B. Diagnosis and treatment of drug induced myocardial disease. In : Muggia FC, Speyer JL, eds. *Cardiotoxicity of anticancer therapy.* 1990.

8. Bristow MR, Mason JW, Bilingham ME, Daniels JR. Dose-effect and structure-function relationship in doxorubicin cardiomyopathy. *Am Heart J* 1981 ; 102 : 709-718.

9. Druck MN, Gulenchyn KY, Evans WK. Radionuclide angiography and endomyocardial biopsy in the assessment of doxorubicin cardiotoxicity. *Cancer* 1984 ; 53 : 1667-1674.

10. Pauwels EKJ, Horning SJ, Goris ML. Sequential equilibrium gated radionuclide angiocardiography for the detection of doxorubicin cardiotoxicity. 1983 ; 1 : 83-87.

Radioactive Isotopes in
Clinical Medicine and Research XXII
ed. by H. Bergmann, A. Kroiss and H. Sinzinger
© 1997 Birkhäuser Verlag Basel/Switzerland

FOLLOW-UP OF HIGH-DOSE CHEMOTHERAPY -TREATED PATIENTS WITH BONE MARROW SCINTIGRAPHY WITH TC99m NANNOCOLL.

S. Gane, W.Pilloy, F. Ries, M. Dicato
Centre Hospitalier Luxembourg, L- 1210 Luxembourg

SUMMARY We assessed bone marrow(BM) hematopoetic capacity before
and after high dose chemotherapy (HDC)by means of Tc99m nannocol
bone marrow scintigraphy (BMS).Quantitative and qualitative BMS
was performed in patients previously treated with standard chemo
therapy and presently submitted to HDC. In this sequential study
the patient is his own standard. 4 stages had been investigated.
All 3 quantification parameters NLU, LU/STU, LU increased from
M0(aplasia)to a higher value in M1(BM recovery) in all patients.

INTRODUCTION

Qualitative study of BM with BMS with Tc99m nannocoll, permits
an earlier diagnosis of malignant bone disease and detects over
20% more malignant bone lesions than BS. Quantitative study of
BM made by Munz(1)on the iliosacral region,showed uptake ratio
dBM,having for adult normal range of 2.66-4.24 Esik(2)quantified
with the same method BM activity in radiochemotherapy-treated
patients,excluding thus patients with abnormal BMS quantification values from further chemotherapy.

The aim of our study is to assess the BM capacity before and
after high dose chemotherapy (HDC) and to quantify BM function
in aplasia (M0)and BM recovery (M1),which are two extreme conditions of BM function,thus following BM kinetics through BMS.

MATERIALS AND METHODS

Group A:8 patients,7 women,1 man,mean age:47 years(36-63) and
group B:6 patients,3 women,3 men;mean age:55 years (43-76).

Group A:Type of tumour:7 breast adenocarcinomas (stII,III,IV) and 1 malignant germ cell tumor of the mediastinum.These patients were submitted to HDC, and were previously treated with standard chemotherapy.We investigated 4 stages of BM activity: 1/after standard chemotherapy:White blood cells(WBC)>4000;6/8 2/after Endoxan priming(D8-D11)2/8;3/during Aplasia(WBC<100);all 8/8 patients; 4/during BM recovery(WBC>500)all 8 patients(8/8). Average interval of BMS execution was 34 days(28-60).Average follow-up of patients after HDC was of 9 months(6-12).

Group B:Type of tumor:1 breast adenocarcinoma stII,1 oat cell pulmonary tumor st IV,1 soft tissue leiomyosarcoma st IV,1 ovarian adenocarcinoma stIII A,1 non-Hodgkin lymphoma stIV,1 esophageal adenocarcinoma stIV. These patients were previously treated with standard chemotherapy. HDC was not performed. BMS was performed only once after standard chemotherapy. This group served as reference for BMS quantification values after standard chemotherapy. Patients either refused HDC (3/6) either were finally not included for HDC by oncologists (3/6).

PROCEDURE
Our measurement equipment a Gamma camera (XRT) General Electric which was connected to a GE computer system. We used a low energy high resolution collimator(LEHR).All acquisitions were made in identical conditions of collimator,with a sweeping speed of 15 cm/mn. Acquisitions were made 30 min.after iv injection of 0.25 μCi/kg body weight Tc99m Nannocoll. Whole body acquisitions were made in anterior and posterior view. The activity of the syringe was measured before and after iv shot.

DATA ANALYSIS
We observed no changes in qualitative distribution of BM during HDC in group A.Qualitative evaluation for group A was for 5 patients without BM metastases,of type I(Munz (1)), which is the normal distribution, and for the remaining 3 patients of type II

(Munz(1)),which means a moderate peripheral extension of BM. Two of these 3 patients had 2-4 BM metastases.

For group B 3 patients had type I BM distribution and had no BM metastases;3 other patients had type II BM distribution,and 2 of them had 2-4 BM metastases.

Quantitative evaluation was made using 3 parameters:

1/ Non liver uptake (NLU) = Whole body activity (WB) background corrected - liver and spleen activity, both background corrected, divided through WB act in % of total activity.

NLU= Marrow act + Extracellular Space (ECS) act + XYZ

2/ Relative Marrow Uptake = Lumbar act/Soft tissue Uptake

LU/STU = LUMB act (ROI) Lkidney act (ROI) act/pix in box ROI of predetermined size and reproductible position.

3/ Specific Marrow Activity= LU= LUMB act (ROI) background corrected in lumbar box ROI of predetermined size and reproductible position= act/ pix /mCi

RESULTS

Results were analysed using Student's test.We considered this a sequential study , where the patient is his own standard. We considered the 2 extreme conditions of BM function in group A.:

1/ Aplasia (WBC<100) timepoint:M0, with low BM function and a baseline value of 100%.

2/ BM recovery (WBC >500) M1 with high BM function; value >100%

NLU increased from baseline value M0 to M1 for all 8 patients. Average increase of 128% (107-179.5).Quantitative values of NLU for 107%:27.29- 29.22; for 179.5%: 23.23- 41.7.Average value for WBC<100:24.28 +/- 4.91.Average value for WBC>500: 30.81 +/-6.69. The significance level was 0.0432.

LU/STU increased from M0 toM1 for all 8 patients. The average increase was of 138%(112.16-173.46).Quantitative value of LU/STU for 112.16%:0.74-0.83; and for 173.46%:0.49-0.85. Average value for WBC<100:0.70+/- 0.16.The average value for WBC >500 was 0.96+/-1.35. The significance level was 0.017.

LU increased from M0 to M1 for all 8 patients.Average increase was 140.7% (120.8- 196.25). Quantitative values LU for

120.8%: 9.13 cts/mCi-11.03 cts/mCi.;for 196.25%: 4-7.85 cts/mCi.
Average value for WBC<100: 6.77 +/- 1.59. The average value for
WBC>500:9.24 +/- 1.35. The significance level was of 0.0048.

All 3 parameters varied between M0 and M1 in a statistical
significant way. LU showed the most significant variations.

DISCUSSION

All 3 parameters of the same patient increased in BM recovery
(M1) with >128% of the initial value in aplasia (M0). The 2d
BMS was possible only in 2 of 8 patients. However the obtained
values suggested BM stimulation after Endoxan priming , as expected for the peripheral blood stem cell (PBSC) collection .
All 8 patients recovered a normal BM hematopoesis after HDC,
pointing out that a correlation could be done between rapidity
of BM recovery from aplasia and the parameters level and between
parameters values as a good prognostic factor of BM recovery,
but further studies are needed on greater samples of patients.

CONCLUSION

Quantitative changes of BMS could be used as a valuable tool to
decide which patient can have HDC.

REFERENCES

1.Munz DL, Voth E,Emrich D:Different approaches to determine the
uptake ratio of bone-marrow seeking radiopharmaceuticals for
classifying the scintigraphic bone marrow status.Nucl Compact
1987; 18:192-194.
2.Esik O,Rajtar M,Naszaly A:Bone marrow scintigraphy for haema-
tological follow-up of radiochemotherapy treated patients.Oncol.
1993; 50:298-302.
3.Reske S.N: Recent advances in bone marrow scanning.Eur.J.Nucl.
Med.1991;18:203-221
4.Ciambellotti E,Cartia GL,Coda C:Scintigrafia del midollo osseo
per la valutazione del danno da farmaci antiblastici.Radiol.Med.
1988; 75:78-82.
5.Bourgeois P,Gassavelis C,Malarme M,Fruhling J:Bone marrow
scintigraphy in breast cancer.Nucl.Med.Commun.1989;10:389-400
6.Linden A, Zancovich R, Theissen P, Diehl V,Schicha H: Malignant lymphoma: Bone marrow imaging versus biopsy.Radiology 1989
173; 335-339

Radioactive Isotopes in
Clinical Medicine and Research XXII
ed. by H. Bergmann, A. Kroiss and H. Sinzinger
© 1997 Birkhäuser Verlag Basel/Switzerland

QUANTITATIVE DETERMINATION OF RENAL ^{99m}Tc-MAG$_3$ CLEARANCE.
A COMPARISON OF RESULTS ACQUIRED SIMULTANEOUSLY IN WHOLE BODY
GEOMETRY AND WITH A GAMMA CAMERA IN ROI-TECHNIQUE.

J. Andreas, D. Sitz, A. Bockisch, D. Eißner.

Department of Nuclear Medicine, Johannes Gutenberg-Universität, Langenbeckstr. 1
D-55101 Mainz.

SUMMARY: 289 patients were simultaneously investigated with a partially shielded whole body counter (Oberhausen) and in camera technique to correlate the values of the MAG3-clearance. Good correlation was found for the often used times schedules of taking blood samples. Late blood samples increase high clearance values in both methods slighly. The shape of the ROI has no influence using camera technique. We conclude, that camera technique can replace the Oberhausen method with a partially shielded whole body counter.

PURPOSE OF THE STUDY:

A good correlation is known between the clearance values gained with the Oberhausen equipment of a partially shielded whole body counter (Fig.1) and those acquired by a "whole body region" out of a gammacamera's field of view (1,2). However, this was only true for clearance values of iodinehippurate higher than 300ml/ min / 1,73 m^2 surface. Postulating this equality à priori for Tc-99m MAG$_3$ seems doubtful for two reasons: The intercompartimental distribution of ^{99m}TcMAG$_3$ differs from that of iodinehippurate and there is a higher binding to plasma proteins. Furthermore, there are continuing discussions about the position of the "whole body region" within the gamma camera's field of view, especially whether the heart should be included or not. Therefore, we want to answer the following questions:

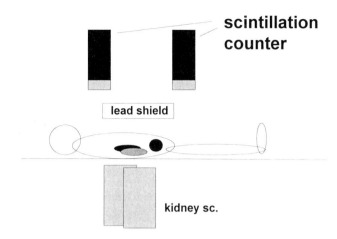

Fig. 1 : Partially shielded whole body counter developed by Oberhausen.

1) What is the the correlation of the MAG$_3$-clearance values (OBHsc, (ml/min/1.73m^2)) measured by the whole body counter developed by Oberhausen and the values gained by camera-technique (OBHcam, (ml/min/1.73m^2)) ?

2) Does the intraindividual MAG$_3$-clearance value differ in each procedures in the same way for different times of taking blood samples as known for iodinehippurate? For this tracer it is well known that late blood sampling times increase the clearance value using OBHsc.

3) Does the positioning of the "whole body region" and the often observed accumulation of MAG$_3$ in the liver influence the clearance value using OBHcam?

METHOD:

In order to investigate the influence of the position of the "whole body region" and a possible intensive accumulation of MAG$_3$ in the liver we evaluated the data of 47 patients in two different ways: First by determining the clearance value using a "whole body region" consisting only liver and spleen (ROI$_{liver}$). Secondly by including all organs above the kidneys within the gamma camera's field of view (ROI$_{liver/heart}$).

After this pre-investigation we recorded data simultaneously with the Oberhausen-method and the gamma camera technique in 289 consecutive patients to determine the clearance values for both methods. Blood samples were drawn after 14 and 16 min in 222 patients and after 14 and 25 min in 67 patients.

The clearance values of both methods were determined by evaluating the median value from the values of the blood samples taken 14 and 16min after injection , and after 14 and 25 min respectively. Additionally the clearance values of the patients with the blood samples taken after 14 and 25 min were correlated for each time of taking blood. This seemed necessary to detect errors, possibly caused by calculating the media values. For all these calculations we used the "whole body region" including all organs above the kidneys.

Finally we investigated whether the clearance values within one method depend on the time of blood sampling. Therefore the clearance values, calculated in one method with blood samples taken after 14 and 25 min were correlated.

RESULTS:

1) A predomination of the liver within the "whole body region" does not change the results of the camera clearance:

$$Cl_{ROI\ heart/liver} = 1.018\ Cl_{ROI\ liver} + 7.3\ ; n = 47,\ r = 0.98$$

2a) The correlation between both methods is good for 14 and 16 min as a time-schedule for taking the blood samples:

OBHsc = 1.002 OBHcam + 4.5, r = 0.98, n = 222

2b) Even for temporary extended times of taking the samples (14 and 25 min p. i.) we

got nearly the identity line:

OBHsc = 0.995 OBHcam + 9.9, r = 0.98, n = 67

2c) Correlating each time of blood sampling we found for 14 and 25 min a good

correlation, too:

1) 14 min: OBHsc = 0.98 OBHcam + 0.63, r = 0.98, n = 67

2) 25 min: OBHsc = 0.97 OBHcam - 0.20, r = 0.98, n = 67

In contrast to iodinehippurate there is a good correlation for all proven patterns of

taking the blood samples even in severe renal dysfunction.

3) Finally we were able to demonstrate that the time of taking the blood samples has the same

influence on the height of the clearance values in both methods: Late blood sampling times

increase the higher clearance values slightly :

$OBHsc_{25}$ = 1.072 $OBHsc_{14}$ - 15.7; r = 0.97; n = 67

$OBHcam_{25}$ = 1.058 $OBHcam_{14}$ - 12.7; r = 0.97; n = 67

CONCLUSION:

The determination of the renal clearance using Tc-99m-MAG$_3$ and a "whole body region" of inter-est within the gamma camera's field of view may replace the Oberhausen-equipment. Different time intervals of blood sampling have no substantial impact on the good correlation for both methods. This applies to low clearance values also. In contrast to iodinehippurate late blood sampling times increase only the higher clearance values in both method in nearly the same way.

Finally, using the gamma camera method, the positioning of the "whole body region" does not have an impact on the height of the resulting clearance values.

REFERENCES:

1)   Rohloff R, Hast B, Leisner B, Heinze HG. Bestimmung der [131]J-Hippuran-Clearance im
        Rahmen der Kamerafunktionsszintigraphie der Nieren nach der vereinfachten Methode
nach Oberhausen. Nucl.-Med. 1974; 13: 303-320.1

2)   Kotzerke J, Walburger N, Gettner U, Buchert W, Hundeshagen, H, Vergleich zweier
Algorithmen zur Bestimmung der renalen Ganzkörperclearance nach simultaner   Acquisition mit
dem teilabgeschirmten Ganzkörperzähler und der Gammakamera. Nucl.-   Med. 1990; 29: 101-108.

Radioactive Isotopes in
Clinical Medicine and Research XXII
ed. by H. Bergmann, A. Kroiss and H. Sinzinger
© 1997 Birkhäuser Verlag Basel/Switzerland

FOLLOW UP OF THE RENAL SCARS IN ASYMPTOMATIC SIBLINGS OF CHILDREN WITH VESICOURETERIC REFLUX

J. Fettich, R. Kenda, Z. Zupancic, A. Meglic

University Medical Centre Ljubljana, 61000 Ljubljana, Slovenia

ABSTRACT: The aim of the study was to evaluate the development of renal scarring, vesicoureteric reflux (VUR) and kidney growth in asymptomatic children with VUR during 3 - 7 years. The results of the study indicate that routine screening for VUR of asymptomatic siblings of children with VUR and other asymptomatic populations at risk is recommended, since high grade sterile VUR seems to be an important factor in development of renal scarring.

INTRODUCTION

The correlation among reflux nephropathy, urinary tract infection (UTI) and vesicoureteric reflux (VUR) is well established. It has been recognised that UTI in the presence of VUR is the most common cause of renal scarring and nephropathy (1). Due to the fact that VUR is usually discovered only after the first or even repeated UTI, when damage to the kidneys, at least to certain extent, might already have been done, little is known about the influence of sterile VUR on kidney development, possible damage to the kidneys and its consequences in asymptomatic children.

While screening of total asymptomatic population for VUR seems unjustified, there are two groups of children, which might benefit from such screening. The first group are neonates in whom dilatation of urinary tract was discovered by ultrasound prenatally or shortly after birth (2) and the second one are asymptomatic siblings of children of with VUR and healthy children of parents with reflux nephropathy or VUR (3,4). In both groups VUR could be discovered early, before the onset of UTI by voiding cystography.

The purpose of the study was to evaluate the development of renal scarring, VUR and kidney growth in asymptomatic children with VUR during 3 - 7 years of follow up.

PATIENTS

105 asymptomatic siblings of children with known VUR were included in the study. There were 56 (53%) boys and 49 (47%) girls, 4 months to 6 years old at the beginning of the study. All had negative history of UTI and were free of symptoms at the time of the study.

VUR was discovered in 47 (45%) of 105 asymptomatic siblings. 43 of the 47 siblings with proven reflux were investigated by 99m-Tc DMSA renal scintigraphy and focal defects suggestive of renal scarring were found in 10 of them, that is in 23% of the siblings with VUR and 10% of all siblings in the study. One child had a solitary kidney (5).

40 of the 43 asymptomatic siblings with VUR and DMSA scintigraphy performed at the onset of the study were followed up. VUR was bilateral in 22 and unilateral in 18, thus representing 62 refluxing units. The children were investigated by repeated direct radionuclide voiding cystography (DRVC), renal ultrasound, and 9 patients with focal defects suggestive of renal scarring on initial DMSA study also by DMSA scintigraphy during 3 - 7 years follow up.

All asymptomatic siblings in whom VUR was detected were on a long term low dose antibiotic prophylaxis, at least one year after VUR disappeared on DRVC.

METHODS

DRVC, usually with multiple voidings and fillings of the bladder was used to detect the presence of VUR (6). VUR was graded as grade 1: radiotracer reaching the ureter only, grade 2: radiotracer reaching the pelvis, and grade 3: radiotracer reaching the pelvis, which was dilated.

Renal ultrasound was performed with real time convex scanner using 3.7 MHz transducer. Kidney size was measured and volume calculated using formula for the ellipsoid. The values were compared to the sonographical growth charts for kidney length and volume (7).

99m-Tc DMSA scintigraphy was performed using a planar gamma camera and parallel hole collimator in three projections (PA, RPO, and LPO), using magnification. Relative kidney function was calculated from the posterior image after background subtraction.

RESULTS

Vesicoureteric reflux: VUR disappeared spontaneously during the period of follow up in 48% of all 62 refluxing units, in 53% of grade 1, 65% of grade 2 and 33% of grade 3 refluxes. 6 (26%) VUR grade 2 and 4 (66%) VUR grade 3 were successfully treated surgically or by endoscopic subureteric collagen injections.

Renal scars: In 7 out of 9 patients with focal defects on the initial DMSA investigation defects persisted, but did not progress and relative kidney function did not deteriorate. In two patients there was progression of focal defects on repeated DMSA scans and relative kidney function decreased. Initially one had VUR grade 3 and the other one grade 2, which progressed to grade 3 during the study. None had evidence of UTI during the follow up period. Both were treated by subureteric collagen injections.

Kidney size and volume: In all children the size and estimated volume related to body height and weight were within 95% margins of tolerance according to the sonographic growth nomograms, except in one child with a solitary kidney, which was enlarged.

Urinary tract infection: Two girls had signs and symptoms of UTI and positive urine cultures, the other 38 were free from UTI. One girl, with VUR grade 1 and normal DMSA scan, had one episode suggestive of lower UTI. One girl with VUR grade 2, which deteriorated to grade 3, and normal DMSA scan, had an UTI and was subsequently treated by subureteric collagen injection.

DISCUSSION

The results of the study indicate that low grade sterile VUR probably does not play a major role in development of renal scarring and reflux nephropathy, while for high grade sterile reflux this may well not be so. The presence of renal scars in asymptomatic siblings with low grade VUR detected at the beginning of the study might be caused by a higher grade VUR at birth which resolved spontaneously, but left renal scars which have not progressed subsequently. Normal renal growth during follow up also indicates that low grade VUR, in the absence of UTI, probably does not play an important role in renal reflux nephropathy.

Routine screening for VUR of asymptomatic siblings of children with VUR and other asymptomatic populations at risk is recommended, since high grade sterile VUR seems to be an important factor in development of renal scarring. Low grade sterile VUR per se probably does not play a major role in reflux nephropathy, therefore it is important to follow up the reflux and to keep it sterile, preferably until it disappears.

REFERENCES

1. Merric MV, Notghi A, Chalmers N, et al. Long term follow up to determine   the prognostic value of imaging after urinary tract infections. Arch Dis   Child 1995; 72: 393-6

2. Marra G, Barbieri G, Moioli C, et al. Mild fetal hydronephrosis indicating   vesicoureteric reflux. Arch DisChild 1994; 70: 147-50

3. Noe HN. The long term results of prospective sibling reflux screening. J   Urol 1992; 148:1739-42

4. Aggarwal VK, Verrier Jones K. Vesicoureteric reflux: screening of first   degree relatives. Arch Dis Child 1989; 64: 1538-41

5. Kenda RB, Fettich JJ. Vesicoureteric reflux and renal scars in   asymptomatic siblings of children with reflux. Arch Dis Child 1992; 67:   506-8

6. Fettich JJ, Kenda RB. Cyclic direct radionuclide voiding cystography: increasing reliability in detecting vesicoureteric reflux in children. Pediatr Radiol 1992; 22: 337-9

7. Dinkel E, Ertel M, Dittrich M, et al. Kidney size in childhood. Sonographical growth charts for kidney length and volume. Pediatr Radiol 1985; 15: 38-43

Poster Session IV:

Immunoscintigraphy; Therapy; Varia

Radioactive Isotopes in
Clinical Medicine and Research XXII
ed. by H. Bergmann, A. Kroiss and H. Sinzinger
© 1997 Birkhäuser Verlag Basel/Switzerland

LABELING OF ANTINEUROBLASTOMA MONOCLONAL ANTIBODY (MoAb) AND FIRST RESULTS OF IN-VIVO DISTRIBUTION IN SCID-MICE

H. Lauterbach, A. Voigt., H. Carlsohn., A. Berndt, M. Hüller, D. Gottschild and F. Zintl

Klinik für Radiologie, Nuklearmedizinische Abteilung; Klinik für Kinder- und Jugendmedizin; und Institut für Pathologie der Friedrich-Schiller-Universität Jena, Germany

Summary: The monoclonal antibody (MoAb 15/7) was labeled with iodine-131 by chloramin-T method (1 minute, ice bath) using excellulose plastic desalting columns (Pierce) to remove free iodine-131. After incubation the labeling mixture was immediately transfered to desalting column without addition of sulfite.
Labeling efficiency was > 80 % and the amount of protein bound iodine was > 95 %.
Labeled antibody (specific activity: 200 kBq/µg) shows an immunoreactivity against cultured neuroblastoma cells (SK-N-MC and SK-PN-DW) of > 80 %.
About 300 kBq labeled antibody were injected into human neuroblastoma transplanted mice.1-4 days after injection principal organs were removed and their I-131-uptake was determined. The highest radioactivity was detected in the tumor expressed as cpm/g tissue.
The calculated tumor/organ ratio ranged from 2.5 (blood) to 41.9 (spleen).
This results indicate the efficacy of this antibody in tumor imaging of neuroblastoma.

INTRODUCTION

Neuroblastoma sympathicum is one of the most malignant tumors of children. The frequency is nearly 10% of all malignant tumors of this age. Yearly fall ill nearly one of 10,000 children in the age to two years (SHIMADA, 1992). In spite of large progress in the field of pediatric oncology the chance of cure for this children above all in stages III and IV is only 5%. For this reason is each endevour to improve diagnosis and treatment of this tumor of large clinical interest.
The animal model SCID-Mouse allowes transplantation of human tumors without antigen-antibody rections because SCID-Mice have a high grade immun deficientcy responsible to absence of both humoral and cellular immundefence.

MATERIALS AND METHODS

- Examination of monoclonal antibodies against human neuroblastoma cells prepared in the field of neuroblastom research in particular MoAb 15/7 in relation to labelling with 131-I preserving a high immun reactivity
- Experimental investigations in xenotransplantated SCID-Mice to demonstrate the possibility to use the antibodies for diagnosis of neuroblastoma in childhood in particular for early detection and localisation of metastases

1.   Optimization of Labelling

- Use of different labelling methods (Beads, Iodogen, classic Chloramin T)
- Optimization of Chloramin T-method (labelling protocol)

The labelling experiments were performed at first with Chloramin T and $Na_2S_2O_3$ and with Iodogen. The obtained products showed only a low immun reactivity in in-vitro cell labelling experiments and were not used for further investigations in animals. To exclude troubling influence of the reductive remedium ($Na_2S_2O_3$) in following experiments we used derivtisated Chloramin T loaded polystyrol spheres IODO-BEADS® (Pierce) as oxydative remedium. This technique substitutes the application of $Na_2S_2O_3$. The parameter immunoreactivity and gain of labelling however showed no main differences to foregoing experiments.
So we worked after all again with Chloramin T in deceased concentration and in homogenic phase without any reductive remedium. In this way the salt removing column has additional the function of separation of the excessive Chloramin T .

In addition to this findings we found references, that the antibody in concentrations about 1 mg/ml showes aggregation and decreasing of original labelling activity.
Therefore we used the antibody for labelling in the optimal dilution of 0,2 to 0,4 mg/ml . The labelled products showed immunoreactivities against neuroblastom cell lines in range of 64 to 90 %. The immunoreactivity increases with increasing dilution (see table 1).

Labeling of MoAb 15/7

- Labeling vial „Reacti-Vial™" (Pierce; Nr.: 13221)
- 50 µl   Antibody (0.33 mg/ml)
- 10 µl   0.25M PBS
- 5 µl   131-I-NaI (Amersham) corresponding 1.3-1.6 MBq 131-I
               after dilution with 0.25M PBS
- 5 µl   Chloramin T (= 2.5 µg) in 0.1M PBS
- after a one minute incubation in an ice bath immediately transfer to desalting column (Extracellulose GF-5, Pierce) without prior addition of sulfite.
- pre-elution of column with 600 µl 0.01M PBS
- elution of column with 500 µl 0.01M PBS (main fraction, contains labeled antibody)

- **Labeling results**
- labeling efficiency: 80-85 %
- radiochemical purity: ≥ 95%
- specific activity: 60-80 MBq/mg (kBq/µg)

RESULTS

1.
The determination of immunoreactively fraction was performed by labelling tests of labelled antibody in relation to different cell concentrations of cultivated tumor cell lines in BSA-containing PBS-buffer. The measurement of cellulary bounded activity was performed in a γ-counter.
The results of immunoreactivities are demonstrated in **Table 1**.

Table 1: Immunoreactivity "**IR**" of labeled MoAb 15/7 and result of animal-experiments

number of labeling procedure	1	2	3	4	5
antibody concentration (mg/ml)	0.2	0.4	0.33	0.33	0.33
IR against cell-line SK-PN-DW (%)	90.1	65.3	86.5	72.2	65.4
IR against cell-line SK-N-MC (%)	-	64.9	84.0	77.5	65.7
transplanted cell-line	SK-N-MC	SK-N-MC	SK-PN-DW	SK-PN-DW	SK-N-MC
mass of tumor	10.1	2.3	18.0	4.5	0.8
specific activity (kBq/µg antibody)	126.2	55.5	83.3	40.0	51.1
injected antibody (µg)	2.7	8.9	5.9	8.4	9.8
organs removed after (days)	1	3	4	3	3
tumorbound activity (%)	20.5	4.0	1.5	4.5	2.5

2.   Results of experiments in animals

The labelled antibody (specific activity 40 to 126 kBq/µg) was in 5 test series intravenously or intraperitonealy applicated with an activity of 347 to 500 kBq adequate 2.7 to 9.8 µg of the antibody per animal. The mass of transplantated tumors ranged from 0.8 to 18.0 g. After 1, **3** or 4 days the animals were killed, the organs extracted, weighted, and the activity calibrated. The main results of the experiments are concluded in the following **Table 2**:

Table 2: Ratio of activity distribution tumor / organ

organ	number of labeling procedure				
	1	2	3	4	5
blood	3.9	-	5.0	2.5	6.5
liver	3.4	7.7	9.8	4.7	4.3
heart	3.6	12.3	7.0	5.4	11.3
spleen	2.8	-	41.9	4.6	4.9
bowel	14.1	21.4	32.0	11.8	19.4
kidney	3.7	9.0	9.5	5.2	6.6
lung	-	-	-	4.2	5.0
stomach	5.9	36.3	12.0	3.4	9.2

Scintigraphic and autoradiographic investigations were only restrictedly possible, because the applicated ranges of activity were too low to get available scintigramms with a small field camera. But orientated investigations with a scintiscanner for small animals (Berthold) showed significant differences between the tumor and the surrounding comparing region.

Autoradiographic investigations showed an increased level of activity in tumor tissue. Correlation to cellular structures was impossible.

CONCLUSION

- The monoclonal antibody MoAb 15/7 can be labelled with 131-I under sparing conditions with a high yield.
- The labelled antibody showes in vitro a high immunoreactivity (to the range of 90% in reaction to cultivated neuroblastom cell lines).
- The acquisition of the labelled antibody in tumor sustaining SCID-Mice results tumor/organ-ratios from >5 (liver) to >30 (stomach). The antibody is principally suitable to idicate tumor tissue in animal experiments. Further investigations are suggestive.
- It must be reviewed, if labelling with other radionuclides (111-In or 99m-Tc) gives similar results.

ACKNOWLEDGEMENT

We thank Mrs. Dr. Lehmann from the company BRAHMs Diagnostica GmbH (yore business division Diagnostika of Henning Berlin GmbH) for her extensive assistance in characterisation of the native antibodies particularly in HPLC investigations.
This paper is supported by DFG (VO 606/1/1).

Radioactive Isotopes in
Clinical Medicine and Research XXII
ed. by H. Bergmann, A. Kroiss and H. Sinzinger
© 1997 Birkhäuser Verlag Basel/Switzerland

RELATIVE Tc-99m-ECD BRAIN UPTAKE UNDER BASELINE CONDITIONS AND AFTER ACETAZOLAMIDE

Barthel H., Dannenberg C., Seese A., Knapp W.H.

Department of Nuclear Medicine, University of Leipzig, Germany

Summary: This study deals with the question whether changes in brain activity uptake produced by vasoactivation differ for control subjects and patients with cerebrovascular disease (CVD). 9 subjects without and 9 patients with CVD underwent Tc-99m-ECD SPET under baseline conditions and after acetazolamide (ACZ). Ratio Q (relative cerebral activity uptake [cts / MBq] at vasoactivation and baseline) differed significantly between control subjects (1.12 ± 0.07) and CVD-patients (0.92 ± 0.03; $p = 0.019$), especially in patients with bilateral CVD or disseminated infarctions ($n = 4$) (0.86 ± 0.02; $p < 0.01$). In conclusion, the hemodynamic relevance of CVD can be evaluated using Tc-99m-ECD SPET with ACZ, even in absence of local perfusion deficits.

INTRODUCTION

Tc-99m ethyl cysteinate dimer (ECD) is a newer cerebral blood flow (CBF) agent that exhibits high first-pass extraction [1]. Therefore, changes of CBF - relative to cardiac output - might be assessed with this agent [2]. ACZ causes a CBF increase of 5 % - 70 % in normal subjects [3,4], in patients with CVD this perfusion reserve may be diminished.

This present study was designed to test the hypothesis that reduced global cerebral perfusion reserve in CVD causes diminished ACZ induced increments in global brain activity uptake as compared with control subjects.

MATERIALS AND METHODS

Subjects:
  (A) Patients: N = 9 (5 female, 4 male). Age: 41-73 years (mean age 56 ± 9 y). Diagnosis: CVD.
  (B) Control group: N = 9 (7 female, 2 male). Age: 36 - 70 years (mean age 56 ± 11 y). Low probability of CVD. Reference methods: doppler-ultrasonography, CT, partly MRT or arteriography.

Protocol:

Each patient underwent a baseline and a vasoactivation study in random sequence (>24 h,< 7d). (1) Baseline-injection: Quiet, dimly lit room; patient's eyes open. Injection of radiopharmaceutical via prefixed butterfly canula. Patients were kept in the same manner for an additional 5 min period.

(2) Vasoactivation: 500 mg ACZ i.v., 25 min prior to injection of radiopharmaceutical. Heart rate and blood pressure were monitored.

SPET:

Acquisition: 1 h after injection of 500 - 600 MBq Tc-99m-ECD. Dual-detector scintillation camera (Vertex, ADAC Lab.) with high-resolution low-energy parallel hole collimator. Collection of 64 projections (64 square matrix) using 30 seconds per projection.

Reconstruction: Standard filtered back projection using Gaussian weighted ramp filter (cutoff 0.38, order 20). Attenuation correction with Chang's first order method (attenuation coefficient $\mu = 0.12$ cm^{-1}).

Quantitation: Calculation of the total counts in all horizontal slices. Separate calculation for each hemisphere. Ratio Q between counts / MBq injected dose under vasoactivation and under baseline conditions.

RESULTS

Sex differences and lateralization: No group differences were found regarding the relative Tc-99m-ECD brain uptake in male and female subjects or in left and right hemispheres, respectively.

Visual patterns: 5 CVD patients had focal activity deficits, 2 patients had equivocal distribution patterns and 2 patients were visually classified as normal by means of Tc-99m-ECD-SPET under vasoactivation.

Quantitation of ACZ response: The change of relative Tc-99m-ECD brain uptake at vasoactivation in comparison to baseline differed significantly between control subjects and patients with CVD (Fig.1, Table1): **Control subjects**: $Q = 1.12 \pm 0.07$

$\qquad\qquad\qquad\qquad$ **CVD patients**: $\qquad Q = 0.92 \pm 0.03 \qquad (p = 0.019)$

In 4 patients with bilateral CVD or disseminated infarctions, respectively, Q decreased to a value as low as 0.86 ± 0.02 ($p < 0.01$).

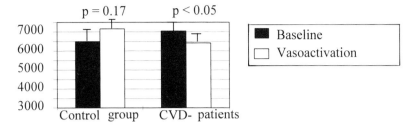

Fig. 1. Tc-99m-ECD uptake [cts / MBq] in patients with CVD and control subjects. Vasoactivation and baseline.

Table 1. Total brain activity related to injected dose [cts / MBq] at baseline and vasoactivation and ratio Q = uptake$_{vasoactivation}$ / uptake$_{baseline}$. Control group and CVD patients:

Nr.	CVD	Baseline	Vasoactivation	Q
1	no	10971	10110	0.92
2	no	5943	8626	1.45
3	no	5969	8245	1.38
4	no	5216	5868	1.13
5	no	5365	4632	0.86
6	no	6940	7351	1.06
7	no	6400	7001	1.09
8	no	6408	5776	0.90
9	no	5337	6768	1.27
Mean Value		6505	7153	1.12
SEM		590	555	0.07
10	yes	4496	3991	0.89
11	yes	6064	5748	0.95
12	yes	7862	6461	0.82
13	yes	6064	5748	0.95
14	yes	10241	9328	0.91
15	yes	8282	7058	0.85
16	yes	8349	7048	0.84
17	yes	5944	6399	1.08
18	yes	6083	6038	0.99
Mean Value		7043	6424	0.92
SEM		585	474	0.03

DISCUSSION AND CONCLUSION

Patients with CVD respond differently from control subjects to ACZ regarding the cerebral Tc-99m-ECD uptake relative to injected dose. This indicates that the fractional cardiac output delivered to the brain under vasoactivation by ACZ is reduced in CVD reflecting diminished global cerebral perfusion reserve capacity. This view is supported by previous findings using Tc-99m-HMPAO and ACZ or CO_2 stimulation [5,6], but it is partly in disagreement with results of CHOKSEY et al [7] who did not find CO_2-induced increase in Tc-99m-HMPAO uptake in normal individuals. The comparison of the actual results with those previous reports, however, is of limited value due to considerable differences in biokinetics (and stability) of Tc-99m-HMPAO and ECD [8].

If routine ECD-SPET with vasoactivation is quantified appropriately, this may improve the diagnostic potential in bilateral stenoses or microvascular disease, since these disorders do not essentially exhibit local perfusion deficits.

ACKNOWLEDGEMENT

This work was supported by a grant from the Bundesministerium für Bildung, Wissenschaft und Forschung to W.H.K. (FKZ 01 ZZ 9103/2.4)

REFERENCES

1.   Vallabhajosula S, Zimmermann RE, Picard M et al. Technetium-99m ECD: A New Brain Imaging Agent: In Vivo Kinetics and Biodistribution Studies in Normal Human Subjects. *J Nucl Med* 1989; 30: 599-604.

2.   Walovitch RC, Hill TC, Garrity ST, et al. Characterization of Tc-99m-L,L-ECD for Brain Perfusion Imaging, Part 1: Pharmacology of Technetium-99m-ECD in Nonhuman Primates. *J Nucl Med* 1989; 30: 1892-1901.

3.   Yudd AP, Van Heertum RL, Masdeu JC. Interventions and functional brain imaging. *Semin Nucl Med* 1991; 21: 153-158.

4.   Bonte F, Devous M, Reisch J et al. The effect of acetazolamide on regional blood flow in normal subjects as measured by single photon emission tomography. *Invest Radiol* 1988; 23: 564-568.

5.   Asenbaum S, Reinprecht A, Brücke T et al. A study od acetazolamide-induced changes in cerebral blood flow using Tc-99m-HMPAO SPECT in patients with cerebrovascular disease. *Neuroradiology* 1995; 37: 13-19.

6.   Knapp WH, Schmidt U, Notohamiprodjo G et al. Response of cerebral Tc-99m-HMPAO uptake and blood flow velocity to CO_2-stimulation - quantitation of perfusion reserve. In: *Radioaktive Isotope in Klinik und Forschung*, (R. Höfer, H. Bergmann, eds.), Schatthauer, Stuttgart - New York, 1991; 19: 230-234.

7.   Choksey MS, Costa DC, Iannotti F et al. Tc-99m-HMPAO SPET and cerebral blood flow: a study of CO_2 reactivity. *Nucl Med Commun* 1989; 10: 609-618.

8.   Tsuchida T, Nishizawa S, Yonekura Y et al. SPECT Images of Technetium-99m-Ethyl Cysteinate Dimer in Cerebrovasculare Diseases: Comparison with Other Cerebral Perfusion Tracers and PET. *J Nucl Med* 1994; 35: 27-31.

Radioactive Isotopes in
Clinical Medicine and Research XXII
ed. by H. Bergmann, A. Kroiss and H. Sinzinger
© 1997 Birkhäuser Verlag Basel/Switzerland

EVALUATION OF REGIONAL CEREBRAL BLOOD FLOW IN PATIENTS WITH MAJOR DEPRESSION USING HMPAO SPECT

R.Junik, D. Baszko-Błaszyk, J.Jaracz, J.Sowinski, A.Rajewski, M.Gembicki

Department of Endocrinology and Department of Psychiatry, University of Medical Sciences, Poznań, Poland

SUMMARY: 99mTc-HMPAO SPECT is a valuable method to demonstrate the functional and structural changes in the brain. The aim of this study was to compare regional cerebral blood flow in patients with major depression before treatment and during remission of the disease. Fourteen patients (9 women and 5 men) who met the DSM-IV criteria for major depressive episode were examined. The subjects were studied using HMPAO and single head gamma camera. After successful therapy regional cerebral blood flow increased in almost all sectors in all patients but one. HMPAO SPECT study seems to be a very useful tool for monitoring the course of major depression.

INTRODUCTION

Studies of regional cerebral blood flow (rCBF) provide interesting information about functional status and structural changes of the brain. Abnormalities in one or more neurotransmitters, neuromodulators and receptors documented in major depression may be resembled in changes of regional blood flow. The results of rCBF studies in patients suffering from major depression have been variable. There are some reports of global reduction (1-5) while a few authors have found no difference from control (6,7). A large number of studies have pointed on an abnormality in topographic distribution of blood flow in depression. A reduction of rCBF during depressive episode was found in basal ganglia, cingulate cortex (8), prefrontal and temporal cortex (5), selective frontal, central, superior temporal and anterior parietal regions (2) when compared to control group. Decreased rCBF all over the cerebral regions in depressive patients turned toward normal in the remitted state following treatment and there was no difference between medicated and unmedicated patients (9,10).

The aim of our study was the comparison of rCBF during depressive episode and in remission.

MATERIALS AND METHODS

In total fourteen patients (9 women and 5 men) who met the DSM-IV criteria for major depressive episode were included in the study. Participation in the study required a minimum score of 18 points on the 17-item Hamilton Rating Scale. Eight patients suffered from bipolar affective disorder, six were diagnosed as unipolar depression.

The patients were studied in a silent, dimly room using HMPAO (Ceretec, Amersham) with 740 MBq (20 mCi) pertechnate 99mTc. Data acquisition were carried out 5-40 min. after injection using a single head rotating gamma camera (Diacam, Siemens) coupled to high resolution collimator. During a $360°$ rotation in a 64x64 matrix, 64x30 sec frames were collected. Image data were processed on Mc Intosh computer (Icon system) provided by the manufacturer. Reconstruction was performed by filtered back projection using a Butterworth filter (cutoff frequency 0.45, order 7). Regional tracer uptake was estimated qualitatively and next measured by a semiquantitative method. Reconstructed brain slices were reorientated according to the orbito-meatal line (approximately OM + 3.5; +4.6, and +6 cm), respectively. Every slice was divided into 6 pieces (sectors). The reference region was delineated on the cerebellum. Relative regional perfusion was expressed as the ratio of cerebral/cereberral activity. Each patient underwent the SPECT study twice- before treatment and after recovery.

All results are presented as the mean +/- SD. The statistical significance between the patients before and after treatment was analysed using the paired t-Student test.

RESULTS AND DISCUSSION

The diagnostic value of rCBF-SPECT in major depression was investigated using both relative quantification and visual estimation. Decreased uptake of HMPAO was observed in all patients before treatment. The cerebral/cereberral ratio ranged 57-77% (+/-5-8%). After successful therapy rCBF increased significantly in all sectors (p<0.05 -p<0.001) except right occipital region (OM +3.5cm) and left frontal region at the same level. After treatment improved rCBF ranged 70-85% and the increase of tracer uptake in comparison to status before therapy was 6-15% (Tab.1). There were no changes in rCBF in one case and the patient relapsed later.

Table 1. The comparison of 99m Tc-HMPAO uptake in sectors of right and left hemisphere

		Right hemisphere				Left hemisphere			
		Depression		Remission		Depression		Remission	
OM +3.5	F	57.8 (8,59)	*	70.3 (7.55)		60.6 (8.40)		70.4 (8.36)	
	T	66.7 (7.69)	*	77.5 (6.70)		66.8 (7.98)	**	81.0 (7.41)	
	O	77.4 (6.71		84.0 (7.29)		77.4 (6.37)	*	85.2 (4.21)	
OM +4.6	F	66.4 (4.41)	*	77.6 (7.48)		68.1 (6.01)	*	77.2 (5.86)	
	T-P	77.2 (3.31)	*	79.9 (4.18)		71.9 (3.42)	**	83.8 (7.35)	
	T-P-O	67.3 (5.04)	*	79.6 (8.35)		67.3 (5.37)	**	77.7 (4.84)	
OM+6.0	F	65.9 (6.67)	*	75.1 (4.09)		63.5 (5.75)	*	72.3 (4.50)	
	P	64.0 (4.60)	**	74.7 (4.71)		65.8 (6.72)	*	75.2 (5.10)	
	P	66.6 (7.21)	*	75.6 (2.24)		68.7 (6.06)	*	76.6 (5.70)	

* p<0.05   ** p<0.001

F-Frontal lobe   O-Occipital lobe   P- Parietal lobe   T- Temporal lobe

The two studies that have reported on blood flow during depression and in remission have indicated blood flow improvement after recovery from depression (9,10) however in both studies N-isopropyl-p-[123I]iodamphetamine (IMP) was used   as a perfusion agent. The lack of significant improvement of rCBF in left frontal and right occipital regions in remitted state found in our study may point on decreased rCBF in these regions as rather state dependent.

CONCLUSION

HMPAO SPECT seems to be very useful tool for monitoring the course of major depression.

REFERENCES

1. Mathew RS, Meyer JS, Francis DJ, Senchuk KM, Morel K, Clarhorn JI. Cerebral blood flow in depression. Am J Psychiatry 1980;137: 1449-1450.

2. Sackeim HA, Prohovnik I, Moeller JR, Brown RP, Apter S, Prudic J, Devanand DP, Mukherjee S. Regional cerebral blood flow in mood disorders I. Comparison of major depressives and normal controls at rest. Arch Gen Psychiatry 1990;47:60-70.

3. Lesser IM, Mena I, Boone KB, Miller BL, Mehringer CM, Wohl M. Reduction of cerebral blood flow in older depressed patients. Arch Gen Psychiatry 1994;51:677-686.

4. Upadhyaya AK, Abou-Saleh MT, Wilson K, Grime SJ, Critchley M. A study of depresion in old age using single photon emission computerised tomography. Brit J Psychiatry. 1990;157(suppl 9):76-81.

5. Yazici KM, Kapucu O, Erbas B, Varoglu E, Gulec C, Bekdik CF. Assessment of changes in regional cerebral blood flow in patients with major depression using the [99m] Tc-HMPAO single photon emission tomography method. Eur J Nucl Med 1992;19:1038-1043.

6. Silfverskiold P, Risberg J. Regional cerebral blood flow in depression and mania. Arch Gen Psychiatry 1989;46:253-259.

7. Gur RE, Skolnick BE, Gur RC, Caroff S, Rieger W, Obrist WD, Younkin D, Reivich M. Brain function in psychiatric disorders II. Regional cerebral blood flow in medicated unipolar depressives. Arch Gen Psytchiatry 1984;41:695-699.

8. Goodwin GM, Austin MP, Dougall N, Ross M, Murray C, O`Carrroll RE, Moffoot A, Prentice N, Ebmeier KP. State changes in brain activity shown by the uptake of 99m Tc-exametazime with single photon emission tomography in major depression before and after treatment. J Affective Disord 1993;29:243-253.

9. Kanaya T, Yonekawa M. Regional cerebral blood flow in depression. Jap J Psych Neurol 1990;44:571-6.

10.Kumar A. Mozley D. Dunham C. Velchik M. Reilley J. Gottlieb G. Alavi A. Semiquantitative I-123 IMP SPECT studies in late onset depression before and after treatment. Int J Geriatr Psychiatry. 1991;6:775-777.

Radioactive Isotopes in
Clinical Medicine and Research XXII
ed. by H. Bergmann, A. Kroiss and H. Sinzinger
© 1997 Birkhäuser Verlag Basel/Switzerland

VENTILATION STUDIES OF THE MIDDLE EAR AND THE PARANASAL SINUSES WITH XENON-133

W. Brenner, K.H. Bohuslavizki, W. Peters*, B. Kroker*, H. Wolf,
M. Clausen, G.S. Godbersen*, E. Henze

Departments of Nuclear Medicine and *Otorhinolaryngology, Head and Neck Surgery,
Christian-Albrechts-University, Kiel, Germany

SUMMARY: This study was designed to quantitatively investigate the ventilation of the middle ear and the paranasal sinuses by using Xe-133 gas. In all patients both maxillary sinuses could be visualized revealing consistent clearance data while only in 19 out of 30 patients tracer accumulation in the tympanum was observed with a large range of clearance half-life. These findings clearly represent the different physiological conditions of the ventilation of the maxillary sinuses and the tympanum. Ventilation studies with Xe-133, therefore, are useful for quantitative evaluation and may be easily obtained for maxillary sinuses, while uptake and clearance in the tympanum are hampered by the involved physiological mechanisms.

INTRODUCTION:

The application of radioactive gas for diagnostic purposes in medicine is mainly used for lung ventilation scintigraphy. Moreover in the ear, nose and throat region many cavities are subject to air ventilation in order to maintain their physiological function. Although many studies of direct and indirect measurement of Eustachian tube function have been published (1, 2) quantitative evaluation of middle ear ventilation has proven difficult. However, up to date only a few attempts have been made to use nuclear medicine procedures to evaluate the ventilation of the tympanic cavity or to quantify ventilation of the paranasal sinuses (3-5), especially due to nasal septum deviation. This would be of great interest for the ENT speciality to improve the management of chronic maxillary sinusitis or chronic middle ear disease.

In this study the non-invasive administration of Xe-133 gas into the middle ear and the paranasal sinuses has been investigated in order to evaluate the physiological and pathophysiological ventilation of these cavities.

PATIENTS AND METHODS:

Studies were performed on 30 ENT patients with a median age of 45 years ranging from 23 to 74 years. 22 patients had clinical symptoms such as nasal septum deviation, sinusitis or vertigo but were considered normal concerning middle ear function by standard ENT tests. In 8 patients one-sided malfunction of the Eustachian tube was proven by impedance measurements.

50 MBq Xe-133 (Amersham-Buchler, Braunschweig, Germany) dissolved in 50 ml air volume was administered into the nasopharyngeal space via a nose olive in the right nostril while the other nostril was closed. Immediately after gas insufflation patients were asked to perform 3 Valsalva maneuvers. Subsequently, sequential planar images of the head were obtained at 60-second intervals for ten minutes followed by 5-minute intervals up to 30 min. A double head gamma camera system with high resolution collimators for low energy was used for simultaneously recording anterior and posterior views (BodyScan, Siemens Gammasonics). For both the tympanic cavities and the maxillary sinuses side-related tracer uptake and clearance half-life were calculated by conventional ROI-technique. Data are given as mean ± one standard deviation.

RESULTS:

Visualization of the tympanum was possible in 19 out of 30 patients corresponding to 63%. In 14 patients with normal middle ear function the clearance half-life was 87 ± 70 min ranging from 9 to 283 min, the side-related uptake was $49.4 \pm 10.4\%$ for the left side to $50.6 \pm 10.4\%$ for the right side. In 5 patients with one-sided tube malfunction clearance half-life was 50 ± 12 min for the side of dysfunction and uptake was $27.1 \pm 12.4\%$ ranging from 15.3 to 31.7%, only one patient had an uptake of 44.9%. The differences between patients with normal function and patients with one-sided tube malfunction were significant ($p = 0.01$) regarding the initial tracer uptake in the middle ear while no significant differences of the widely scattering clearance half-lives between both subsets could be demonstrated. However, all patients with one-sided tube malfunction revealed half-lives of less than 64 min while about 40% of the values of patients without tube dysfunction were higher than 100 min.

Tracer ventilation and clearance from both maxillary sinuses was observed in all 30 patients from anterior view, even in those patients with no gas trapping within the tympanic cavities. Due to the way of tracer application via the right nostril quantification yielded a significant higher tracer uptake of $59.7 \pm 19.7\%$ on the right side as compared to $40.3 \pm 19.7\%$ on the left side ($p = 0.05$). The clearance half-life was 17 ± 9 min for both the left and the right maxillary sinuses. No significant correlation of nasal septum deviation and initial tracer uptake or clearance half-life could be found most probably due to the way of gas insufflation.

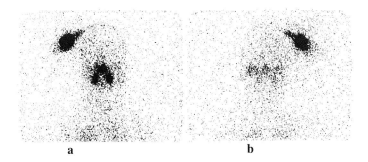

Figure 1: Planar scintigrams of the head 3 min after insufflation of 50 MBq Xe-133 gas. **a:** Anterior view with tracer accumulation in the nasopharyngeal cavity, in the ethmoidal cells, and in both maxillary sinuses. **b:** From posterior view tracer uptake can be seen in both tympanic cavities, in the nasopharynx, and only faint in the maxillary sinuses. There is still activity in the syringe on top right of the patient.

DISCUSSION:

Based on our experience most of the patients were able to perform correct Valsalva maneuvers yielding a success rate of visualizing the tympanum of about 63%. However, in 11 out of 30 patients no tracer trapping in the tympanic cavities was observed although the patients seemed to perform well. In these subjects the physiological conditions of the middle ear ventilation via the Eustachian tube were most probably responsible for the lack of tracer trapping. There is no continuous and free gas exchange between the middle ear and the nasopharynx, because the tubes normally open only during swallowing, and not necessarily during each act of swallowing (6). Even performing Valsalva maneuvers the tubes do not open in all cases to let air into the tympanum (6). Furthermore, the opening of the tube depends on the patient's position: In an upright position the opening occurs more regularly than in a supine position (6). Therefore, to increase the success rate a combination of Valsalva maneuver and Toynbee's test including swallowing should be considered and application should take place in an upright position and not in a supine position on the camera table as done in this study.

The side-related uptake in the tympanum as a measure of tube function ranged from 32.4 to 67.6% in normal subjects, while the uptake in patients with one-sided tube dysfunction was less than 32% in all cases but one. Thus, uptake values revealed significant differences between normals and patients with one-sided tube dysfunction confirming the findings of Yamashita et al. (4), who reported a reduced Xenon inflation into the middle ear in patients with occluded tubes when using direct tracer application into the orifice of the Eustachian tube.

Another parameter for tube function might be the tracer clearance. Tympanum clearance half-lives scattered widely with a range from 9 to 283 min in patients with normal tube function. Since most gases including Xenon are continuously absorbed by the mucosa of the middle ear (4), the Xenon clearance is mainly to be considered a function of resorption into the blood and should be faster in patients with inflammatory middle ear disease according to an increased blood flow. Our findings suggest such a - not significant - trend to increased washout from the affected tympanum revealing maximum half-lives of 64 min while about 40% of the values in normals were higher than 100 min.

In contrast to middle ear ventilation a constantly open airway passage between nasopharynx and maxillary sinuses (1) enables visualization of the maxillary sinuses in all patients investigated. Consistent clearance data with a small range of clearance half-life and a quick washout compared to the tympanum clearly represent these physiological conditions.

The significant higher uptake of the right maxillary sinuses depends most probably on the way of tracer application via the right nostril. This methodologically caused shift also may be the reason for the missing correlation of maxillary sinus affections or nasal septum deviation and initial tracer uptake as would be expected according to the results of middle ear ventilation. Further ventilation studies, therefore, encouraged by a clear visualization of the maxillary sinuses in all patients, have to be performed under physiological conditions of ventilation via both nostrils in order to quantify pathophysiological changes.

In conclusion, quantitative assessment of physiological and pathophysiological maxillary sinus ventilation may be easily obtained, while uptake and clearance in the tympanum are hampered by the involved physiological mechanisms.

REFERENCES:

1. Ingelstedt S, Örtegren U. Qualitative testing of the Eustachian tube function. Acta Otolaryng (Stockholm) 1963; Suppl 182: 7-23

2. Guillerm R, Riu R, Badre R, Le Den R, Le Mouel C. Une nouvelle technique d´exploration fonctionelle de la trompe d´eustache. Ann Oto-Laryng 1966; 83: 523-542

3. Kirchner FR, Robinson R, Smith RF. Study of the ventilation of middle ear using radioactive Xenon. Ann Otol Rhinol Laryngol 1976; Suppl 25: 165-168

4. Yamashita T, Maeda N, Tomoda K, Kumazawa T. Middle ear ventilation mechanism. Acta Otolaryng (Stockholm) 1990; Suppl 471: 33-38

5. Paulsson B, Bende M, Larsson I, Ohlin P. Ventilation of the paranasal sinuses studied with dynamic emission computer tomography. Laryngoscope 1992; 102: 451-457

6. Thullen A. Prüfung von Tubenfunktion und Paukendruck. In: Berende J, Link R, Zöllner F, eds. Hals-Nasen-Ohren-Heilkunde. Band 5: Ohr I. Thieme, Stuttgart 1979: 15.1-15.36

Radioactive Isotopes in
Clinical Medicine and Research XXII
ed. by H. Bergmann, A. Kroiss and H. Sinzinger
© 1997 Birkhäuser Verlag Basel/Switzerland

OXIDATIVE STRESS AND FREE RADICAL FORMATION: MODIFICATION OF
PROTEINS AND THEIR GLYCOSYLATED PRODUCTS DURING OXIDATIVE
CONDITIONS. LABELING OF AGE-ALBUMIN WITH 125-IODINE.

Sobal G., Menzel E.J.
Department of Nuclear Medicine, University of Vienna; Institute of Immunology, University of
Vienna, Austria

SUMMARY: The oxidation reaction was performed using a modified method by R.Levine(1)
in which BSA at a concentration of 2 mg/ml in 50 mM Hepes buffer pH 7.4 was oxidized by
Fe^{3+} or Cu^{2+} at concentrations from 1 μM to 1 mM in the presence of 25 mM ascorbate. The
maximal effect of oxidation in the Fe^{3+} system (1mM) was 339% of the basal value. In the
Cu^{2+} system it was 407%. In the case of native BSA the oxidation rate in presence of 20 μM
Fe^{3+}, corresponding to the physiological Fe^{3+} level, amounted to 137% of the basal va-
lue.Interestingly, glycation of BSA resulted in the formation of a very high content of carbonyl
groups amounting to 758% of the native, nonglycated BSA. Further oxidation under the same
conditions as used for native BSA (20 μM Fe^{+3}) resulted only in a small increase amounting to
115% of the glycated BSA value.

INTRODUCTION

Free radicals are species that contain unpaired or free electrons.They can be generated in cells
by normal biological processes and bioenergetic electron transfer. Normally, a balance between
oxidative events and antioxidative forces maintains the status quo within living cells. When the
normal balance is disturbed by the loss of reducing agents or protective enzymes or by increased production of oxidizing species the organism is exposed to "oxidant stress".
Under these uncontrolled conditions generated radicals can cause reversible or irreversible
damage to macromolecules such as proteins, DNA and essential enzymes. In addition lipid
peroxidation and nonenzymatic glycation of proteins takes place.Metal catalyzed oxidation
leads to introduction of carbonyl groups into amino acid residues of proteins.Also glucose can
react with protein bound amino groups to form Schiff's base which may then undergo the
Amadori rearragement to form ketoamine(2)

METHODS:

PROTEIN OXIDATION: Protein oxidation in vitro can be performed by Fe^{+2}/H_2O_2 in the
Fenton or Fe^{+3}/ascorbate in the Udenfriend reaction .The oxidation reaction of BSA was performed using a modified method of protein oxidation by Rodney Levine (1).

We used BSA (bovine serum albumin) as model protein at a concentration of 2mg/ml in 50 mM HEPES buffer pH 7.4, iron as $FeCl_3$ 20µM and ascorbate at 50µM, 100µM, 200µM, 400µM or 25mM concentration. The reaction was started by adding ascorbate and transfer every 15 sec of the Eppendorf tubes into 37°C shaking water bath. The tubes were open during the incubation because the reaction needs oxygen.After the incubation time of 25 minutes ,the derivatisation reaction was performed by addition of 20mM DNPH (2,4-Dinitrophenylhydrazine).The reaction may be stopped by the addition of EDTA to 1 mM.Then the derivatisation by DNPH was performed.

DERIVATISATION:

Reaction with 2,4-dinitrophenylhydrazine by Rodney Levine et al(3) is the most convenient method for quantitation of the oxidative modification of protein.To 500 µl BSA in HEPES containing 1mg of protein 500 µl of 20 mM 2,4-dinitrophenylhydrazine in 2M HCL was added The mixture was incubated at room temperature for 1 hour,with vortexing every 10-15 min. After that 500µl of 20% trichloroacetic acid was added ,the tubes were centrifugated in table-top microcentrifuge (11000 g) for 3 min, and the supernatant was discarded.The pellets were washed 3 times with 1ml ethanol-ethyl acetate (1:1) to remove free reagent, allowing the sample to stand 10 min before centrifugation. The precipitated product was dissolved in 0,6 ml guanidine solution and incubated 15 min at 37°C.

The carbonyl content was measured by spectrophotometer at the maximal absorbance (360-390 nm) using molar absorption coefficient of 22000/ M /cm.

GLYCATION :

Bovine serum albumine (BSA) was incubated in 0,2 M phosphate buffer pH 7,4 at a concentration of 100 mg/ml with 0,5 M glucose -6-phosphate for 10 weeks at 37°C.The fluorescence of the advanced glycosylation end product AGE-BSA was determined (370 nm excitation and 440 nm emission).Some glycation experiments were performed in the presence of 0.3 mM EDTA.

RADIOIODINE LABELLING:

The labelling of AGE-BSA was performed with iodine-125 (Amersham) and Chloramine-T(Merck) as oxidans according to the method of Mc Conahey and Dixon(4). Reaction time was one minute.
The final specific radioactivity of AGE-albumin was 6,4 mCi/µmol protein.

RESULTS

The results show that oxidation of BSA (2mg/ml) by Fe^{3+} or Cu^{2+} at concentrations from 1 µM to 1 mM in the presence of 25 mM ascorbate results in the introduction of carbonyl groups. The maximal effect of oxidation in the Fe^{3+} system at 1mM metal ion concentration was 339% of the basal value. In the Cu^{2+} system it was 407% (figure1).

Figure 1. Influence of Fe 3+, Cu 2+ concentration on oxidation.

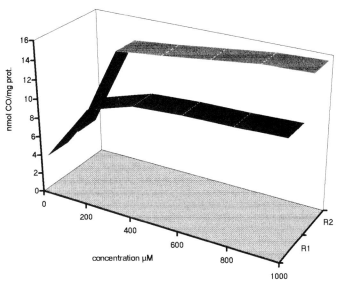

R1=Fe/ascorbate system. R2=Cu/ ascorbate system.

The influence of ascorbate concentration on oxidation of BSA in the presence of 20 μM Fe^{+3} was less pronounced, especially in case of glycated BSA.(Tables 1,2).

Table 1:Influence of ascorbate on the oxidation rate of native BSA.

Concentration of Ascorbate	Absorpt. 360-390 nm	Conc in μM CO	Protein content mg	Concentr. CO nM	Amount CO nM/ mg Prot	Amount CO/BSA
0 μM	0,131	5,955	1	2,978	2,978	0,199
50μM	0,108	4,909	"	2,455	2,445	0,164
100μM	0,119	5,409	"	2,705	2,705	0,181
200μM	0,137	6,227	"	3,114	3,114	0,219
400μM	0,171	7,773	"	3,886	3,886	0,260
25mM	0,180	8,182	"	4,091	4,091	0,274

The maximal oxidation rate in this case at 25 mM ascorbate is represented by 137% of the basal value.

Table 2: Influence of ascorbate on the oxidation rate of glycated BSA.

Concentration of Ascorbate	Absorpt. 360-390 nm	Conc in µM CO	Protein content mg	Concentr. CO nM	Amount CO nM/ mg Prot	Amount CO/BSA
0 µM	0,511	23,230	1,185	23,230	19,603	1,313
50µM	0,564	25,636	"	25,636	21,634	1,450
100µM	0,568	25,818	"	25,818	21,787	1,460
200µM	0,593	26,955	"	26,955	22,746	1,524
400µM	0,568	25,818	"	25,818	21,787	1,460
25mM	0,589	26,773	"	26,773	22,593	1,514

The concentration of Fe^{+3} was 20 µM in both systems.

The effect of oxidation in the case of glycated protein ranged up to 115% of the basal value.

Interestingly, glycation of BSA results in the formation of a high amount of carbonyl groups represented by 758% (22,593 vs 2,978) of the basal value. The further oxidation then results in only a small increase by 115%. This finding indicates, that in case of competitive conditions between glycation and oxidation, the first one should play the greater role (Figure2).

Figure 2.Native and glycated protein oxidation.

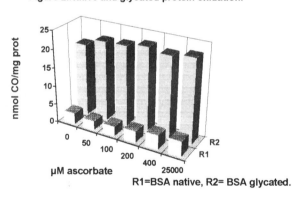

R1=BSA native, R2= BSA glycated.

Fig. 3 shows that glycation of BSA by glucose-6-phosphate is much stronger than by glucose. Addition of EDTA at a concentration of 0.3 mM resulted in a clearcut reduction of the glycation rate.

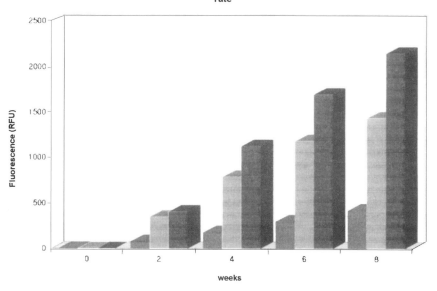

Figure3. Influence of metal chelators and glycating agents on the glycation rate

R!=glycation with glucose R2=glycation with glucose 6-phoshate (+EDTA) R3=glycation with glucose 6-phosphate(-EDTA)

DISCUSSION

The results show, that glycation of BSA results in the formation of a very high content of carbonyl groups amounting to 758% of the native, nonglycated BSA. Further oxidation under the same conditions as used for native BSA ($20\mu M$ Fe+3) then resulted only in a small increase by 115% of the glycated BSA value. These findings indicate, that in case of competition between glycation and oxidation, the first one should play the greater role.It is known that non enzymatic glycosylation of proteins leads to the formation of AGEs.They acumulate in increased amounts in hyperglycemia and can act as toxic agents that contribute to atherosclerotic lesions of diabetes. Glycation leading eventually to AGE formation is increased by metal-catalysed oxidation, as shown by comparing AGE formation in the presence or absence of EDTA (Figure 3). In general, glycation is much accelerated by the use of glucose-6-phosphate instead of glucose. The task for nuclear medicine in the future should be to develop a method for imaging of AGE-receptors (RAGEs) on endothelial cells of large arteries and/or vasa vasorum in patients with diabetes mellitus or non-diabetic nephropathy.

REFERENCES

1.Levine R. Mixed Function Oxidation of Histidine Residues. Meth Enzym 1984; 107:370-376

2.Kortlandt W,Van Rijn HJM, Erkelens DW. Glycation and lipoproteins. Diab Nutr Metab 1993; 6:231-23

3. Levine R, Garland D, Oliver S, Amici A, Climent I, Lenz AG, Ahn BW, Shaltier S, Stadtman ER.Determination of carbonyl content in oxidatively modified proteins. Meth Enzym 1990; 186:464-478.

4.McConahey PJ, Dixon FJ. A method of trace iodination of proteins for immunologic studies. Int Arch Allergy 1966; 29: 185-187

Radioactive Isotopes in
Clinical Medicine and Research XXII
ed. by H. Bergmann, A. Kroiss and H. Sinzinger
© 1997 Birkhäuser Verlag Basel/Switzerland

THERAPY TRIALS IN CANCER PATIENTS USING AN IMPROVED 3-STEP PRETARGETING APPROACH.

G. Paganelli, M. Chinol, C. Grana, M. Fiorenza, M. Cremonesi, R. Franceschini*, L. Tarditi*, A. Pecorale*, C. Meares**, A. Corti*** and A.G. Siccardi***.

European Institute of Oncology, Milan, Italy; * Sorin Biomedica Diagnostics SpA, Saluggia, Italy; **Dept. of Chemistry, University of California, Davis, CA, USA; ***DIBIT, H.S. Raffaele, University of Milan, Milan, Italy.

SUMMARY: Three-step monoclonal antibody tumor targeting using the avidin-biotin system has been successfully applied to the detection of a variety of solid tumors. We have adopted the same protocol in a pilot therapy trial introducing the therapeutic radionuclide yttrium-90 (Y-90). Eleven patients with various tumors were administered with Y-90 doses ranging from 1.85 to 5.55 GBq. Treatment was well tolerated and no acute toxicity was observed. One patient with brain tumor achieved over 50% regression while another showed a total regression of one of his metastases. Overall 4 out of 11 pts are still in partial remission 1-5 months after therapy. The work is still in progress, however, these preliminary data are encouraging and warrant further studies.

INTRODUCTION

The use of radiolabeled monoclonal antibodies (MoAbs) or their fragments, specific for tumor associated antigens, has allowed the detection of neoplastic foci by external imaging (1). However, only a relatively small amount of the injected dose is bound by the tumor, while radiolabeled MoAbs keep circulating in the blood stream and in normal tissues resulting in a high blood pool activity and poor target to non-target ratios. An alternative approach to increase the tumor to non-tumor ratios, by decreasing the normal tissue concentration of the radiolabeled MoAbs, is based on the "pre-targeting" of the tumor. By delaying the delivery of the radionuclide to a time when the ratio of tumor-bound to tumor-unbound antibody is at its highest, one may markedly improve tumor visualization (2). A method based on similar principles but with distinct advantages is the one that exploits the high affinity (Kd = 10^{-15} M) that exists between avidin and biotin (3). Due to the flexibility of this system, several protocols have been envisaged (4-5). In this work, we have improved the so called three-step pretargeting protocol and, by introducing the pure beta emitter radionuclide Y-90, we have treated eleven patients with various tumors.

MATERIALS AND METHODS

Reagents. Monoclonal antibodies: FO23C5, specific for the protein portion of the CEA molecule; B72.3, raised against the tumor-associated glycoprotein TAG-72 and BC4, raised against tenascin, were supplied by Sorin Biomedica (Saluggia, Italy) and biotinylated with biotinyl-aminocapronic acid N-hydroxysuccinimide ester according to a procedure described elsewhere (5). At the end of the reaction the immunoreactivity of the biotinylated MoAbs was tested in a standard ELISA system. Clinical grade avidin and streptavidin were obtained from Società Prodotti Antibiotici (Milan, Italy). Biotin conjugated to the macrocyclic chelating agent DOTA through an extended spacer arm was provided by the Dept. of Chemistry, University of California (Davis, CA, USA).

Radiolabeling. DOTA-conjugated biotin was dissolved in ammonium acetate 1.0 M (pH=7.0) and labeled with 1850-5550 MBq of Y-90-chloride (MAP, Finland) by reacting 1 hr at room temperature under stirring. Labeling efficiency was determined by thin-layer chromatography (TLC) run on plastic backed silica gel plates using a 10% (w/v) aqueous ammonium acetate/methanol (1:1 v/v) solution as the eluent. The developed TLCs were scanned for radioactivity using a radioactive chromato-scanner (Bioscan System 200, Camberra Packard, USA). In this system, unchelated yttrium remains at the origin while labeled biotin migrates to Rf 0.5. No purification was performed after labeling. The ability to bind avidin after labeling was verified by FPLC by mixing Y-90-conjugated biotin with an appropriate amount of avidin.
The final preparation was spiked with a little amount of biotin-DOTA labeled with 74-111 MBq of Indium-111 to follow the in-vivo biodistribution.

Patients and administration protocol. Eleven patients with advanced metastatic tumors (breast, brain, colon) were enrolled in the study. All patients had lesion assessment by conventional radiographic techniques. They received i.v. 30-50 mg of biotinylated MoAbs (1st step) followed, after 36 hr, by 20-30 mg of avidin and 50 mg of streptavidin (2nd step). 18-24 hr later, a second chase of 5-10 mg of biotinylated HSA was administered 10 min prior the injection of 5 mg of radiolabeled biotin.

Imaging and biodistribution protocol. Urine and blood samples were obtained at different time points up to 48 hr post-injection. The percent of the injected dose was determined by gamma-counter measurements of the samples along with a standard of the injection mixture. The biodistribution was determined by drawing regions of interest in static, whole body and SPECT images, acquired at 1, 15, 24, 40 h after injection. Absorbed dose in critical organs (kidney, liver, lung, brain) and, whenever possible, in tumor was determined considering the activity integrated over time, the considered mass, evaluated by CT or MRI, and the "S" values of the MIRD formalism properly modified from standard to specific situations. The bone marrow mean dose was calculated from the activity in the blood samples with the conservative assumption that the bone marrow and blood pool activities are equivalent.

RESULTS

The treatment was well tolerated and no acute toxicity was observed. None of the patients developed HAMA and only one showed anti-avidin immunoresponse. However, an immunoresponse to streptavidin was observed in all patients. Hematologic toxicity up to six weeks was negligible with mean values of PTL, RBC, and WBC within normal ranges. The blood clearance of Y-90-DOTA-biotin was biexponential with a faster componenet of $t_{1/2} = 1.4 \pm 0.4$ hr. About 70% of the injected dose was cleared through the kidneys in the first 16 hr. Bone marrow, kidney and liver mean absorbed doses were 1.1±0.6, 4.5±2.1, 1.5±1.0 cGy/37 MBq while the dose to the tumor was 15.2±8.7 cGy/37 MBq (Figure 1).

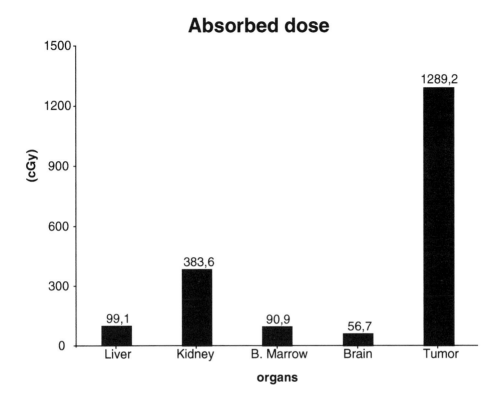

Figure 1: Mean absorbed dose (N=5 pts) in tumor and normal organs following therapy with ^{90}Y-biotin using the three-step pretargeting approach.

One patient with multiple lung and liver lesions showed a normalization of CEA level in 4 weeks after treatment (from 60 to 2.6 ng/ml). One patient with brain tumor (graded III astrocitoma), in progression after radiotherapy, obtained a partial remission with over 50% regression 60 days after therapy (Figure 2).

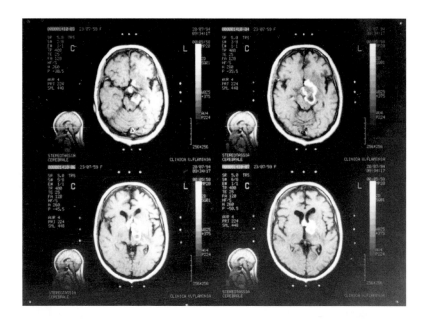

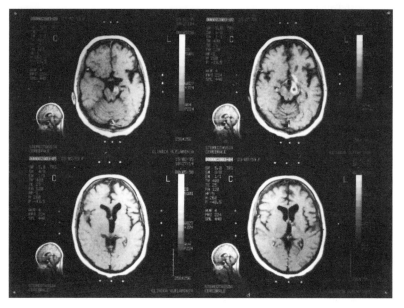

Figure 2 : MRI of a 30y old patient with grade III astrocitoma before (2a) and 60 days after treatment (2b) with 3-step [90] Y-biotin. The study shows over 50% regression after pretargeted therapy.

One patient with colon cancer showed a complete regression of one liver lesion of 1.5 cm. Five patients with widespread disease progressed and two are still under evaluation.

DISCUSSION

Pretargeting strategies have overcome many drawbacks associated with the use of directly labeled MoAbs. In particular, the 3-step protocol is designed to remove the excess circulating biotinylated antibodies as cold complexes, which are taken up and metabolized by the liver. This results in a drastic reduction of background levels in a short time since the radioactive label, being a small molecule, is rapidly excreted. The potential advantage in cancer therapy of this pretargeting strategy has been the low toxicity observed which has allowed to administer high doses of therapeutic radionuclides, such as Y-90, without bone marrow toxicity. The entire procedure has also shown to be non-toxic to the patients based not only on the absence of clinical manifestations but also on the absence of changes in blood profiles. However, all patients developed antibodies against streptavidin. Despite its immunogenicity, streptavidin was preferred to avidin in the second step due to its slower blood clearance and higher organ retention (6). Methods to block this response are currently under evaluation and it is anticipated that advances in molecular biology and recombinant DNA technology will contribute to circumvent this potential problem. Refinements of clinical protocols, such as the use of genetically engineered avidins and the introduction of the second chase, already under evaluation in our institution, may play an important role in the future success of this technique in cancer therapy.

REFERENCES

1. Larson SM. Clinical radioimmunodetection, 1978-1988: overview and suggestions for standardization of clinical trials. Cancer Res 1990; 50: 892-898.

2. Goodwin DA, Meares CF, McCall MJ, McTigue M, Chaovapong W. Pretargeted immunoscintigraphy of murine tumors with indium-111-labeled bifunctional haptens. J Nucl Med 1988; 29: 226-232.

3. Hnatowich DJ, Virzi F, Rusckowski M. Investigations of avidin and biotin for imaging applications. J Nucl Med 1987; 28: 1294-1302.

4. Paganelli G, Belloni C, Magnani P, Zito F, Pasini A et al. Two-step tumour targetting in ovarian cancer patients using biotinylated monoclonal antibodies and radioactive streptavidin. Eur J Nucl Med 1992; 19: 322-329.

5. Paganelli G, Magnani P, Zito F, Villa E, Sudati F et al. Three-step monoclonal antibody tumor targeting in carcinoembryonic antigen-positive patients. Cancer Res 1991; 51: 5960-5966.

6. Schechter B, Silberman R, Arnon R, Wilchek M. Tissue distribution of avidin and streptavidin injected to mice. Effect of avidin carbohydrate, streptavidin truncation and exogenous biotin. Eur J Biochem 1990; 189: 327-331.

Radioactive Isotopes in
Clinical Medicine and Research XXII
ed. by H. Bergmann, A. Kroiss and H. Sinzinger
© 1997 Birkhäuser Verlag Basel/Switzerland

COURSE OF TIME AND EXTENT OF THE THYROID VOLUME REDUCTION AFTER RADIOIODINE THERAPY IN GRAVES DISEASE AND AUTONOMOUS GOITRE.

B. Dederichs, J. E. Klink, R. Otte and H. Schicha

Klinik und Poliklinik für Nuklearmedizin, Joseph-Stelzmann Straße 9, 50924 Köln, D

SUMMARY: It is well known that radioiodine therapy (RITh) leads to a significant thyroid volume reduction (TVR). The analysis of the data of 33 patients with Graves disease (GD) and 36 patients with autonomous goitre (AG) showed a highly significant TVR for both groups, which continued up to 1 year after RITh. Receiving equal effective radiation doses, the extent of TVR was significantly greater for GD than for AG. This difference developed within six weeks up to 3 months after RITh. This observation suggests that the underlying thyroid disease affects the therapeutic effect of RITh and may be partially explained by the total suppression of non-autonomous thyroid tissue in AG at the time of RITh.

INTRODUCTION:

The radioiodine therapy (RITh) is a standard procedure for treatment of hyperthyroidism caused by autonomous goitre (AG) or Graves disease (GD) (1, 2). In addition to the normalization of the thyroid function, the thyroid volume reduction (TVR) is another criterion of a successful RITh. Until now only few data (3 - 6) has been presented due to the course of time and extent of TVR. The aim of this study was to answer the following questions: Does RITh of AG and GD achieve a significant TVR in both groups ? Is the quantitative extent of the TVR identical for AG and GD ? Are there differences between the two patient groups due to the course of time of the TVR after RITh ?

PATIENTS AND METHODS

The data of 33 patients with GD (mean age 46 ± 12 years, 24 women, 9 men) and of 36 patients with multifocal AG (mean age 61 ± 9 years, 30 women, 6 men) were analyzed retrospectively. Patients were only included into the study, if they received the first RITh and had not undergone a previous subtotal or total thyroidectomy. Baseline TSH was totally suppressed at the time of RITh. The intended radiation doses were 150 Gy for both patient groups. The achieved effective radiation doses were calculated by means of the measurement of radioiodine kinetics during therapy. For GD and AG the mean effective radiation doses were 163 ± 95 Gy and 161 ± 66 Gy respectively. Patients, in whom a successful elimination of hyperthyroidism during the first year after RITh could not be achieved, were excluded from the study.

All follow-up examinations were performed by the same observer - before, 6 weeks, 3, 6 and 12 months after RITh. For sonography of the thyroid, a real time sector scanner with a 7.5 MHz transducer (Philips SDR 1550) was used. The breadth (b), length (l) and depth (d) of each lobe of the thyroid were measured and the volume was calculated by the formula: $b \times l \times d \times 0,5$. The sum of the volume of both lobes was taken as the total thyroid volume. Results were analyzed using Student's "t" test.

RESULTS:

For patients with GD and AG the thyroid volume reduction after RITh was highly significant ($p < 0,001$) at all follow-up intervals as compared to the pretherapeutic thyroid volume. The differences between all follow-up intervals were significant ($p < 0,001$) as well (table 1).

Table 1. Thyroid volume (ml) and volume reduction (%)

		Before RITh	After RITh			
			6 weeks	3 months	6 months	12 months
AG	(ml)	59 ± 20	48 ± 17	43 ± 16	37 ± 15	33 ± 15
	(%)		-17 ± 18	-26 ± 18	-35 ± 17	-44 ± 18
GD	(ml)	43 ± 22	33 ± 19	25 ± 14	21 ± 14	16 ± 11
	(%)		-24 ± 22	-41 ± 23	-51 ± 26	-61 ± 22

The greatest extent of volume reduction was already observed within the first 6 weeks up to 3 months after RITh (figure 1). During these follow-up intervals Patients with GD showed a significantly greater total extent of thyroid volume reduction than patients with AG (41 % versus 26 %), although the mean effective radiation doses were not significantly different.

At 3 months up to 6 and 12 months after RITh the amount of further volume reduction became equal for both groups and was about 10 % for each interval (table 1).

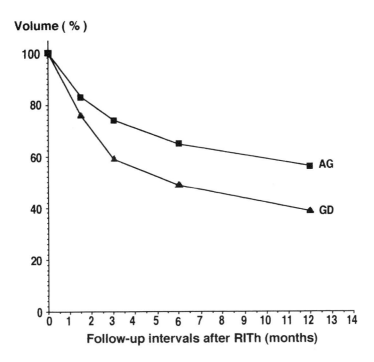

Figure 1. The thyroid volume is expressed as the percentage of the pretherapeutic volume and shows a gradual decrease at every follow - up interval for AG and GD

DISCUSSION:

In concordance with other authors we could confirm, that RITh is an effective method to achieve a significant thyroid volume reduction (3 - 6). Luster et al. (5) reported about a volume reduction of 39 % at 6 months after RITh for multifocal AG, which was slightly greater than in our study. This may be explained by the fact that the mean effective radiation dose in this study was greater than in our patients (226 ± 98 Gy).

The fact that equal effective radiation doses lead to a significantly different extent of thyroid volume reduction between GD and AG, suggests that the underlying thyroid disease affects the therapeutic effect of RITh. This may partially be explained by the suppression of the non-autonomous thyroid tissue of the patients with AG at the time of RITh, whereas GD involves the total thyroid tissue. Although Goldstein and Hart (7) did not examine the volume reduction of the thyroid after RITh, they observed a higher incidence of hypothyroidism if extranodular tissue suppression was incomplete. In contrast Hegedüs et al. (4) found a volume reduction even of the extranodular tissue in patients with a solitary autonomous nodule. But the suppression of the extranodular tissue was only confirmed by scintigraphy of the thyroid. Baseline TSH or TSH response to TRH were not stated in this study.

Our data do not answer the question whether the thyroid volume reduction finally terminates after more than 1 year after RITh. This has to be examined by further studies with a longer observation period.

REFERENCES:

1. Moser E, Pickardt CR, Mann K, Engelhardt D, Kirsch CM, Knesewitsch P, Tatsch K, Kreisig T, Kurz C , Saller B. Results of radioiodine therapy of patients with immunogenic and non-immunogenic hyperthyroidism using different radiation doses. Nucl-Med 1988; 27: 98-104.

2. Schicha H. Radioactive iodine therapy - updated: Non-immunogenic hyperthyreosis. Akt Endokr Stoffw 1992; 13: 71-79.

3. Hegedüs L, Hansen BM, Knudsen N , Hansen JM. Reduction of size of thyroid with radioactive iodine in multinodular non-toxic goitre. Br Med J 1988; 297: 661-663.

4. Hegedüs L, Veiergang D, Karstrup S , Hansen JM. Compensated 131I-therapy of solitary autonomous thyroid nodules: effect on thyroid size and early hypothyroidism. Acta Endocrin (Copenh) 1986; 113: 226-232.

5. Luster M, Jacob M, Thelen MH, Michalowski U, Deutsch U , Reiners C. Reduction of thyroid volume following radioiodine therapy for functional autonomy. Nucl-Med 1995; 34: 57-60.

6. Nygaard B, Hegedüs L, Gervil M, Hjalgrim H, Søe-Jensen P , Hansen JM. Radioiodine treatment of multinodular non-toxic goitre. Br Med J 1993; 307: 828-833.

7. Goldstein R, Hart IR. Follow-up of solitary autonomous thyroid nodules treated with 131I. N Engl J Med 1983; 309: 1477-1480.

Author Index

Subject index